CURRENT
PRACTICE
of
MEDICINE

CURRENT PRACTICE of MEDICINE

editor
Roger C. Bone, MD

President
Medical College of Ohio
Toledo, Ohio

VOLUME I

Dermatology

volume editor
Jeffrey P. Callen, MD

Professor of Medicine
Chief, Division of Dermatology
Department of Medicine
University of Louisville
Louisville, Kentucky

CURRENT MEDICINE

400 MARKET STREET, SUITE 700
PHILADELPHIA, PA 19106

Managing Editor: **Lori J. Bainbridge**

Developmental Editors: **Peter Stevenson, Jim Slade, Karen Nevers, Barbara Cohen-Kligerman**

Editorial Assistants: **Charlene French, Danielle Shaw**

Art Director: **Paul Fennessy**

Layout: **Patrick Whelan**

Cover Design: **Robert LeBrun**

Illustration Director: **Ann Saydlowski**

Illustrator: **Gary Welch**

Production Manager: **David Myers**

Assistant Production Manager: **Wendy Feinstein**

Typesetting Director: **Colleen Ward**

Printed in Spain by T.G. Hostench, S.A.

Current Practice of Medicine Series: ISBN 1-85922-687-6

ISBN: 1-85922-688-4
ISSN: 1079-980X

10 9 8 7 6 5 4 3 2 1

Series Preface

There are more things in heaven and earth...
Than are dreamt of in your philosophy.
—Shakespeare, *Hamlet,* I.v

It has been stated that medical knowledge doubles approximately every five years. Complicated diagnostic tools, emerging pharmaceuticals, and innovative treatment protocols continually challenge today's physician. To provide the highest quality health care to patients, the general practitioner must use every available resource to keep pace with the burgeoning medical literature.

Today's physicians have access to many good sources of information, including continuing education courses, journals and textbooks, and interactive computer software. However, until now a complete information source that is always within an arm's reach has been lacking. As Editor-in-Chief of the *Current Practice of Medicine* series, I am proud to introduce a comprehensive medical reference source that will satisfy the substantial informational needs of the general practitioner. The series is designed to provide the general practitioner with accessible, in-depth commentary on contemporary medicine. Each volume is filled with hundreds of photographs, tables, and detailed medical illustrations, covering every aspect of internal medicine:

- Allergy & Immunology
- Cardiology
- Dermatology
- Endocrinology & Metabolic Diseases
- Gastroenterology
- General Internal Medicine
- Hematology
- Hepatology
- Infectious Diseases
- Nephrology
- Neurology
- Oncology
- Psychiatry
- Pulmonary Medicine & Critical Care
- Rheumatology

The Volume Editors have asked the premiere specialists of their respective fields to contribute up-to-date and reliable chapters specifically intended for the general practitioner.

Current Practice of Medicine is an ambitious series. It is a valuable addition to the reference libraries of all physicians who deal with the complicated mysteries presented by patients. I am proud to oversee the important and essential information that each of these volumes contributes to medical knowledge.

I would like to thank all of the contributing authors and the Volume Editors, whose efforts are central to the great success of this series. I also offer my sincere thanks to Abe Krieger, President of Current Medicine; Lori J. Bainbridge, Managing Editor; Pete Stevenson and Jim Slade, Developmental Editors; Gary Welch, Illustrator; Paul Fennessy, Art Director; Patrick Whelan and Robert LeBrun, Designers; and everyone on the staff of Current Medicine who helped to make this project possible.

Roger C. Bone, MD
Medical College of Ohio
Toledo, Ohio

Preface

As an educator, I have always strived to effect patient care in a positive manner. When Dr. Roger Bone invited me to serve as Editor of the Dermatology volume of *Current Practice of Medicine,* I saw an opportunity to design a text that would aid practitioners in the daily care of patients.

This volume presents common and complex areas of the field in a format that makes diagnosis, treatment, and referral decisions easier for the practitioner. Chapter topics ranging from *Common Bacterial Infections of the Skin* to *Life-Threatening Dermatoses* are presented in a practical format using a list of key points at the start of each chapter. Easy-to-follow algorithms and tables throughout the text offer a practical approach to diagnostic evaluation and therapeutic interventions. Color photographs are an important part of any dermatologic text, and this volume is liberally illustrated.

As Volume Editor, it was my pleasure to recruit recognized specialists in the field to write these chapters. Many of these authors have published extensively on their given topics, several have written texts, and many are department chairs or division heads at their respective medical schools and hospitals.

I believe that the practical approach this book offers will increase the knowledge base of generalists and specialists alike, ultimately improving patient care.

Jeffrey P. Callen, MD
University of Louisville
Louisville, Kentucky

Contributors

JAMIE A. ALPERT, MD
Assistant Professor
Division of Dermatology
University of Vermont
Burlington, Vermont

GRANT J. ANHALT, MD
Professor and Vice Chairman
Department of Dermatology
School of Medicine
Johns Hopkins University
Baltimore, Maryland

KENNETH A. ARNDT, MD
Professor of Dermatology
Harvard Medical School;
Dermatologist-in-Chief
Beth Israel Hospital
Boston, Massachusetts

RAYMOND L. BARNHILL, MD
Associate Professor of Pathology
Harvard Medical School;
Director, Dermatopathology Division
Brigham and Women's and Children's Hospital;
Attending Dermatologist
Brigham and Women's Hospital
Boston, Massachusetts

JEFFREY D. BERNHARD, MD
Professor of Medicine
Director, Dermatology Division
University of Massachusetts Medical Center
Worcester, Massachusetts

JEFFREY P. CALLEN, MD
Professor of Medicine
Chief, Division of Dermatology
Department of Medicine
University of Louisville
Louisville, Kentucky

RICHARD A.F. CLARK, MD
Professor and Chairman
Department of Dermatology
State University of New York at Stony Brook
Stony Brook, New York

PHILIP R. COHEN, MD
Assistant Professor
Departments of Dermatology and Pathology
The University of Texas-Houston Medical School;
Department of Medical Specialties (Section of Dermatology)
University of Texas M.D. Anderson Cancer Center
Houston, Texas

BONI E. ELEWSKI, MD
Associate Professor
Department of Dermatology
Case Western Reserve University
Cleveland, Ohio

VINCENT FALANGA, MD, FACP
Associate Professor of Dermatology and Medicine
Department of Dermatology and Cutaneous Surgery
University of Miami School of Medicine
Miami, Florida

FRANKLIN P. FLOWERS, MD
Professor and Chief
Division of Dermatology
Department of Medicine
University of Florida
Gainesville, Florida

STEVEN M. HACKER, MD
Assistant Clinical Professor
Department of Medicine
Division of Dermatology
University of Florida
Gainesville, Florida

TISSA R. HATA, MD
Chief Resident
Department of Dermatology
Harvard Medical School
Boston, Massachusetts

TERRENCE HOPKINS, MD
Clinical Assistant Professor
Department of Dermatology
State University of New York at Stony Brook
Stony Brook, New York

JOSEPH L. JORIZZO, MD
Professor and Chairman
Department of Dermatology
Bowman Gray School of Medicine
Wake Forest University
Winston-Salem, North Carolina

SETH G. KATES, MD
Chairman
Department of Dermatology
Fallon Clinic
Worcester, Massachusetts

FRANCISCO A. KERDEL, BSc, MBBS
Associate Professor of Dermatology
Department of Dermatology and Cutaneous Surgery
University of Miami School of Medicine
Miami, Florida

PAUL A. KRUSINSKI, MD

Professor of Medicine
Director, Division of Dermatology
University of Vermont School of Medicine
Burlington, Vermont

CAROL L. KULP-SHORTEN, MD

Assistant Clinical Professor of Medicine
University of Louisville
Louisville, Kentucky

GRACE S. LIANG-FEDERMAN, MD

Department of Dermatology and Cutaneous Surgery
University of Miami School of Medicine
Miami, Florida

HENRY W. LIM, MD

Professor of Dermatology
The Ronald O. Perelman Department of Dermatology
New York University School of Medicine;
Chief of Staff
Veterans Affairs Medical Center
New York, New York

DONALD P. LOOKINGBILL, MD

Professor of Medicine
Chief of Dermatology
College of Medicine
Pennsylvania State University
Milton S. Hershey Medical Center
Hershey, Pennsylvania

NICHOLAS J. LOWE, MD

Clinical Professor of Dermatology
University of California at Los Angeles School of Medicine
Los Angeles, California

LYNN MCKINLEY-GRANT, MD

Department of Dermatology
Washington Hospital Center
Washington, DC;
Chief, Division of Dermatology
Veterans Affairs Medical Center
Washington, DC

RONALD L. MOY, MD

Assistant Clinical Professor
Division of Dermatology
University of California at Los Angeles School of Medicine
Los Angeles, California

PAUL I. OH, MD, FRCPC

Research Fellow in Clinical Pharmacology
Sunnybrook Health Science Centre
University of Toronto
Toronto, Ontario, Canada

JEFFREY B. PARDES, MD

Wound Healing Fellow
Department of Dermatology and Cutaneous Surgery
University of Miami School of Medicine
Miami, Florida

DANIEL RIVLIN, MD

Director, Mohs Microsurgery Unit
Mount Sinai Medical Center
Miami Beach, Florida

LISA M. SEUNG, MD

Research Fellow
Division of Dermatology
University of California at Los Angeles School of Medicine
Los Angeles, California

NEIL H. SHEAR, MD, FRCPC, FACP

Director, Clinical Pharmacology
University of Toronto;
Deputy Director, Dermatology
University of Toronto;
Director, Drug Safety Research Group
University of Toronto;
Associate Professor of Medicine, Pharmacology, Pediatrics and
*   Pharmacy*
Sunnybrook Health Science Centre
Toronto, Ontario, Canada

KAREN SIMPSON, MD

Research Fellow
Department of Dermatology
University of California at Irvine
Irvine, California

ARTHUR J. SOBER, MD

Associate Professor of Dermatology
Harvard Medical School;
Associate Chief of Dermatology
Massachusetts General Hospital
Boston, Massachusetts

YARDY TSE, MD

Clinical Instructor
The Ronald O. Perelman Department of Dermatology
New York University School of Medicine
New York, New York

GUY F. WEBSTER, MD, PhD

Associate Professor of Dermatology and Internal Medicine
Thomas Jefferson University
Jefferson Medical College
Philadelphia, Pennsylvania

VICTORIA P. WERTH, MD

Associate Professor of Dermatology and Internal Medicine
Department of Dermatology
University of Pennsylvania
Philadelphia, Pennsylvania;
Chief, Division of Dermatology
Veterans Affairs Medical Center
Philadelphia, Pennsylvania

Contents

ix

Principles of Diagnosis
Donald P. Lookingbill

1

Key Points

- Dermatologic diagnosis is based upon the history of the patient, skin examination, and laboratory testing as necessary.
- In new patients the complete skin surface should be examined.
- Dermatologic disorders are divided into growths and rashes.
- Growths are subdivided into epidermal, pigmented or dermal processes.
- Rashes are first separated according to the presence or absence of epidermal involvement, and then further subdivided according to the nature of the epidermal change or the type of dermal inflammation.
- The configuration and distribution of rashes may serve as secondary diagnostic considerations.
- If a clinical diagnosis cannot be made, a dermatologist should be consulted.

To diagnose a skin disease, the physician must 1) take a history, 2) carefully examine the skin, and 3) occasionally perform laboratory testing. In the skin examination, particular attention is given to identifying the nature of the primary lesion. By correlating the clinical appearance of the primary lesion with the responsible pathologic change, an algorithmic approach to diagnosis can be developed. Two algorithms have been developed: one for growths (Fig. 1-1) and one for rashes (Fig. 1-2). In diagnosing rashes, it is sometimes also helpful to note the way in which the lesions are arranged and their distribution on the body surface. Laboratory tests are less often employed in dermatologic diagnosis than in many other fields of medicine, but a few simple skin tests are invaluable in diagnosing some skin conditions.

HISTORY

For many skin disorders, a brief history will suffice. For nearly every patient, the physician should obtain at least three pieces of historical information: 1) the duration and progression of the problem, 2) associated symptoms, and 3) prior treatment. For skin disorders, the most important symptom is itch. In regard to therapy, careful and often repeated inquiry is necessary to elicit all the topical and systemic medications that the patient may have used. This obviously includes over-the-counter as well as prescription products.

Following the brief preliminary history-taking, the physical examination should be performed. After this, additional history will sometimes be needed. For example, if during the physical examination the physician notes a butterfly rash suggestive of cutaneous lupus erythematosus, the patient should be asked about other signs or symptoms associated with systemic lupus erythematosus.

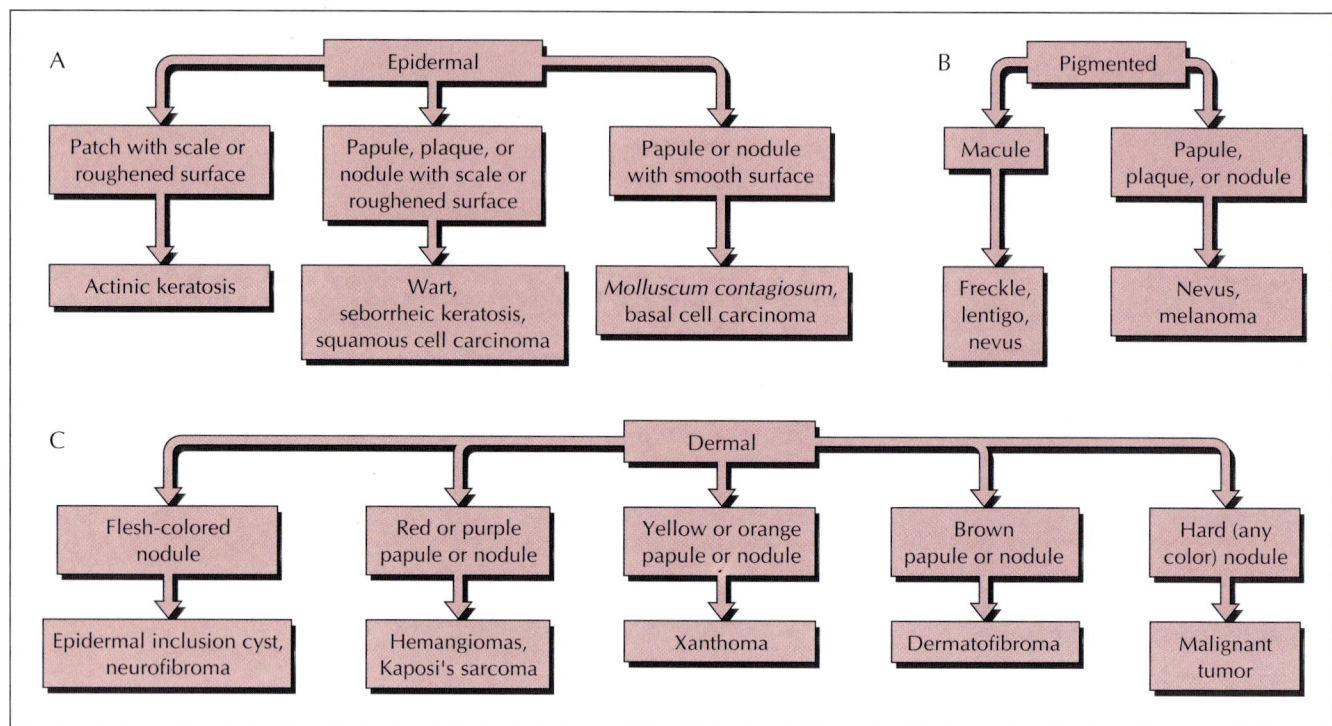

FIGURE 1-1 Algorithm of (*panel A*) epidermal, (*panel B*) pigmented and (*panel C*) dermal growths.

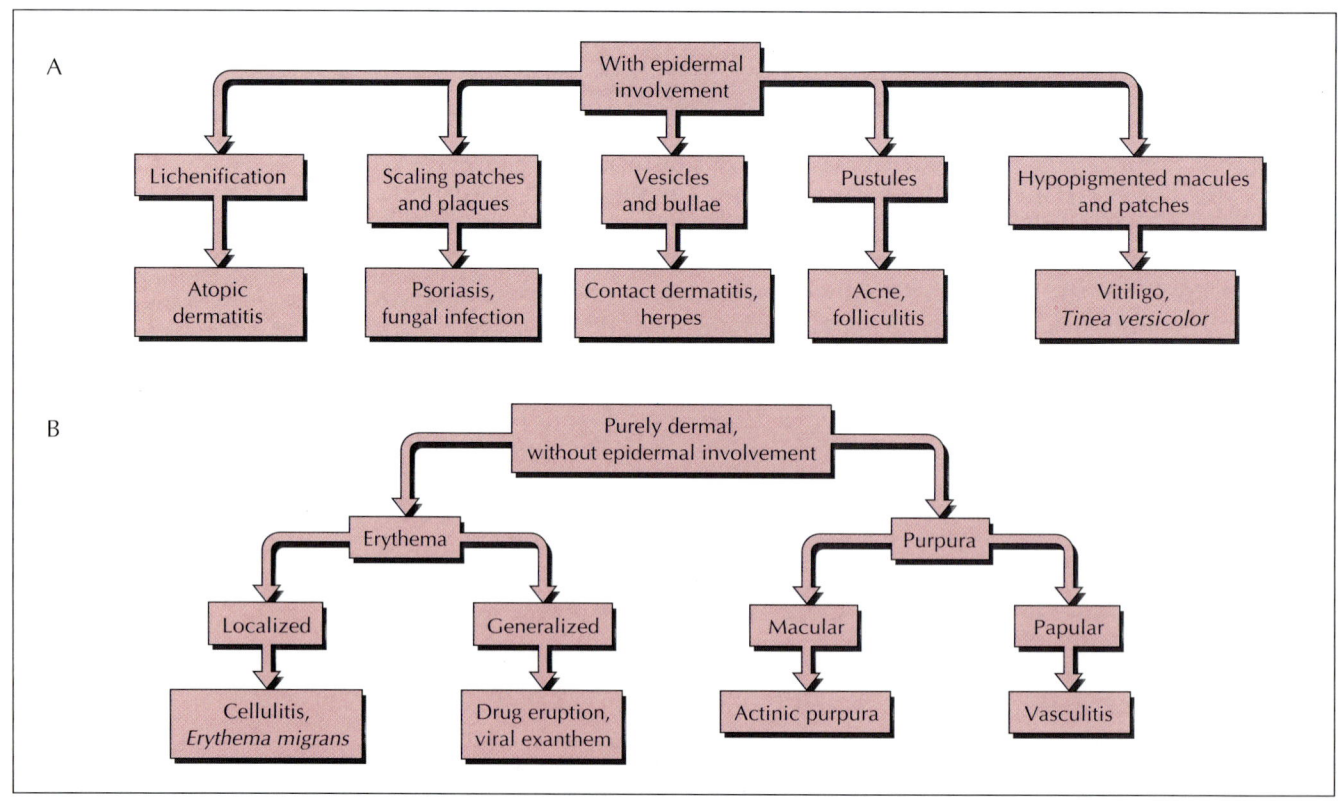

FIGURE 1-2 Algorithm of rashes (*panel A*) with epidermal, and (*panel B*) with purely dermal involvement.

If the physical examination suggests a diagnosis of contact dermatitis, the patient should be questioned regarding exposures to possible contact allergens. Because the nature of a responsible environmental allergen is not always obvious, this type of history-taking is often painstaking and can tax the skills of even the most seasoned dermatologic detective [1•].

PHYSICAL EXAMINATION

For new patients, a complete skin examination is strongly recommended. The reasons for this are twofold: 1) the physician may discover that a rash involves more areas than the patient realized (or admitted) and this can help in making the diagnosis; and 2) an incidental important growth might be found, for example, an early melanoma, detection of which could be lifesaving. In two studies that determined the frequency of finding an incidental skin cancer from a complete examination, the yield in the first was 1.9%, and in the second, 3.4% [2,3]. One of the cancers detected in the first study was Kaposi's sarcoma, and this represented the initial finding that led to a diagnosis of AIDS in that patient.

Environment

To properly examine a patient's skin, the patient should be disrobed, gowned, and examined under adequate light. Ideally, this should include bright overhead lighting, as well as a movable incandescent light for bright local illumination. A penlight is particularly helpful for "sidelighting" lesions in order to determine whether they are flat or elevated. A Wood's light is a black light that has been used in the past to diagnose *tinea capitis*. The Wood's light is not useful for diagnosing fungal infection in any other body location, and in recent years even most of the cases of *tinea capitis* are of the type that do not fluoresce with Wood's light. Wood's light can be helpful, however, in accentuating pigment changes in the skin (*eg*, hypopigmented spots in patients of light complexion).

Examination

Inspection of skin lesions can sometimes be enhanced with the use of a hand lens, but for the diagnosis of most skin lesions magnification is not required. *Palpation* of skin lesions, however, is almost always a useful maneuver. With palpation, the physician can determine the texture and consistency of the skin lesions. For example, if a nodule feels hard, the physician should suspect the possibility of malignancy. Even in these days of AIDS, gloves need not be worn for palpation of dry skin lesions. Gloves should be worn for examining exudative, mucosal, and genital lesions.

In addition to examining the skin, the physician should look at the nails and the mouth, where irregularities may be detected that will aid in the dermatologic diagnosis (*eg*, oral hairy leukoplakia on the sides of the tongue strongly suggests a diagnosis of AIDS).

TERMINOLOGY OF SKIN LESIONS

In determining a dermatologic diagnosis, the physician must first be prepared to describe what is seen. Dermatologic vocabulary terms are used to describe the morphology of the primary lesion (Table 1-1). Proceeding from description to diagnosis, the physician will find it helpful to employ clinical pathologic considerations. An algorithmic approach can then be used (*eg*, it is critical to distinguish a vesicle from a papule because the differential diagnosis for each of these is entirely different). Similarly, erythema must be distinguished from purpura; this distinction is made by determining whether or not the redness is blanchable. As a

TABLE 1-1 TERMINOLOGY OF SKIN LESIONS	
Lesion	**Appearance**
Macule	Flat with color (*eg*, red, brown)
Patch	Flat with color and surface change (*eg*, scale)
Papule	Elevated <0.5 cm in diameter
Plaque	Elevated >0.5 cm in diameter, but without depth
Nodule	Elevated *and* indurated, >0.5 cm in diameter and depth
Cyst	A nodule filled with fluid or semisolid content
Vesicle	A small blister, filled with visible clear fluid, <0.5 cm
Bullae	Same as vesicle but >0.5 cm
Pustule	Same as vesicle except fluid is yellow
Wheal	Edematuous plaque (hive)
Erosion	Shallow sore from partial denudation of the epidermis
Ulcer	Deeper wound with loss of all of the epidermis and part or all of dermis
Descriptive terms	
Colors	
Erythema	Blanchable redness from dilated blood vessels
Purpura	Nonblanchable, deep red or purple color from extravasated blood
Hyperpigmented	Increased brown pigment, usually melanin
Hypopigmented	Whiter than normal
Surface change	
Crust	Dried serum, pus or blood on surface of skin (scab)
Scale	White or whitish flakes on surface of skin from thickened stratum corneum
Lichenification	Thickened skin with accentuated surface markings

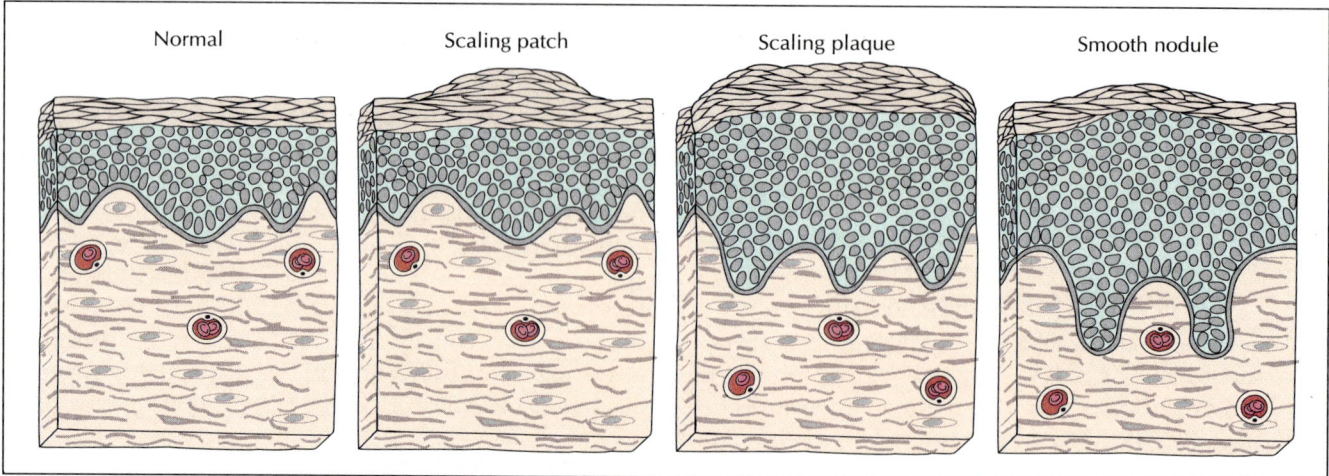

FIGURE 1-3 Epidermal growths. These growths arise from thickening of the stratum corneum and/or the epidermis.

final example, crust and scale must be distinguished from each other. A crust represents dried blood or serum on the surface of the skin, and hence indicates the preexistence of a vesicle, bulla, or pustule. Scale, on the other hand, represents thickened stratum corneum and suggests an entirely different differential diagnosis.

ALGORITHMIC APPROACH TO DIAGNOSIS

It is useful to divide dermatologic disorders into growths and rashes [4•]. This is often the way patients describe their complaint (*eg*, "I'm concerned about this bump on my skin," or "I have developed this itchy rash").

Growths

Growths can be subdivided into those that arise from the epidermis, those that are pigmented, and those that are derived from processes confined to the dermis (Fig. 1-1).

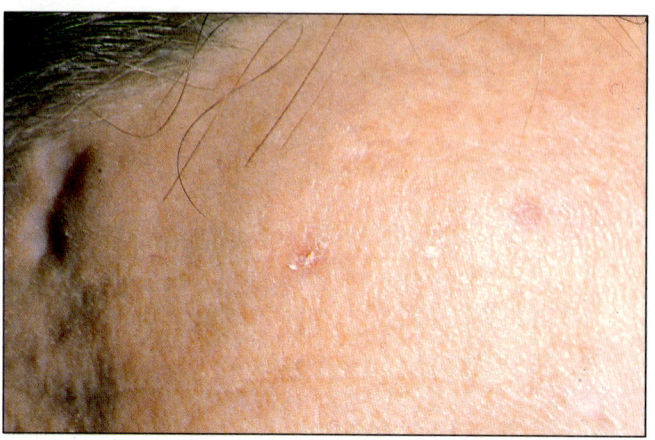

FIGURE 1-4 Actinic keratosis. Epidermal growth appearing as a (often subtle) scaling patch.

The clinicopathologic correlation for epidermal growths is demonstrated in Figure 1-3, and illustrated with the examples in Figures 1-4 through 1-6. The clinicopathologic correlation for pigmented growths is illustrated in Figure 1-7, and exemplified by Figures 1-8 and 1-9. Dermal growths represent proliferation of cellular elements in the dermis (Fig. 1-10), and examples of such growths are shown in Figures 1-11 through 1-15. Most dermal growths appear as nodules in the skin. If a nodule cannot be clinically diagnosed, a biopsy should be done to rule out malignancy.

Rashes

The algorithmic approach for the diagnosis of rashes is shown in Figure 1-2. Rashes are inflammatory processes, so by definition there is vascular involvement, and this therefore always involves the dermis, as there are no blood vessels in the epidermis. The physician must first decide whether there is also epidermal involvement. The possible types of epidermal involvement are depicted in Figure 1-16 with specific examples shown in Figures 1-17 through 1-21. Correctly identifying the type of epidermal involvement will lead to selection of the proper differential diagnosis and ultimately the correct final diagnosis of a rash. If, for example, the physician mistakes crust for scale, the chances of determining a correct final diagnosis are very remote.

If a rash has no surface change, then it is described as purely dermal (Fig. 1-22). For these rashes, the physician must determine whether the redness from the inflammation is blanchable. Erythema represents blanchable redness (Fig. 1-23). Common causes for these types of rashes are listed in Figure 1-2. Purpura represents extravasated blood in the dermis. (Figs. 1-24 and 1-25). If purpura is elevated, it is termed palpable purpura, an important finding that indicates necrotizing vasculitis in the skin.

The algorithmic approaches place emphasis on correctly describing and identifying the primary process affecting the skin in terms of its morphology.

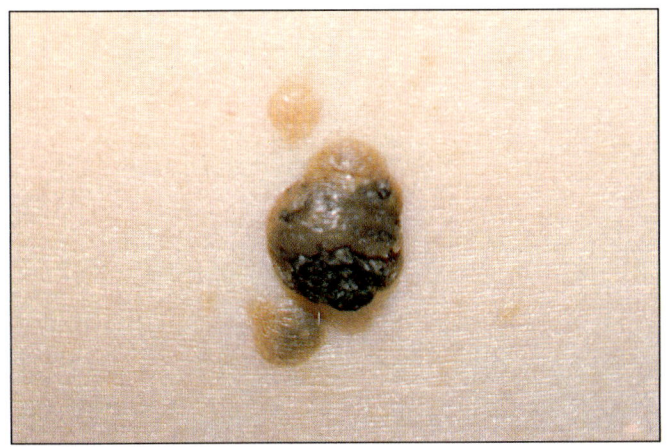

FIGURE 1-5 Seborrheic keratosis. Epidermal growth appearing as a plaque with scale, a rough surface, or both.

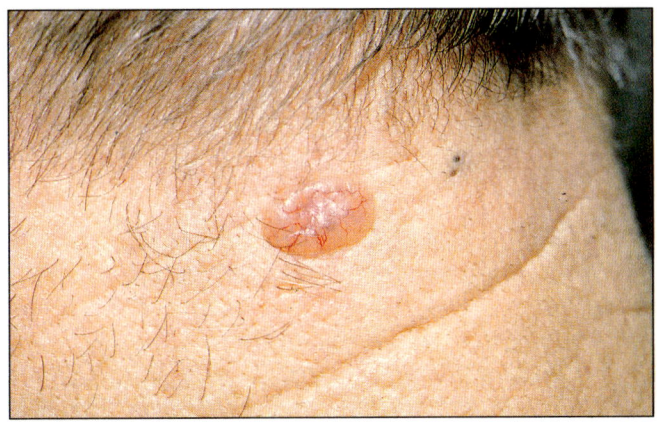

FIGURE 1-6 Basal cell carcinoma. Epidermal growth appearing as a smooth, "pearly" nodule. (*From* Lookingbill and Marks [4•]; with permission.)

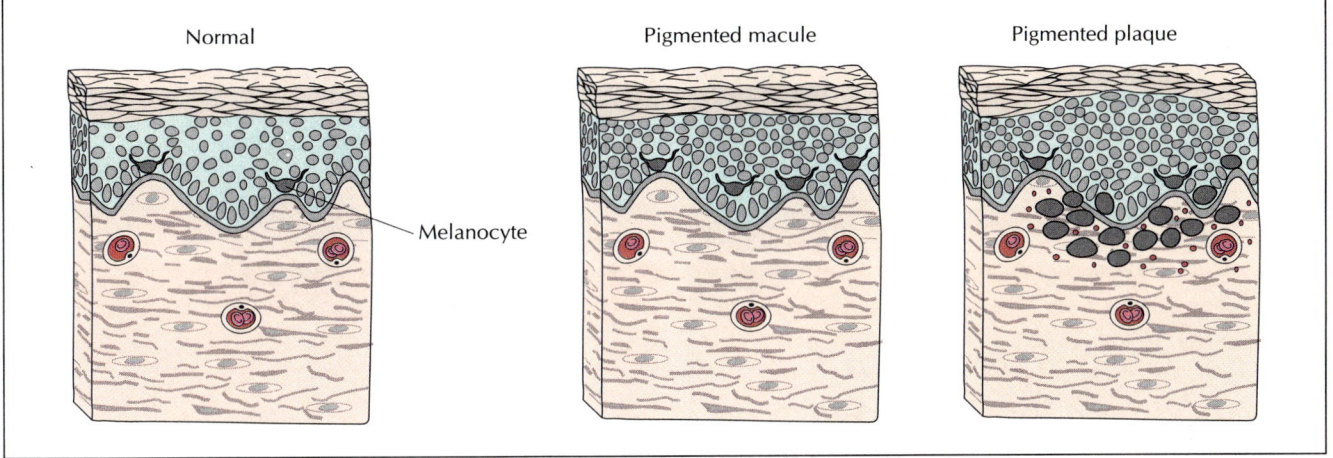

Normal   Pigmented macule   Pigmented plaque

Melanocyte

FIGURE 1-7 Pigmented growths. These growths are due to increased pigment with or without an increase in pigment-producing cells.

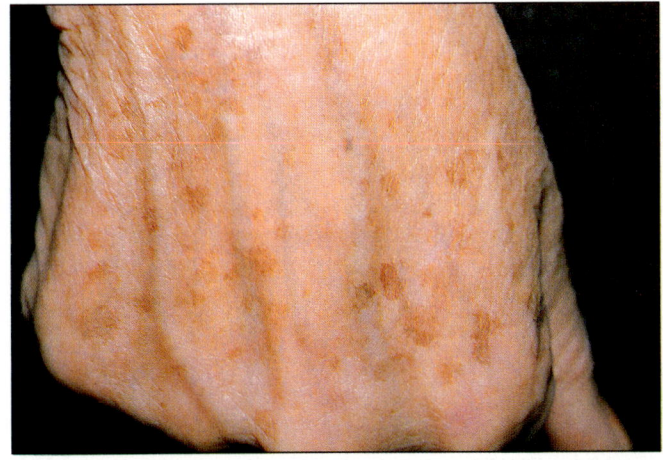

FIGURE 1-8 Lentigines (liver spots). Pigmented growths appearing as macules. (*From* Lookingbill and Marks [4•]; with permission.)

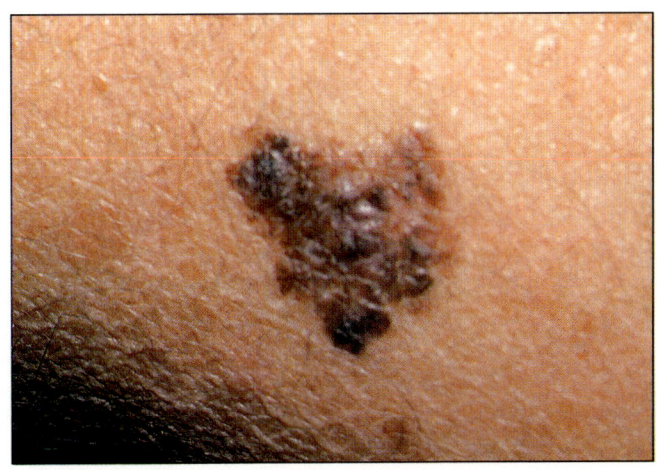

FIGURE 1-9 Melanoma. Pigmented growth appearing as plaque.

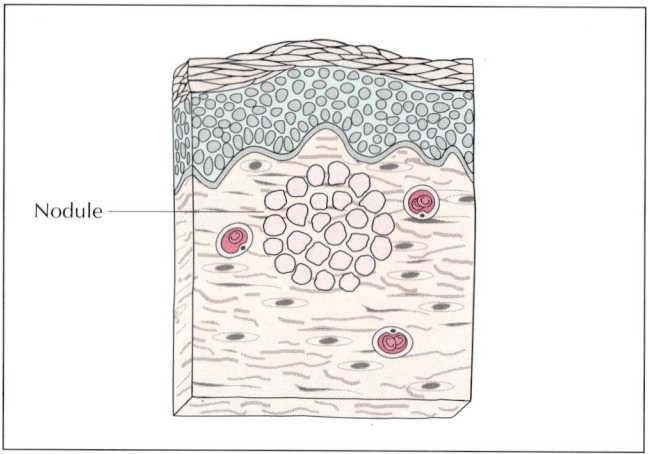

FIGURE 1-10 Dermal growths. These nodules result from proliferation of cells in the dermis.

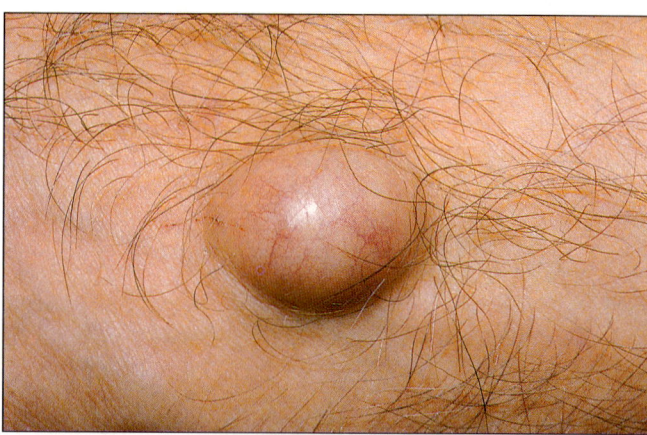

FIGURE 1-11 Epidermal inclusion cyst. Dermal growth appearing as a flesh-colored nodule resulting from an epidermal-lined, keratin-containing cyst in the dermis.

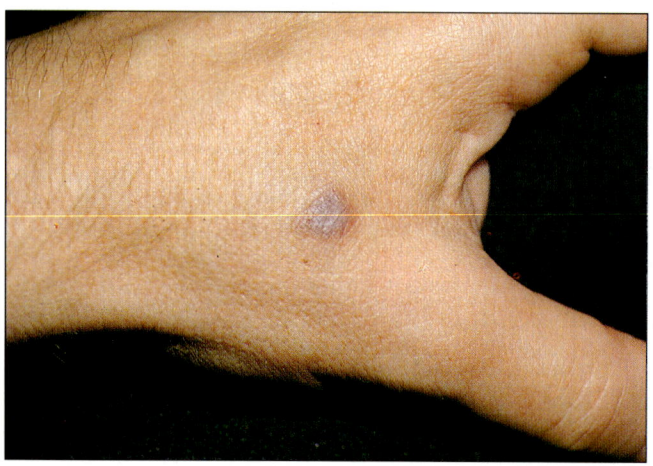

FIGURE 1-12 Kaposi's sarcoma. Dermal growth appearing as a purple nodule that results from a proliferation of vascular elements in the dermis.

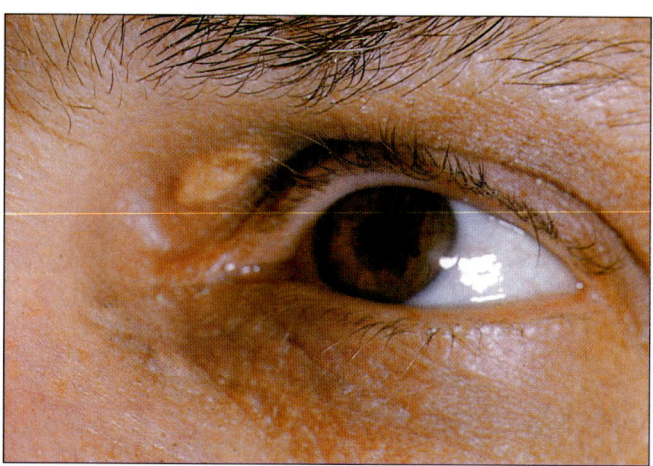

FIGURE 1-13 Xanthelasma. Dermal growth appearing as a yellow plaque derived from a collection of lipid-laden cells in the dermis.

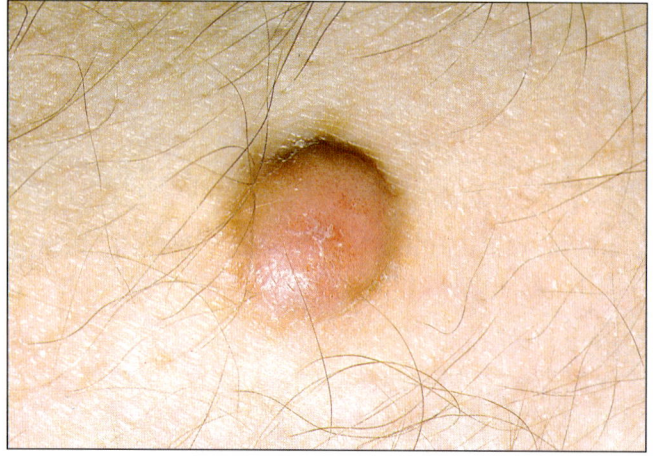

FIGURE 1-14 Dermatofibroma. Dermal growth due to increased number of fibroblasts in the dermis. The pigment, however, is epidermal.

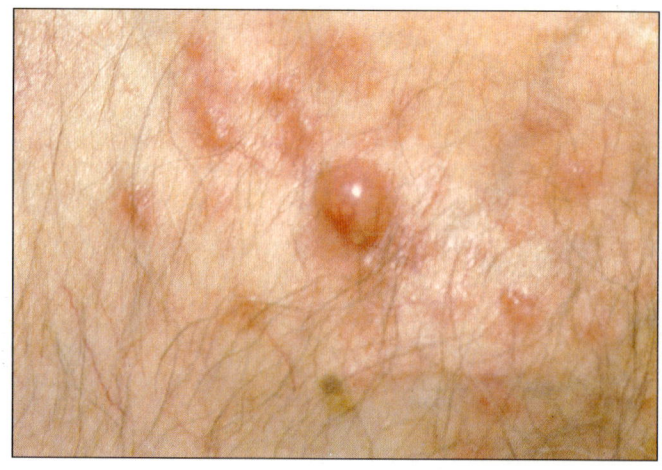

FIGURE 1-15 Metastatic adenocarcinoma. Dermal growth forming a hard nodule from malignant cells that have aggregated in the dermis.

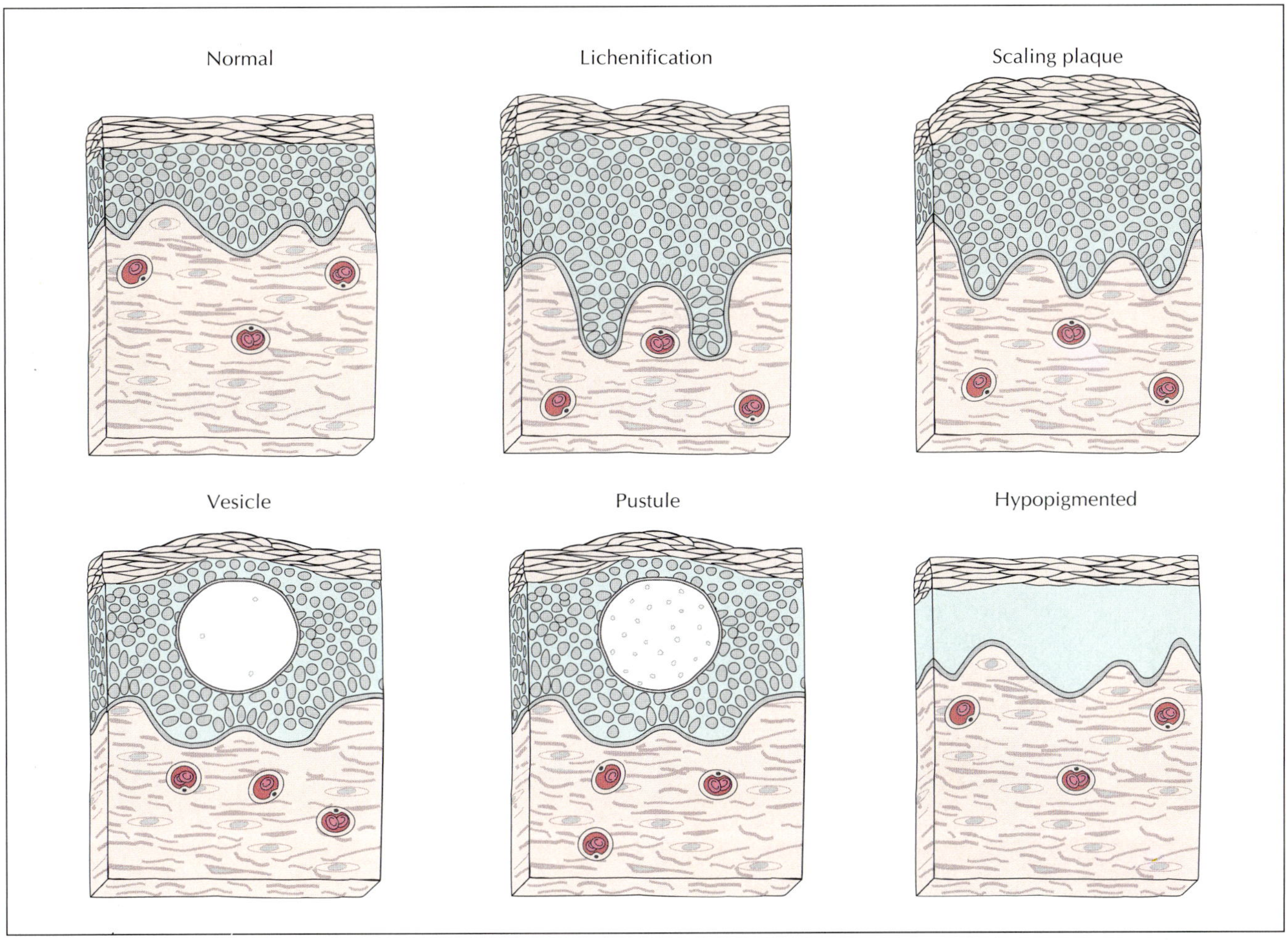

Normal	Lichenification	Scaling plaque

Vesicle	Pustule	Hypopigmented

FIGURE 1-16 Rashes with epidermal involvement. These rashes are characterized by epidermal thickening (lichenification), scaling, disruption (vesicles and pustules), or hypopigmentation.

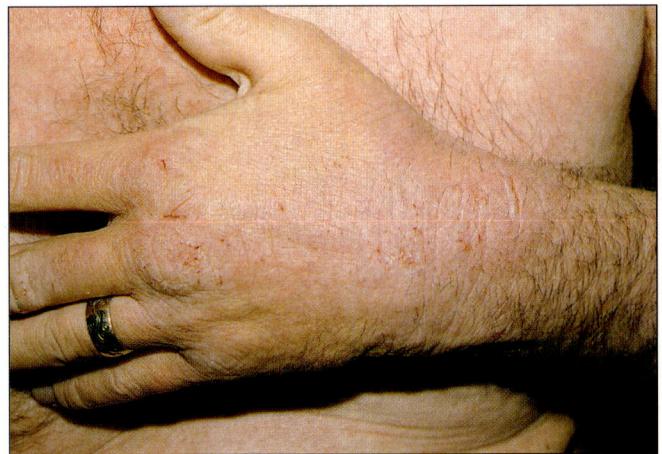

FIGURE 1-17 Atopic dermatis. Rash with epidermal involvement—lichenification.

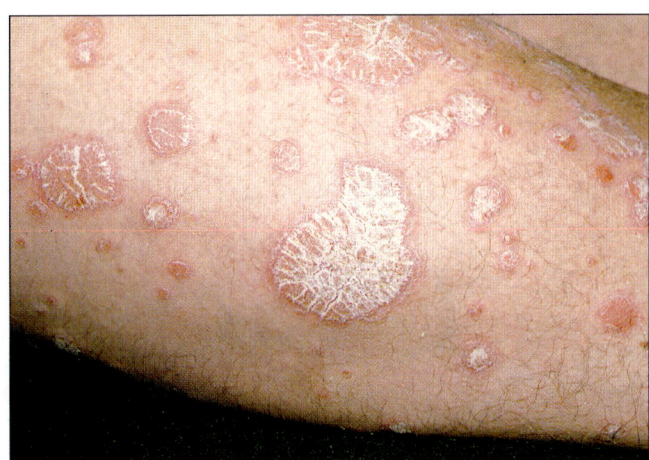

FIGURE 1-18 Psoriasis. Rash with epidermal involvement—scaling plaques.

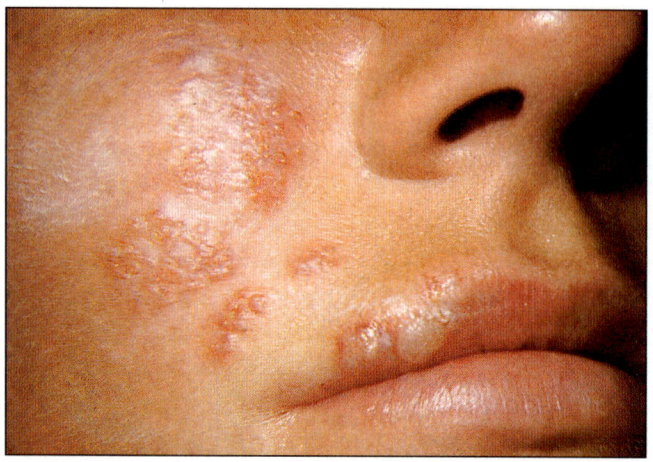

FIGURE 1-19 Herpes simplex. Rash with epidermal involvement—vesicles.

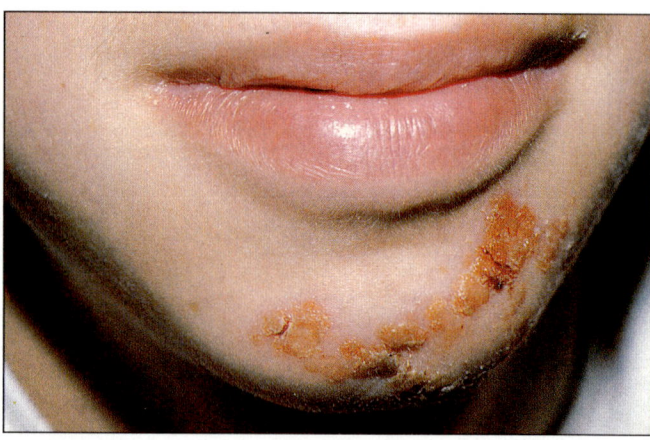

FIGURE 1-20 Impetigo. Rash with epidermal involvement—pustules. The pustules have ruptured and dried to form honey-colored crusts.

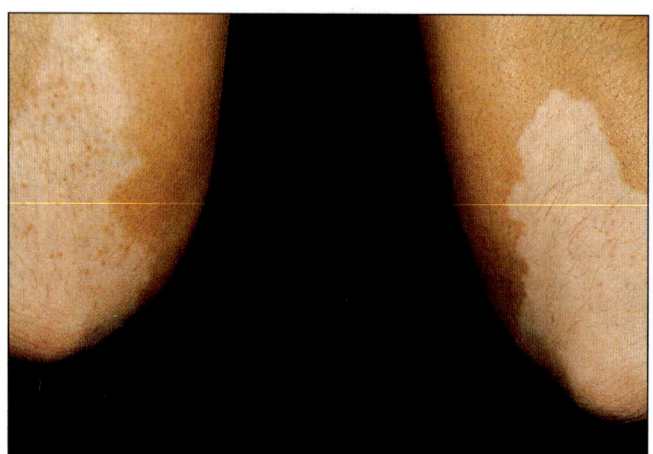

FIGURE 1-21 Vitiligo. Rash with epidermal involvement—hypopigmentation.

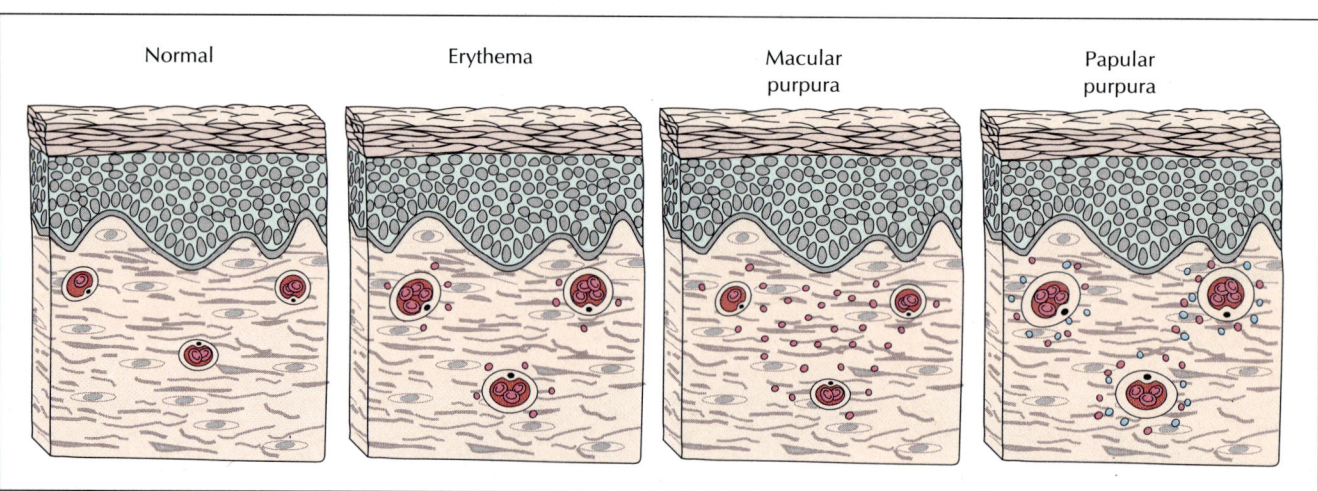

FIGURE 1-22 Rashes, purely dermal. These rashes have no epidermal involvement. They are characterized by dermal vascular changes resulting in erythema (blanchable redness) or purpura (purple that is not blanchable). Noninflammatory purpura is macular; inflammatory purpura is papular (palpable).

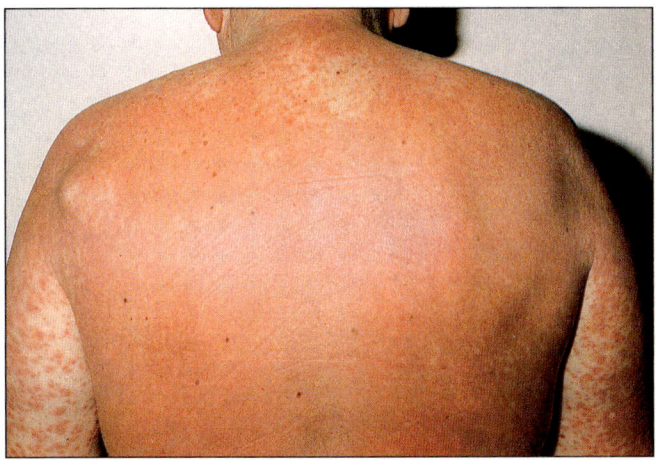

FIGURE 1-23 Drug eruption. Purely dermal rash characterized by erythematous macules and papules, confluent and generalized.

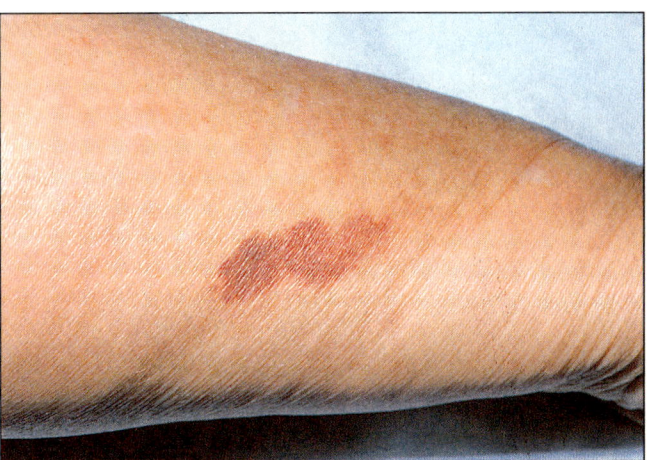

FIGURE 1-24 Actinic purpura. Purely dermal rash from non-inflammatory extravasation of blood from fragile blood vessels. (*From* Lookingbill and Marks [4•]; with permission.)

CONFIGURATION AND DISTRIBUTION OF RASHES

Occasionally, additional diagnostic information can be obtained for rashes if the lesions are arranged in a special way or distributed in particular locations (Table 1-2, Figs. 1-26 and 1-27). As is shown in these common configurations, when vesicles appear in streaks, a contact dermatitis is virtually always the cause. Streaks of papules can be seen in patients with psoriasis or lichen planus.

The distribution of a rash can sometimes help with the diagnosis (*eg*, scaling plaques in psoriasis commonly occur on the scalp, elbows, knees, and intergluteal cleft, and scabies frequently involves the finger webs and genital areas, but rarely involves the head).

LABORATORY TESTS

For the majority of patients with skin disease, laboratory tests are not needed. In some circumstances, however, dermatologic testing is invaluable [5]. The tests most frequently employed are office microscopic examinations and skin biopsies. Patch tests, which are also useful, are done by dermatologists (*see* When to Refer section).

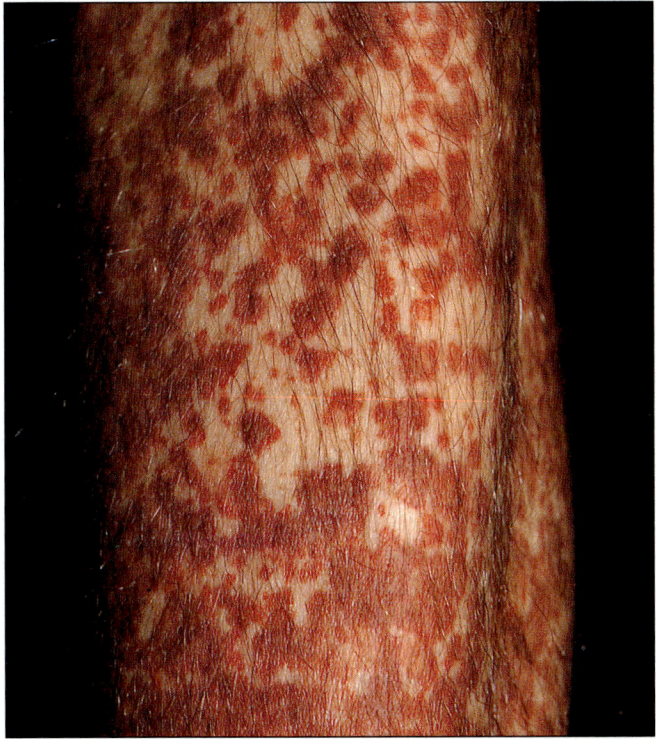

FIGURE 1-25 Necrotizing vasculitis. Purely dermal rash due to inflammatory necrosis of dermal blood vessels, resulting in palpable purpura.

TABLE 1-2 RASHES ASSOCIATED WITH SPECIFIC CONFIGURATIONS	
Configuration	**Disease**
Vesicles	
Linear	Contact dermatitis
Grouped	Herpes simplex
Grouped and dermatomal	Herpes zoster
Papules, scaling	
Linear	Psoriasis
	Lichen planus
Papules, nonscaling	
Grouped	Insect bites
Annular scaling patches and plaques	*Tinea corporis*

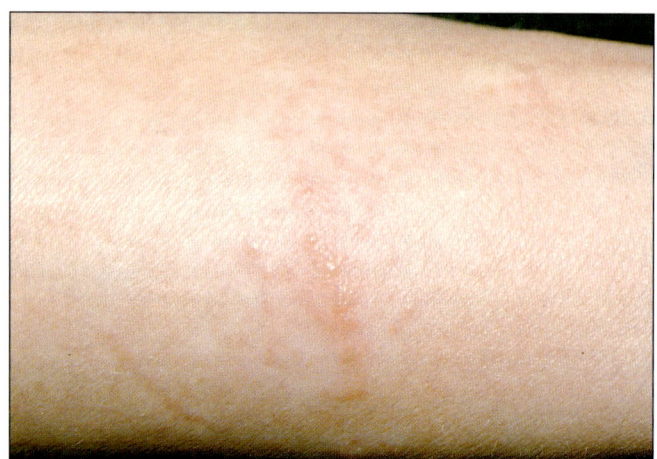

FIGURE 1-26 Vesicles in linear configuration. Streaks of vesicles signify a dermatitis to an external contactant, for example poison ivy.

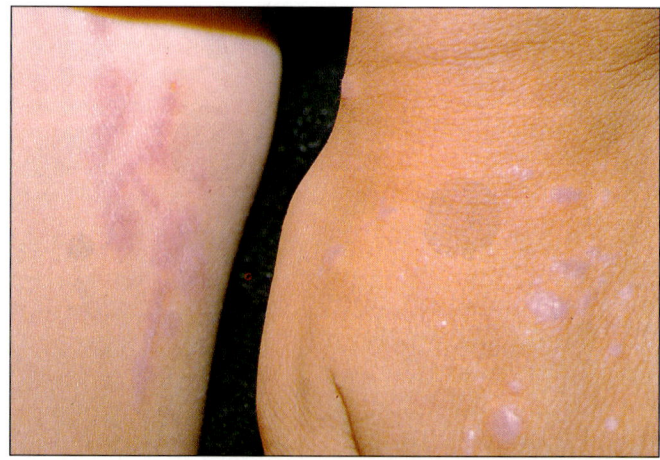

FIGURE 1-27 Koebner phenomenon. In psoriasis and lichen planus (*shown here*), external trauma such as scratching may precipitate streaks of papules.

Office Microscopic Examination

For dermatologic diagnosis, the microscope is most frequently used for examining potassium hydroxide preparations. For scaling rashes, if the diagnosis is uncertain, the physician should follow the admonition that "if it scales, scrape it." A #15 scalpel blade is used to scrape scale from the edge of a lesion onto a glass slide, to which one drop of 10% or 20% potassium hydroxide is applied, covered with a coverslip, gently heated, blotted, and microscopically examined under low power and low illumination. Suspicious elements are examined under high power to confirm whether or not they represent fungal hyphae. The finding of even one definite hypha is diagnostic for cutaneous fungal infection.

Other microscopic examinations sometimes employed for dermatologic diagnosis include the Gram stain, Tzanck preparation for diagnosis of herpes infections, and scabies scrapings. For a scabies scraping, a #15 scalpel blade is moistened with oil, and a suspicious lesion (preferably a burrow) is vigorously scraped at right angles to the skin. The material is transferred to a drop of oil on a glass slide, covered with the coverslip, and examined for presence of mites, eggs, or mite feces.

Skin Biopsy

Skin biopsies are sometimes necessary to determine the diagnosis of a growth or rash. Since the skin is an external organ, a biopsy is a simple procedure. Two common methods for performing a skin biopsy are with shave or punch. For either procedure, the skin is first prepped with an antiseptic and numbed with an injection of xylocaine. A shave biopsy can be used for diagnosing a superficial process, while a punch biopsy is needed to reach the depth of a nodular growth or deep inflammatory process. Biopsies of growths are usually diagnostic, while biopsy results from rashes may often be nonspecific. Accordingly, a physician performing a biopsy of a rash, should provide the pathologist with a meaningful differential diagnosis and also be prepared to place the pathology report into a clinicopathologic correlation context. If the clinician seeing the patient is unequipped to provide the forgoing, a random biopsy of an undiagnosed rash is unlikely to be helpful to that physician. A dermatologist should be consulted instead.

WHEN TO REFER

Referral to a dermatologist is recommended when the primary physician is unable to make a diagnosis, or not equipped for or not successful with therapy. A dermatologist will also be needed if patch testing is indicated.

Patch testing, an invaluable method for determining allergens that might be responsible for contact dermatitis, is done almost exclusively by dermatologists and requires the necessary materials and careful attention to detail. Because patch testing is used for the detection of delayed hypersensitivity to specific allergens, the method differs from that of scratch testing, which detects immediate hypersensitivity reactions to systemic (inhaled and ingested) allergens. In patch testing, the materials are placed on the skin under a patch for 48 hours, at which point the patches are removed and an initial reading is taken. A second reading is taken at 96 hours, and any positive results must be interpreted in light of the patient's history: that is, it must be determined whether a positive result is relevant to the patient's dermatitis [6].

References and Recommended Reading

Recently published papers of particular interest have been highlighted as:

• Of interest

1.• Marks JG, DeLeo VA: *Contact and Occupational Dermatology.* St. Louis: Mosby Yearbook; 1992.

2. Lookingbill DP: Yield from a complete skin examination: findings in 1157 new dermatology patients. *J Am Acad Dermatol* 1988, 18:31–37.

3. Lee G, Massa MC, Welykyj S, *et al.*: Yield from total skin examination and effectiveness of skin cancer awareness program. Findings in 874 new dermatology patients. *Cancer* 1991, 67:202–205.

4.• Lookingbill DP, Marks JGM: *Principles of Dermatology*, edn 2. Philadelphia: WB Saunders; 1993.

5. McBurney EI: Diagnostic dermatologic methods. *Ped Clin North Am* 1983, 30:419–434.

6. Adams RM: Patch testing—a recapitulation. *J Am Acad Dermatol* 1981, 5:629–643.

2 Common Bacterial Infections of the Skin

Steven M. Hacker
Franklin P. Flowers

Key Points

- One of the most important mechanisms of prevention of cutaneous infection is an intact stratum corneum.
- The most common cutaneous infections tend to be caused by gram-positive cocci such as *Staphylococcus aureus*.
- Diagnosis of cutaneous infections is based on characteristic clinical presentation and history. It is confirmed by Gram stain and culture.
- The therapeutic approach to cutaneous infection may involve local measures, systemic measures, or both.
- Local therapy should always include good basic skin hygiene with antibacterial soaps and topical antibiotics.
- Systemic therapy should be based on antibiotic sensitivity for the causative organisms.

Resident and transient flora harmlessly colonize the skin; their numbers and distribution varying with site, age, climate, underlying disease, and medication. By contrast, pathogenic organisms are normally prevented from invading and colonizing the skin by an intact stratum corneum, rapid cell turnover, skin surface lipids, and skin surface pH. Moreover, normal skin flora elaborate protein-complex antibiotics in the presence of potential pathogens [1].

Impetigo, folliculitis, furuncles, and other skin infections are almost all caused by β-hemolytic organisms—either group A streptococci or *Staphylococcus aureus*. Less common infections are caused by gram-negative microbes and by *Pseudomonas aeruginosa*.

IMPETIGO

Impetigo occurs in a vesiculo-pustular form with thick golden crusts and in a bullous form (Table 2-1). Although it is seen in all age groups, it is one of the most common skin infections in children. Impetigo may spread rapidly when left untreated, and it may take several weeks before spontaneous healing occurs.

Diagnosis

The diagnosis of impetigo is based on clinical presentation with laboratory confirmation. Nonbullous impetigo begins as superficial vesicles that may become pustular or develop a honey-colored crust (Fig. 2-1). These crusts can be easily removed, and doing so leaves a smooth, red, moist surface that may produce fresh exudate. At times, a halo of erythema surrounds the lesion. Typically, the lesions

TABLE 2-1 TYPES OF IMPETIGO

Type	Characteristic lesion	Most common site	Most common causative organism	Treatment
Nonbullous impetigo (*impetigo contagiosa*)	Honey-colored crusting at site of previous vesicle or pustule	Legs then arms, face, and trunk	*Staphylococcus aureus* group A β-hemolytic streptococcus	If mild, topical antibiotics and good hygiene; if severe, systemic antibiotics
Bullous impetigo	Bulla, and ruptured bulla that leave an inflamed red base with thin varnish-like crust	Face	Group II *S. aureus*, usually plaque type 71	Systemic antibiotics
Ecthyma	Thick crust that when removed reveals a superficial ulceration; scars may occur	Lower legs	Group A β-hemolytic streptococcus	If mild, removal of crust followed by topical antibiotic; if severe, systemic antibiotics

are not painful but on occasion may itch, especially those that are preceeded by a bug bite. Nonbullous impetigo commonly occurs on such exposed surfaces as the extremities and the face where minor trauma, insect bites, contact dermatitis, or abrasions may occur.

Laboratory evaluation includes a Gram stain and culture of an early lesion or a base of a crust. A Gram stain reveals gram-positive cocci. A bacterial culture yields *S. aureus*, streptococci, or both.

A serious complication of nonbullous impetigo is acute glomerulonephritis (AGN). It is most often associated with the nephrotigenic strains of streptococci (types 49, 55, 57, 60 and strand M-type 2). The incidence of AGN with impetigo varies from 2% to 15% depending upon the strain of streptococcus. It is a complication most commonly seen in children under 6 years old. The prognosis is better for children than adults. Treatment of the impetigo does not alter the risk for the development of AGN. There is no evidence suggesting that bullous impetigo is associated with the development of AGN. Other disorders associated with

streptococcal skin infections include scarlet fever, lymphangitis, and transient postinflammatory pigmentary changes. Rheumatic fever has not been reported following nonbullous impetigo.

Bullous impetigo classically represents a toxin-induced lesion that remains nonpurulent. It is unusual to find bullous lesions that are secondarily infected by streptococci or other bacteria. This may be a result of the production of bacteriocins produced by group II *S. aureus*. Clinically, the lesions of bullous impetigo begin as small vesicles which quickly enlarge to form bullae (Fig. 2-2). The bullae will usually rupture within 24 to 48 hours and leave a thin varnish-like brown to black crust. Bullous impetigo frequently begins on nontraumatized skin of the buttocks, perineum, trunk, or face. However, these lesions may be found anywhere on the body. They are shallow lesions that are rarely associated with regional lymphadenopathy. The group II strains of *S. aureus* are also associated with neonatal bullous impetigo, staphylococcal scalded skin syndrome, and staphylococcal scarlet fever.

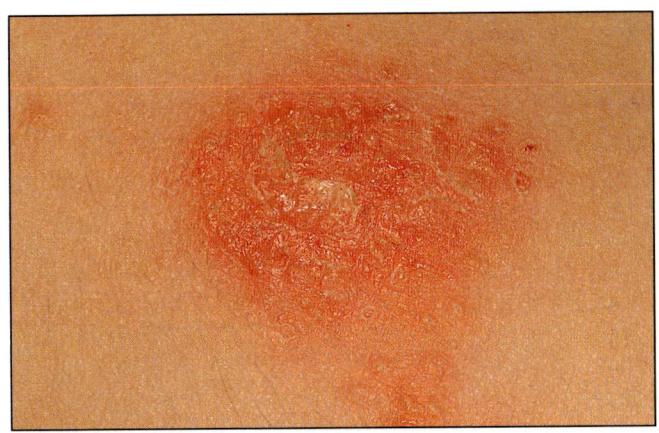

FIGURE 2-1 Nonbullous impetigo (note the honey-colored crusting).

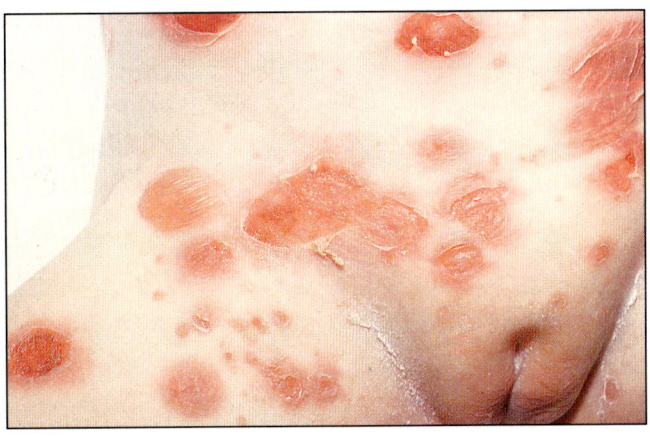

FIGURE 2-2 Bullous impetigo.

TABLE 2-2 TOPICAL ANTIBIOTICS USED FOR SKIN INFECTIONS

Agent	Dose	Duration	Indication
Bacitracin ointment Mupirocin ointment Neomycin-bacitracin-polymyxin B	bid to tid	2–3 wk, or 1 wk after lesion has healed	Impetigo, ecthyma
Erythromycin 2%	bid	2–3 wk or 1 wk after lesion has healed	Folliculitis

bid—twice daily; tid—three times daily.

Treatment

Topical therapy should be reserved for those cases where only a few lesions are present (Table 2-2). It would be impractical to treat dozens of lesions topically when systemic therapy would be equally efficacious and probably provide better compliance. Also, a patient using topical therapy should be able to demonstrate reasonably good hygiene and reliability in applying the medication. Some disadvantages of topical therapy are slower rates of healing, continued development of new lesions, inability to eradicate streptococci concomitantly present in the respiratory tract, and practical difficulties in applying medication for numerous lesions. Topical therapy is not effective in bullous impetigo.

Probably the two most effective topical therapies for nonbullous impetigo are mupirocin and neomycin-bacitracin-polymyxin B [2]. Mupirocin is highly effective against all species of staphylococci, including methicillin-resistant *S. aureus* and most species of *Streptococcus pyogenes* [3]. It is ineffective against most gram-positive bacilli, anaerobes, and aerobic gram-negative bacilli. It is as efficacious as oral erythromycin for the treatment of impetigo [4•].

Neomycin is active against staphylococci but less so against streptococci and gram-negative bacilli. It does, however, have activity against *P. aeruginosa* and obligate anaerobe bacteria. Bacitracin inhibits both staphylococci and streptococci as well as other gram-positive bacilli. Bacitracin ointment alone has been shown to be effective in the treatment of nonbullous impetigo [5]. Polymyxin B is active against aerobic gram-negative bacilli, including *P. aeruginosa*. Combining these medications into one topical medication thus provides a spectrum of activity that may be adequate for the treatment of pyoderma.

Systemic therapy combined with topical therapy is advised in more severe cases (Table 2-3). Treatment with dicloxacillin, erythromycin, or cephalexin rather than with penicillin has been suggested because of the recent emergence of *S. aureus* as the primary pathogen. However, because of an increase in the number of erythromycin-resistant strains of *S. aureus* [6,7], cephalexin or dicloxacillin should be the initial treatment. A comparison of twice daily cephalexin versus four times daily dicloxacillin revealed the cephalexin to be equally efficacious to dicloxacillin in the treatment of impetigo [8]. Recently, 5 days of azithromycin

TABLE 2-3 SYSTEMIC ANTIBIOTICS USED FOR SKIN INFECTIONS

Type	Dose/frequency	Duration	Indication
Penicillin-VK	50 mg/kg/d in four divided doses	7–10 d	Erysipelas
Erythromycin ethylsuccinate	30–40 mg/kg/d in three divided doses	7–10 d	Impetigo, folliculitis, ecthyma, paronychia, furuncles, cellulitis
Dicloxacillin	15 mg/kg/d in four divided doses	7–10 d	Impetigo, folliculitis, ecthyma, paronychia, furuncles, cellulitis
Cephalexin	50 mg/kg/d in two divided doses	7–10 d	Impetigo, folliculitis, ecthyma, paronychia, furuncles, cellulitis
Azithromycin	500 mg orally on d 1, then 250 mg oraly once daily x 4 d	5 d	Impetigo, folliculitis, ecthyma, paronychia, furuncles, cellulitis
Ciprofloxacin	500–750 mg orally twice daily	7–10 d	Impetigo, folliculitis, ecthyma, paronychia, furuncles, cellulitis
Amoxicillin clavulanate	500 mg orally three times daily	7–10 d	Impetigo, folliculitis, ecthyma, paronychia, furuncles, cellulitis, deep nodular gram-negative folliculitis

was shown to be as or more effective than 7 days of erythromycin or cloxacillin in the treatment of impetigo as well as carbuncles, furuncles, paronychia, folliculitis, and erysipelas [9•].

Prevention

Good hygiene and appropriate clothing that covers exposed skin in those patients susceptible to insect bites is recommended as a preventive measure. Topical antibiotics applied prophylactically to areas of minor skin trauma in children in a daycare center significantly reduced the development of cutaneous infections [3]. Additionally, eradication of nasal carriers of *S. aureus* by the administration of 5 days of topical mupirocin four times a day was shown to be effective [10].

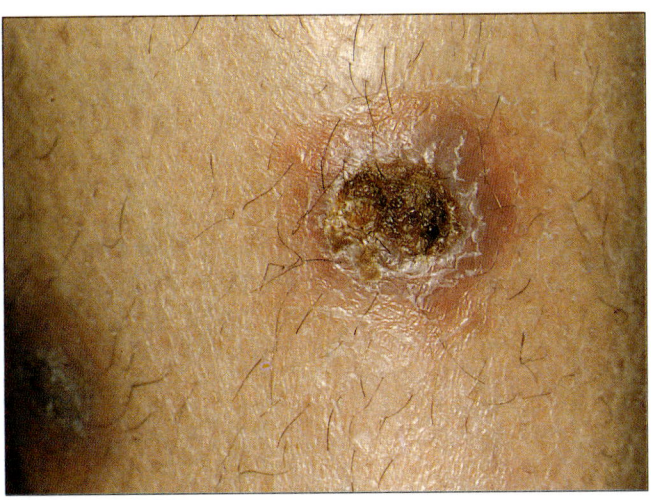

FIGURE 2-3 Ecthyma on the leg.

ECTHYMA

Ecthyma is a form of impetigo that involves deeper layers of the skin. In this disorder the process erodes through the epidermis and results in a shallow ulcer. The lesions typically begin as vesiculopustules that quickly crust over (Fig. 2-3). The crust of ecthyma differs from the crust of impetigo because it is larger, heaped up, and harder. Upon removal, it reveals an ulcer. An individual lesion will usually heal within a few weeks and may or may not form a scar. The most common area of the body affected is the lower extremities. The most common organism is β-hemolytic streptococci.

The disease is more common in children, due to trauma that occurs during normal recreational activity. Other predisposing factors include insect bites, scratches, pediculosis, scabies, and eczema, especially in those patients with underlying poor hygiene in warm, humid environments.

Treatment

The treatment of ecthyma includes removal of the overlying crust and application of a topical antibiotic to the ulcer base (Table 2-2). The removal of the crust may be facilitated by prior softening with warm, gentle soap compresses. A topical antibiotic such as mupirocin may be used. In more severe cases oral antibiotics such as dicloxacillin, erythromycin, or azithromycin should be instituted (Table 2-3). Encouragement of proper skin hygiene is paramount.

FOLLICULITIS

Folliculitis is classified according to depth of involvement and etiology (Table 2-4). All types involve the hair follicle in some manner.

Superficial Folliculitis

Superficial folliculitis (Bockhart's impetigo, superficial pustular perifolliculitis, impetigo follicularis) is caused by coagulase-positive *S. aureus*. Predisposing conditions include poor hygiene, maceration, and occlusive therapies

| | | | **Most common** | |
Type	**Characteristic lesion**	**Most common site**	**organism**	**Treatment**
Superficial folliculitis (Bockhart's impetigo)	Small dome-shaped pustule at the follicular orifice	In children, the scalp; adults—scalp, back, and extremities	*Staphylococcus aureus*	Topical erythromycin 2% solution
Gram-negative folliculitis Superficial variant	Superficial pustules	Centrofacial, perinasal area	Enterobacter, klebsiella	If mild, topical antibiotics
Deep variant	Fluctuant, deep-seated nodules	Centrofacial, perinasal area	Proteus	If severe, systemic antibiotics or isotretinoin
Hot tub folliculitis	Follicularly oriented erythematous papules topped by a small pustule	Buttocks, axilla, lateral aspects of trunk	*Pseudomonas aeruginosa* (serotype 0:11)	Discontinue use of hot tub

TABLE 2-4 TYPES OF FOLLICULITIS

and dressings. Occupational exposures to cutting oils, solvents and tar preparations may also induce this disorder.

Superficial folliculitis is a clinical diagnosis supported by Gram stain and culture. Characteristically, the lesion is approximately a 1- to 4-mm dome-shaped yellow pustule located at the follicular orifice. There may be multiple or single lesions. The usual sites of involvement are the scalp, back, and extremities (Figs. 2-4 and 2-5). Any hair-bearing area, however, may be involved. In children, the most common site of involvement is the scalp. The course of individual lesions typically reveals a pustule that may rupture or become excoriated and leave a crust in its wake. A bacterial culture of the lesion will usually yield coagulase-positive staphylococci.

Treatment

Superficial folliculitis may spontaneously resolve without therapy. However, appropriate antibiotic therapy will accelerate the clearing process. Local care is usually both effective and sufficient for the treatment of superficial folliculitis. Soap and water cleansing should be performed routinely prior to the application of topical antibiotics (Table 2-2). Erythromycin 2% solution applied twice a day to affected areas can also be useful. This treatment is empiric, and culturing pustules to determine antibiotic sensitivities for the causative organism is usually unnecessary except in severe resistant cases.

Gram-Negative Folliculitis

Another variant, gram-negative folliculitis, presents in two forms: superficial pustules around the nose, and deep nodular or cystic lesions. It predominantly occurs as a superinfection in a patient who has received long-term antibiotics for acne vulgaris. The usual cause of the superficial variant is klebsiella or enterobacter. The deep nodular type is associated with proteus. Although Gram stain is usually nega-

tive, cultures will often be positive. The superficial variant may be treated with topical antibiotics while the deep nodular variant often requires oral antibiotics such as ampicillin-clavulanate, trimethoprim-sulfamethoxazole or ciprofloxacin (Table 2-3). In severe cases, the treatment of choice is isotretinoin [6].

Hot Tub Folliculitis

Hot tub folliculitis is a variant of folliculitis caused by *P. aeruginosa*. Although *Pseudomonas* has been associated with folliculitis after prolonged therapy of topical corticosteroids under occlusion, it is being increasingly recognized after the recreational use of whirlpools and hot tubs [11]. *Pseudomonas* species tend to flourish in pools that have low chloride levels, high pH, and high water temperatures.

Clinically, the skin lesions are erythematous papules topped by a pustule ranging from 2 to 10 mm in size that occurs in a follicular distribution. The lesions are often very pruritic and are characteristically found on the buttocks, hips, axilla, and lateral aspects of the trunk. Those areas that are not submerged in the hot tub are typically spared and include the head, neck, and mucous membranes. The eruption may begin anywhere from 6 hours to 5 days after the exposure; however, the incubation period is typically 2 days. The diagnosis is made clinically and supported by bacterial culture. The organism may be cultured from a pustule as well as the pool water. Serotype O:11 is most often affiliated with hot tub folliculitis.

Hot tub folliculitis is a self-limited disease and does not require therapy. However, hot tub use should be discontinued until the water source is appropriately adjusted. Topical corticosteroids should also be avoided. Serious infections have occurred in immunosuppressed patients infected with *P. aeruginosa* O–11 [12]. Thus, it may be prudent to advise immunosuppressed patients to avoid recreational hot tub use because of the theoretical possibility of serious infection.

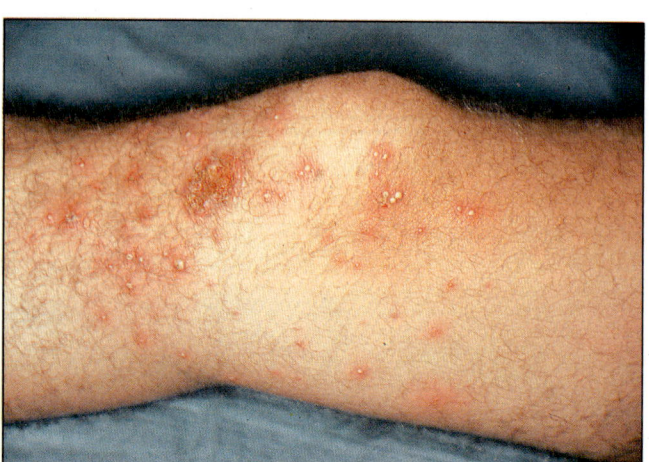

FIGURE 2-4 Superficial folliculitis on the leg.

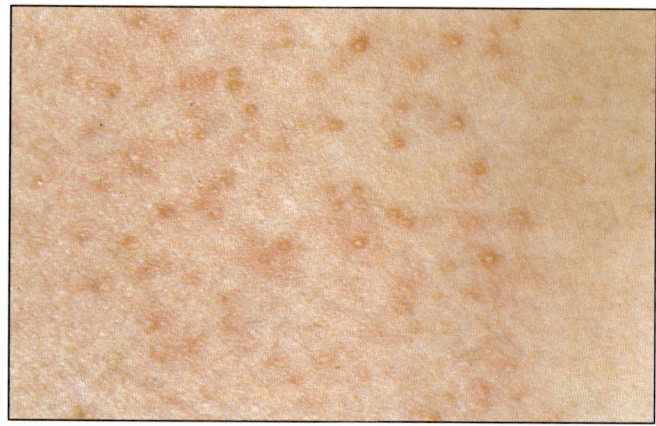

FIGURE 2-5 Folliculitis (note the dome-shaped pustules in a follicular distribution).

FURUNCLES AND CARBUNCLES

A furuncle or a boil is an acute perifollicular staphylococcal abscess of the skin and subcutaneous tissue. A carbuncle is an aggregation of interconnected furuncles that drain through a number of points in the skin surface. The lesions always begin near a hair follicle or a sebaceous gland. True furuncles are not thought to occur in hairless areas. Although the exact cause of furuncles is unknown, sebaceous gland obstruction or ingrown hairs probably play an important role.

Diagnosis

Predisposing factors to furunculosis or multiple recurrent furuncles include poor hygiene, occupational exposure to grease and oil, infection of preexisting dermatoses, malnutrition, alcoholism, and underlying hypogammoglobulonemia or leukopenia. Furuncles also tend to be more common in participants in contact sports. However, most cases do not have any predisposing local or systemic cause. Although furuncleosis tends to be more severe in diabetics, it is felt that diabetes alone does not predispose to furunculosis.

Clinically, furuncles prefer the following sites: nape, face, buttocks, thighs, perineum, breasts, and axillae (Fig. 2-6). Carbuncles occur in thick skin since these areas tend to favor lateral extension of subcutaneous abscesses (Fig. 2-7). These areas include the nape, shoulders, buttocks, outer thighs, and hips. Carbuncles develop more slowly than furuncles but attain larger sizes and are more painful. Because of the overlying thick skin, the drainage of the suppurative process is delayed and favors formation of necrosis within the abscess. This necrotic process extends laterally along the fibrous trabeculae to other follicles and produces more abscesses. The surface of the overlying skin often reveals a dull red color and indurated texture. It is tense with sieve-like changes that allow pus drainage from multiple follicular orifices. Furuncles are painful when they occur in skin that is tightly bound down, such as over the external auditory canal or nasal cartilage, while carbuncles are almost always painful, regardless of location.

Treatment

The initial treatment of furuncles and carbuncles should be warm compresses and good hygiene. Also, an oral semisynthetic penicillinase-resistant penicillin such as dicloxacillin, cephalosporin, or azithromycin [8,9•] should be prescribed, for at least a 2-week minimum (Table 2-3). In the event that furunculosis is severe and associated with systemic symptoms and lymphadenitis, intravenous antibiotics may be indicated. If drainage has already occurred and only a few lesions are present, local therapy is indicated. Surgical excision should be avoided in early lesions. Additionally, squeezing the lesion to extract hair or pus should not be performed. Both of these maneuvers may cause local or systemic extension.

When it begins to suppurate and become boggy, the lesion may be drained by "nicking" with a #11 blade. Draining lesions should be covered with topical antibiotics (Table 2-2) and loose dressings that are changed frequently to prevent autoinoculation. Medicated wicks or rubber drains should not be used as they prevent healing and may lead to scarring. Typically, after a lesion has been drained it will completely resolve after 2 weeks. However, the overlying violaceous color of the skin may not resolve for weeks to months.

Prevention

Prevention of recurrences may be difficult and unrewarding. Avoidance of skin irritants, good personal hygiene, and daily antibiotic washes may be attempted but are often ineffective. Topical washes that have shown some success in preventing furunculosis include chlorhexidine. Attempts to

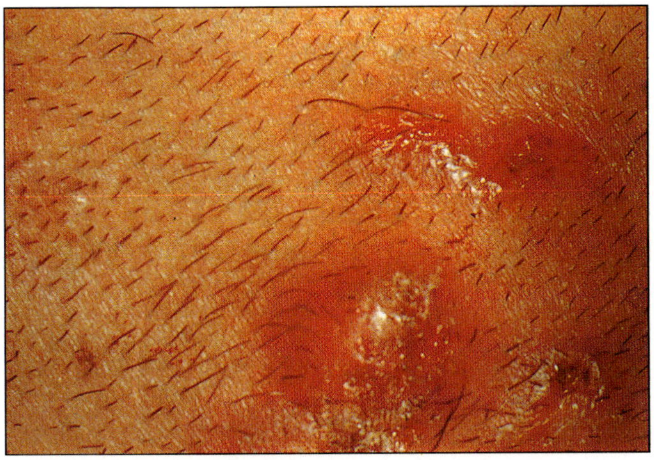

FIGURE 2-6 Furuncle (note the discrete hard subcutaneous nodule with an overlying erythematous hue).

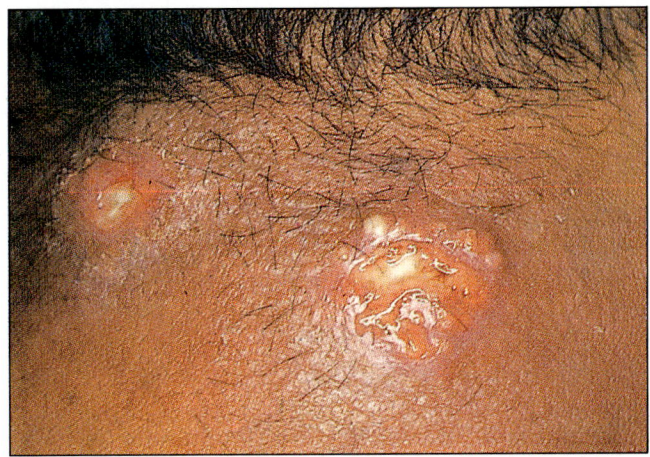

FIGURE 2-7 Carbuncle on the nape (notice the multiple number of drainage points through the skin).

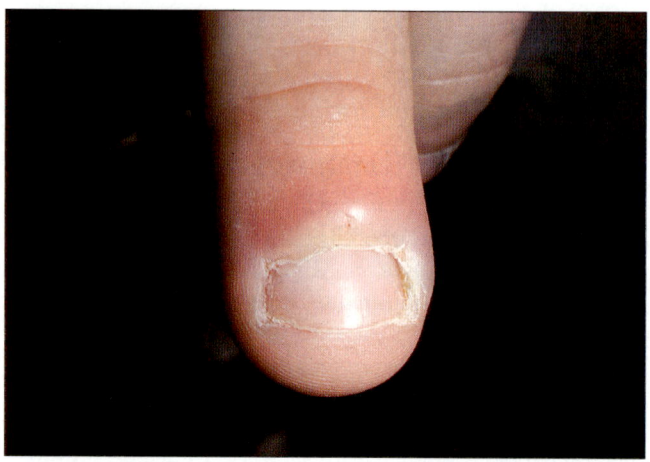

FIGURE 2-8 Acute staphylococcal paronychia (note the acute swollen, inflamed erythematous paronychial folds).

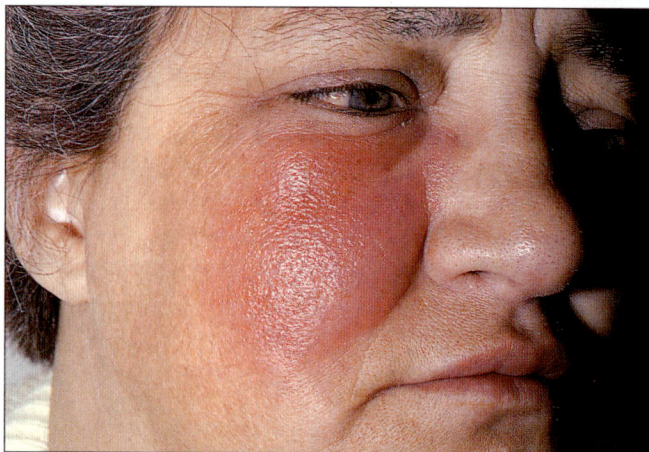

FIGURE 2-9 Erysipelas (note the erythematous and edematous skin with a sharply demarcated margin).

eliminate the *S. aureus* carrier state with nasal mupirocin have been effective [10].

PARONYCHIA

Paronychia is inflammation of the nail folds. The potential space surrounding the nail fold provides an excellent setting for infection. The infection begins in the paronychium at the site of the nail and usually manifests as swelling, local redness, and pain (Fig. 2-8). Pyonychia is a term that is used to refer to pyoderma involving the perionychium. In acute paronychia, the most common causative bacteria include staphylococci, beta-hemolytic streptococci, and gram-negative enteric bacteria. Chronic paronychia is usually caused by *Candida*.

Gentle pressure on the tender swollen paronychium will usually express a drop of pus. It is also not unusual to see pus through the nail or at the paronychial fold. As the syndrome progresses, the tender red swollen area extends around the nail fold and spares the distal edge. Resolution typically occurs within a few days. However, if it does not occur rapidly, the nail matrix may become disturbed and a permanent dystrophy of the nail plate may occur.

Common predisposing factors include minor trauma that results in a break of the skin, such as a hangnail, a splinter lodged under the distal edge of the nail, or a prick from a thorn. Paronychia may be secondary to hematoma.

Treatment

Medical treatment includes wet compresses (Burow's solution) or hot bland soaks combined with appropriate systemic antibiotic therapy. Topical antibiotics are of limited value because of poor penetration throughout the nail plate to the affected area. If medical treatment does not resolve these measures and a pocket of pus remains, then surgical drainage of the loculation is indicated.

ERYSIPELAS

Erysipelas or superficial cellulitis is characterized by an edematous, brawny, infiltrated, well-demarcated plaque that is bright red and warm (Fig. 2-9). It spreads peripherally without central clearing. Although the infection may occur anywhere, the most common sites are the face and scalp. The characteristic leading border is often palpable and distinct from the uninvolved skin. Clinically, the patient with erysipelas is febrile and appears ill.

The most common causative organism is group A β-hemolytic streptococci. Other less common causes include group B, group C, or group G streptococci. Predisposing factors include poor skin hygiene, prior wounds and injuries, and preexisting ulcers or suppurative cutaneous processes. Additionally, underlying conditions that lower the host's resistance and predispose to erysipelas include: cachexia, malnutrition, and underlying systemic disease.

The diagnosis is made clinically since diagnostic techniques such as culture and Gram stain are frequently unrewarding. The treatment of choice is penicillin either via oral, intramuscular, or intravenous routes continued for at least 10 days. It is very effective and rapid improvement may be seen within 24 to 48 hours. Local treatment should include elevation of the affected body part, rest, and cold compresses.

Complications of erysipelas include *elephantiasis verrucosa nostra* in those patients in whom recurrent erysipelas of the lower extremity occurs. Other complications include septicemia or deep cellulitis and these are more common in the elderly and newborn.

CELLULITIS

Cellulitis is a diffuse suppurative inflammation involving the subcutaneous tissue. Clinically there is local erythema and warmth. The cutaneous erythema is poorly demarcated

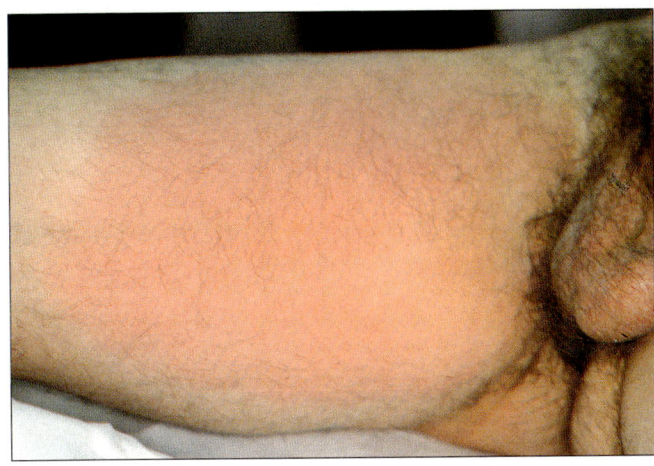

FIGURE 2-10 Cellulitis on the inner thigh (note the vague demarcation between normal and affected skin).

from uninvolved areas and thus presents a contrasting clinical picture to that of the distinct palpable margin of erysipelas (Fig. 2-10). Associated with cellulitis are systemic symptoms such as malaise, fever, and chills. The most common causes of cellulitis are beta-hemolytic streptococci and *S. aureus*.

Cellulitis is a clinical diagnosis since the causative organism is often very difficult to recover. Nonetheless, attempts to retrieve the causative organisms by skin biopsy, blood culture, or aspiration of the advancing edge have been positive on occasion.

Treatment should include bed rest, elevation of the affected parts, and systemic antibiotic therapy that will provide adequate coverage for either streptococci or staphylococci (Table 2-3). Complications of cellulitis include gangrene, metastatic abscess, and sepsis. These are more common in immunocompromized adults or very young children.

REFERENCES AND RECOMMENDED READING

Recently published papers of particular interest have been highlighted as:

• Of interest

•• Of outstanding interest

1. Roth R, James W: Microbiology of the skin: resident flora, ecology, infection. *J Am Acad Dermatol* 1989, 20:367–390.

2. Hirschmann JV: Topical antibiotics in dermatology. *Arch Dermatol* 1988, 124:1691–1700.

3. Leyden J: Mupirocin: A new topical antibiotic. *J Am Acad Dermatol* 1990, 22:879–883.

4.• McLin S: A bacteriologically controlled randomized study comparing the efficacy of 2% mupirocin ointment (Bactroban) with oral erythromycin in the treatment of patients with impetigo. *J Am Acad Dermatol* 1990, 22:883–885.

5. Dillon H: Topical and systemic therapy for pyodermas. *Int J Dermatol* 1980, 19:443–451.

6. James WD, Leyden JJ: Treatment of gram-negative folliculitis with isotretinoin: positive clinical and microbiologic response. *J Am Acad Dermatol* 1985, 12:319.

7. Grossman KL, Rasmussen JE: Recent advances in pediatric infectious disease and their impact on dermatology. *J Am Acad Dermatol* 1991, 24:379–389.

8. Dillon H: Treatment of staphylococcal skin infections: a comparison of cephalexin and dicloxacillin. *J Am Acad Dermatol* 1983, 8:177–181.

9.• Daniel R: Azithromycin, erythromycin and cloxacillin in the treatment of infections of skin and associated soft tissues. *J Int Med Res* 1991, 19:433–445.

10. Casewell MW, Hill LR: Elimination of nasal carriage of staphylococcus aureus with mupirocin "pseudomonic acid"—a control trial. *J Antimicrob Chemother* 1986, 17:365–372.

11. Fox A, Hambrick G: Recreationally associated pseudomonas aeruginosa folliculitis. *Arch Dermatol* 1984, 120:1304–1307.

12. Aze P, Thyss A, Caldani C, *et al.*: Pseudomonas aeruginosa O–11 folliculitis: development into ecthyma gangrenosum in immunosuppressed patients. *Arch Dermatol* 1985, 121:873–876.

3 Common Viral Infections of the Skin

Paul A. Krusinski

Key Points

- Genital molluscum contagiosum, in spite of its banal nature, implies unprotected sexual exposure, and testing for syphilis, hepatitis B, and HIV may be necessary.
- Recently published Centers for Disease Control and Prevention guidelines for the treatment of recurrent genital herpes simplex with acyclovir suggest a 5-day course of 200 mg five times daily, 400 mg three times daily, or 800 mg twice daily.
- Zoster therapy now includes a choice of either acyclovir or famciclovir. Additional agents will become available in the next few years.
- Post-herpetic neuralgia is no longer considered separately, but is a category of all "zoster-associated pain."
- The viral etiologies of erythema infectiosum (Fifth disease) and roseola (exantheum subitum) have now been elucidated. Exposure to these agents may have serious consequences for some patients.

Even though the primary emphasis of this chapter is on the manifestations, diagnosis, and treatment of cutaneous viral infections, these do not occur in a vacuum. Infected skin envelops a human being, and even the most banal cutaneous viral skin lesions have systemic implications. For example, some forms of papillomavirus that cause warts are associated with the development of carcinoma of the cervix and squamous cell carcinoma. Genital molluscum contagiosum implies unprotected sex, and questions about syphilis, hepatitis B, and HIV must be discussed. Herpes simplex and zoster infections may become life-threatening in the immunocompromised individual. This chapter discusses common viral infections of the skin and points out when the clinician must be on the lookout for more serious complications and systemic effects.

HUMAN PAPILLOMAVIRUS INFECTIONS

Warts are extremely common, usually banal, and characteristically fall into the category of a clinical nuisance. The various clinical types include: common warts (*verrucae vulgaris*), plantar warts (*verrucae plantaris*), flat warts (*verrucae plana*), and genital warts (*condyloma acuminata*). These types are described as separate clinical entities because their appearance and treatment sometimes vary considerably.

Common Warts

This condition can occur on almost any area of the body, most often in children but also in any age group, and many warts may persist for years. However, in children one half of all warts will spontaneously regress in 1 year and two thirds of all warts will clear in 2 years without therapy. The verrucous papules are so common that recognition and diagnosis are usually easy (Fig. 3-1). For treatment, one may use keratolytic acid paintings that are available over the counter

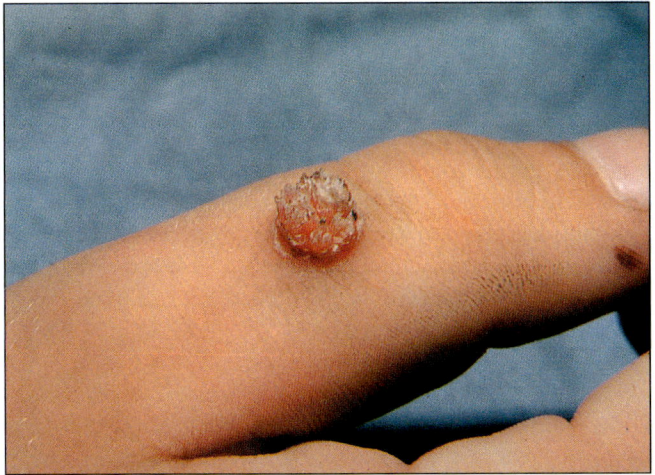

FIGURE 3-1 Verrucous papule of a common wart. (*From* Flowers and Krusinski [24]; with permission.)

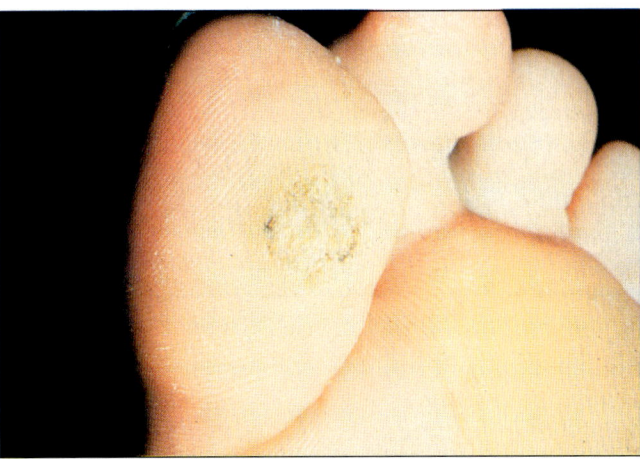

FIGURE 3-2 Planter warts interrupt the skin lines and have dark dots (thrombosed vessels) within them. (*From* Flowers and Krusinski [24]; with permission.)

under a variety of names. Each contains 17% salicylic acid, and should be applied twice daily (Table 3-1). For warts that are few in number or fail to be relieved by topical keratolytic acids, liquid nitrogen cryosurgery is successful 70% to 80% of the time. This procedure should be performed at monthly intervals and may take three or four applications to achieve clearing on areas of thicker skin.

Plantar Warts

Plantar warts, appearing on the soles of the feet, are particularly recalcitrant to therapy. They occur most frequently on weight-bearing prominences, and at times are extremely painful. They must be differentiated from calluses that have increased skin lines and also from hard corns. Dark dots that represent thrombosed blood vessels are usually present in plantar warts (Fig. 3-2). The differential diagnosis

includes verrucous carcinoma and amelanotic melanoma that can also occur on the sole. Plantar warts may be treated with the same modalities used for common warts (Table 3-1) [1•]. However, liquid nitrogen cryosurgery may be painful when used on the sole and is usually only effective for plantar warts of very small diameter and thickness. It can be combined with paring and topical chemodestruction to enhance its effectiveness. Topical formalin and glutaraldehyde represent alternatives to keratolytic acid paintings for persistent plantar warts. CO_2 laser vaporization has a 90% success rate and should be used in place of electrodesiccation and curettage because it usually causes less scarring.

Flat Warts

Flat warts are found most often on the face in children, the beard region in men, and on the legs in women where shaving causes inoculation along the minor nicks from a razor. They are asymptomatic flat papules and plaques that may be pink, flesh-colored, or slightly hyperpigmented (Fig. 3-3). They range in size from 1 mm to greater than

TABLE 3-1 TREATMENT OF COMMON AND PLANTAR WARTS
Keratolytic acid paintings
File with emery board after bath or shower
Apply 17% salicylic acid twice daily
If irritation develops, apply castor oil in place of acid twice daily
Resume acid paintings twice daily
Liquid nitrogen cryosurgery
Freeze 3–4 mm around wart
Curettage and electrodesiccation
May lead to substantial scarring
CO_2 laser vaporization
For periungual or recalcitrant warts

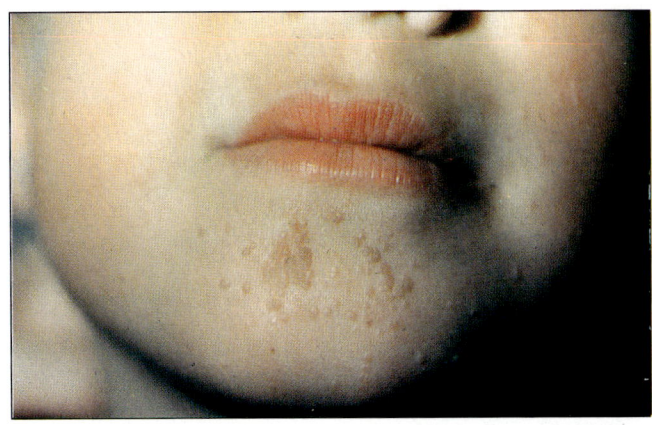

FIGURE 3-3 Flat warts.

1 cm and are often multiple. As with warts in general, they will spontaneously clear in many patients. When clearing occurs, it is frequently heralded by pruritus and erythema. The treatment of choice for verrucae plana is topical tretinoin cream, Retin-A (Ortho Pharmaceuticals, Raritan, NJ), applied twice daily, with application of 0.5% for facial and 0.1% for hands or legs. The condition may take several months to clear.

GENITAL WARTS

Genital warts are one of the most common sexually transmissible diseases. Most patients have asymptomatic flesh-colored or pink verrucous papules that are easily diagnosed (Fig. 3-4). However, in some patients they may be extensive, persistent, and resistant to treatment. In patients with condyloma acuminata, questions regarding unprotected sex and the possibility of other diseases (eg, syphilis, hepatitis B, and HIV) need to be discussed and ruled out. Some human papillomavirus types associated with condyloma acuminata have been shown to be oncogenic but the vast majority of venereal warts are caused by nononcogenic strains [2]. There is no question that carcinoma of the cervix, carcinoma of the head of the penis, and intraanal squamous cell carcinomas have been linked to oncogenic strains of papillomavirus [3]. This extremely common epidemiologic problem is compounded by the existence of subclinical human papillomavirus infection of the genitals in both men and women, which is very difficult to diagnose and treat.

Genital warts need to be differentiated from molluscum contagiosum, folliculitis, nevi, and skin tags. Sometimes this can be accomplished through the use of acetowhitening. Five percent acetic acid (white vinegar) is applied by compresses over the genital region for 3 to 5 minutes. The typical white appearance of condyloma acuminata aids in the diagnosis. One should realize that many false-positive and false-negative reactions occur with this method. Occasionally biopsies of genital warts may be helpful, but histo-logically this may sometimes be confounding. The use of monoclonal antibody immunohistochemical stains to characterize the human papillomavirus type are not readily available in most clinical laboratories at the present time. Women who have external genital condylomata should have frequent pap smears and colposcopy examinations. Likewise, women who come in contact with men with genital warts should have frequent pap smears even if clinical examination is negative for warts. The frequency of sexual abuse as a cause of childhood genital or perianal warts is controversial, but issues relating to abuse need to be raised when the diagnosis is made [4].

There are many different treatments available for condyloma acuminata (Table 3-2). Careful follow-up is necessary as recurrences or newly developing warts will occur during the course of treatment.

HERPES SIMPLEX VIRUS INFECTIONS

Herpes simplex virus infections can occur anywhere on the body. Type I infections will occur above the waist 70% to 90% of the time, and type II below the waist 70% to 90% of the time. The primary infection of herpes simplex type 1 (HSV 1) manifests itself as a painful, erosive gingivostomatitis. The patient appears febrile and extremely toxic, but in the immunocompetent host it will resolve in 2 to 3 weeks. Primary HSV 1 gingivostomatitis is extremely rare, and most infected individuals have a subclinical infection that is never clinically diagnosed. The most frequently observed manifestation of HSV 1 infection is recurrent herpes labialis. It typically occurs at the mucocutaneous junction frequently in or around the same location after a 12 to 24 hour prodrome of itching and tingling (Fig. 3-5). Precipitating factors of a febrile illness or upper respiratory infections have led to the term cold sore or fever blister. Other precipitating events include exposure to ultraviolet

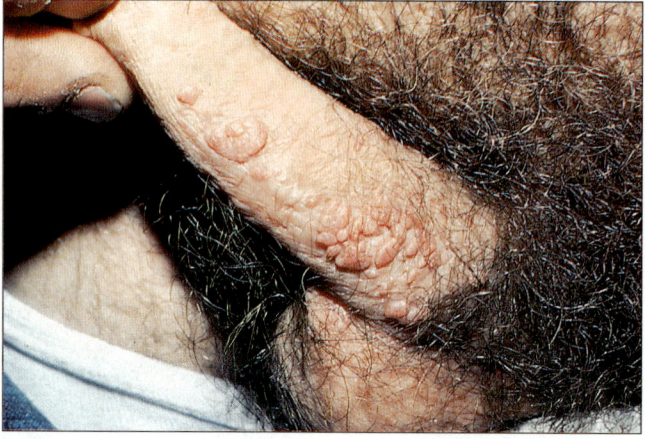

FIGURE 3-4 Condyloma acuminata. (*From* Flowers and Krusinski [24]; with permission.)

TABLE 3-2 TREATMENT OF GENITAL WARTS
Podophyllin 25% in tincture of benzoin
Apply once weekly (by physician)
Wash off as tolerated in 4–6 h
Podophyllotoxin (Condylox*) [5]
Apply twice daily 3 d/wk (by patient)
Use for 1 mo
Liquid nitrogen cryocautery
5-Fluorouracil cream, 5%
Apply daily or twice daily 4 d/wk
Use for 2 mo
CO₂ laser vaporization
*Oclassen Pharmaceuticals, San Rafael, CA.

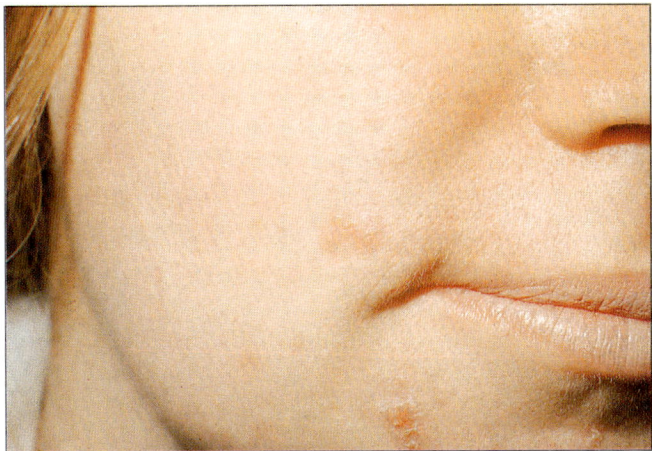

FIGURE 3-5 Grouped vesicles on an erythematous base that recur in the same location are characteristic of herpes simplex.

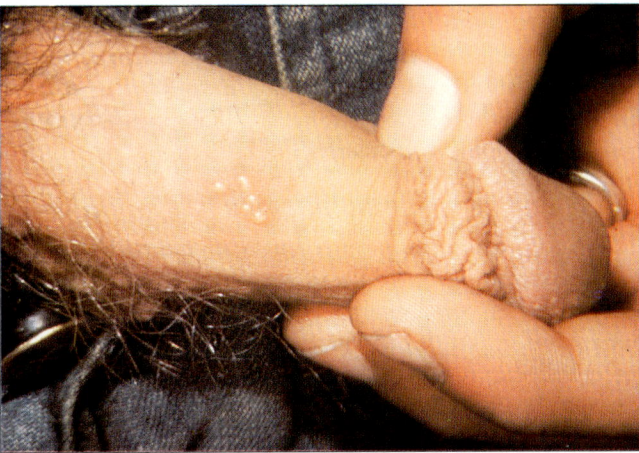

FIGURE 3-6 Recurrent genital herpes. (*From* Flowers and Krusinski [24]; with permission.)

light, trauma, and psychological stress. Recurrent cold sores typically last 7 to 10 days, and may cause considerable discomfort as well as cosmetic concern.

As in orolabial herpes simplex, primary genital infection may be subclinical. When infection does occur, multiple discreet bilateral vesicles and erosions may appear on the external genitalia. This may be associated with systemic symptoms of fever, malaise, and acute toxicity in both sexes, but healing will occur spontaneously in 2 to 3 weeks in the immunocompetent individual. In women with vaginal and cervical involvement, additional symptoms of vaginal discharge, dysuria, urinary retention, and lumbosacral reticulopathy may occur. Men may have bilateral inguinal lymphadenopathy. Primary genital herpes simplex may be due to HSV 1 or HSV 2. Genital herpes is almost always due to HSV 2. The typical morphology of recurrent genital herpes simplex consists of tightly clustered vesicles on an erythematous base, which occur in and around the same location before healing spontaneously in 7 to 10 days (Fig. 3-6). Fifty percent of patients will experience a prodrome of itching, burning, or tingling. This sexually transmitted disease is the source of potentially life-threatening neonatal herpes simplex infection. Maternal asymptomatic shedding may occur 1% of the time and accounts for most neonatal infections [6•]. Also, there is possible increased susceptibility to HIV infection if mucosal erosions are present during sexual intercourse.

Localized herpes simplex infection of the fingertip is called herpetic whitlow. In 10% of patients, usually children, it is caused by HSV 1 related to thumb and finger sucking. The remaining 90% of patients have HSV 2 obtained through sexual contact [7]. The usual herpes morphology of grouped vesicles on a red base helps distinguish herpetic whitlow from a felon or other digital inflammatory conditions (Fig. 3-7). Considerable edema is associated with the lesion and the pain is frequently quite severe.

Herpes gladiatorum is the term for herpes simplex lesions on the torso of competitive wrestlers, caused by HSV 1 infection [8]. Both herpes simplex and molluscum contagiosum skin infections may disqualify athletes from competitive wrestling.

Perianal erosions of herpetic proctitis may be present with or without the usual morphology of herpes simplex. It is often associated with pain, discharge, and tenesmus. It is most frequently seen in homosexual men and heterosexual women.

Diagnosis

The diagnosis of herpes simplex on the skin is usually easily made on clinical grounds. However, before using expensive antiviral chemotherapeutic agents one should obtain laboratory confirmation. A Tzanck smear is taken from scrapings from the floor of a herpetic vesicle. It may be stained with Wright stain in the examiner's office or sent to the laboratory for a Papanicolaou's stain. The results are positive approximately 50% of the time in active vesicular lesions.

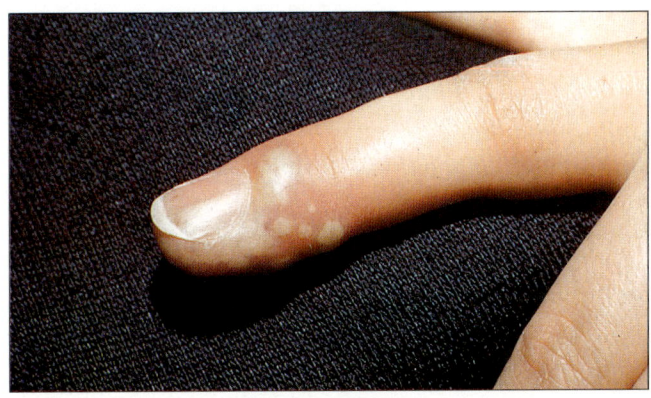

FIGURE 3-7 Herpetic whitlow. (*From* Flowers and Krusinski [24]; with permission.)

Viral culture early in the course of a recurrence will yield positive results 80% to 90% of the time. Current serologic assays are only helpful in identifying individuals at risk for reactivation who are about to undergo organ transplantation. However, they are otherwise of little clinical use.

Complications

A banal cold sore may represent a severe and possibly life-threatening problem in selected individuals. Specifically, patients undergoing organ transplantation and patients with AIDS may develop severe chronic herpetic infections that may lack the usual morphology (Fig. 3-8), and may lead to disseminated infection. Herpes simplex is also the most common infectious cause of erythema multiforme (*see* Kulp-Shorten, Urticaria and Reactive Dermatoses). Patients with severe atopic dermatitis, Darier's disease, and mycosis fungoides may get Kaposi's varicelliform eruption caused by herpes simplex (Fig. 3-9). Prompt diagnosis and early, aggressive treatment is necessary for these serious complications.

Treatment

Topical, oral, and intravenous acyclovir or Zovirax (Burroughs-Wellcome Laboratories, Research Triangle Park, NC) are effective against herpes simplex virus infections. However, topical acyclovir is only slightly more beneficial than placebo when evaluated in clinical trials. Its only clinical utility is in the treatment of cutaneous infections in immunocompromised individuals, where it has definitely been shown to shorten the clinical course of their disease. For primary and recurrent herpetic infections that are not very frequent, episodic treatment with oral acyclovir is indicated (Table 3-3). Those patients who have frequently recurring genital herpes simplex may wish to take a suppressive regimen of acyclovir 200 mg orally three times daily or 400 mg orally twice daily for 1 year prophylactically. Immunocompromised individuals, those with disseminated infection, or complications of herpes simplex infec-

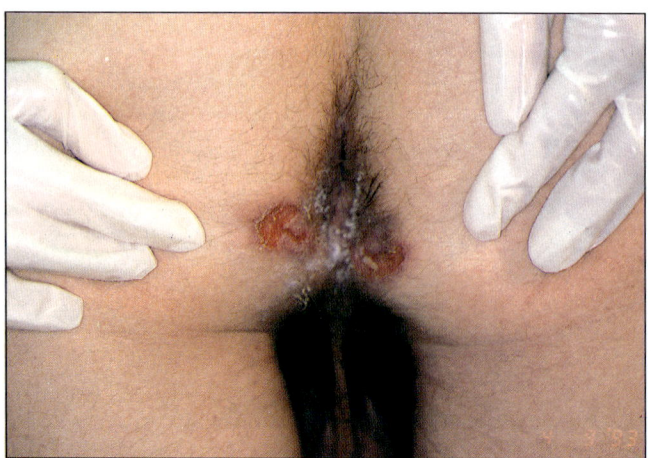

FIGURE 3-8 Chronic ulceration in an AIDS patient with herpes simplex virus.

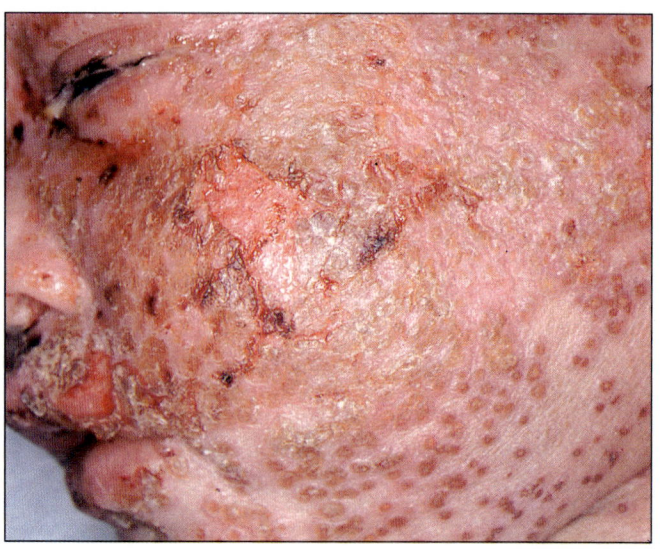

FIGURE 3-9 Kaposi's varicelliform eruption.

TABLE 3-3   TREATMENT OF HERPES SIMPLEX INFECTIONS

Orolabial

Primary
   Toxic patient: acyclovir 10 mg/kg i.v. every 8 h for 5 d
Recurrent
   Infrequent: topical antibiotic cream or ointment 3 times daily (placebo therapy)
   Frequent, severe, or immunocompromised: acyclovir 200 mg orally 5 times daily for 5 d

Herpes gladiatorum or herpetic whitlow

Acyclovir 200 mg orally 5 times daily for 5 d

Genital herpes

Primary: acyclovir 200 mg orally 5 times daily for 7–10 d
Recurrent
   Infrequent: acyclovir 200 mg orally 5 times daily for 5 d
   Or acyclovir 400 mg orally 3 times daily for 5 d
   Or acyclovir 800 mg orally 2 times daily for 5 d
   Acyclovir 200 mg orally 3 times daily for 1 y or
   Acyclovir 400 mg orally twice daily for 1 y

Complications of herpes simplex

Recurrent erythema multiforme and Stevens-Johnson syndrome
Suppressive regimen (*see above* Genital herpes)
Disseminated herpes simplex (immunocompromised or eczema herpeticum): acyclovir 200–400 mg orally 5 times daily for 10–14 d or longer, or in severe cases acyclovir i.v. (*see above* Primary)
Acyclovir 10 mg/kg i.v. every 8 h for 10 d
Foscarnet 60 mg/kg every 8 h i.v. (in patients with AIDS with acyclovir-resistant infection)

tion may need intravenous therapy. Immunocompromised individuals may also need to be treated for much longer periods of time to achieve clinical clearing. Patients with AIDS may need to be treated frequently or continuously with oral acyclovir. Thymidine kinase-negative strains of herpes simplex resistant to acyclovir have been isolated from patients with AIDS after intravenous courses of acyclovir. These patients may be treated successfully with intravenous foscarnet therapy [9].

VARICELLA ZOSTER VIRUS INFECTIONS

Varicella

Varicella or chickenpox is usually a banal infection, most often occurring in children aged between 5 and 15 years old [10]. Mild symptoms consist of fever and a pruritic, polymorphic skin eruption that begins on the torso and spreads centrifugally (Fig. 3-10). Eruptions begin as macules and papules that develop into vesicles, pustules, and frequently, hemorrhagic erosions. Punched-out, pocklike scars may occur, especially after secondary bacterial infection. The eruption usually occurs 14 to 21 days after exposure to another individual who has chickenpox, and is spread in expired respiratory droplets [11].

Diagnosis

The Tzanck smear may be very helpful in the diagnosis of varicella zoster virus (VZV) infections. Results are positive 80% of the time when taken from a varicella or zoster vesicle. Viral culture for this virus takes at least 2 weeks, is expensive, and is only positive approximately 50% of the time. Serologic testing for VZV is only helpful in determining susceptibility to varicella.

Treatment

Acyclovir has been shown to be helpful for the treatment of varicella in healthy children [12•]. Its use decreases fever and duration of illness, and also decreases the number of cutaneous lesions. However, complications of chickenpox have not been reduced in these early studies. It is reported that perhaps 20% of all patients with chickenpox who have a more severe course might benefit substantially from this therapy. However, in most children it is a banal disease, and therapy may not be necessary. The Oka vaccine for varicella may soon be available in the United States [13]. It is to be given with the measles, mumps, and rubella immunizations at 18 months and 5 years of age. It has been shown to diminish life-threatening varicella infections in children with leukemia.

Zoster or Shingles

Reactivation of the varicella virus from its latent state in the dorsal root ganglia with migration along sensory nerves to the adjacent skin dermatome leads to the clinical development of zoster [14]. A prodrome of 5 to 7 days of hyperesthesia or radicular pain in the same dermatome is quite common. Clinically, one sees tightly grouped vesicles on an erythematous base in a dermatomal pattern (Fig. 3-11). However, occasionally two or three adjacent dermatomes may be involved. In otherwise healthy individuals zoster will resolve in 2 to 3 weeks. It is felt that zoster is more frequent in the elderly and in patients with decreasing cell-mediated immunity, Hodgkin's disease, and AIDS. Disseminated zoster may occur in severely immunosuppressed patients. It is diagnosed when the patient has ten or more extradermatomal vesicles. Pneumonitis, hepatitis, and meningoencephalitis represent life-threatening visceral complications.

Treatment

Oral or intravenous acyclovir decreases viral shedding and acute pain associated with zoster. Acyclovir should be used in patients with ophthalmic involvement to prevent the occurrence of blindness. Acute pain from zoster is usually well controlled with oral acyclovir, and some studies suggest a decrease in the incidence of postzoster neuralgia with the

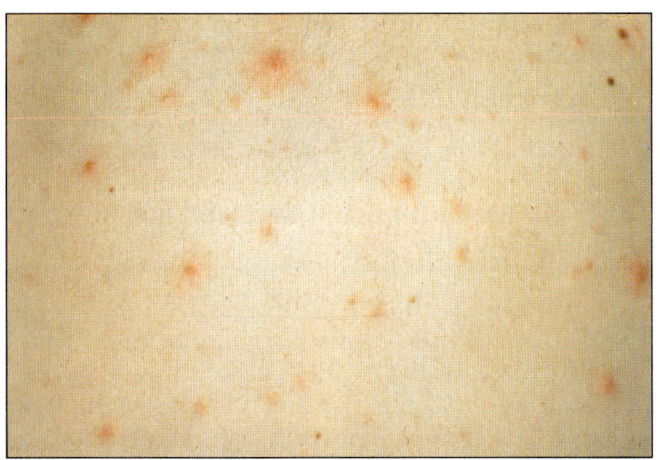

FIGURE 3-10 The lesions of chickenpox (varicella) are polymorphous and congregate on the torso.

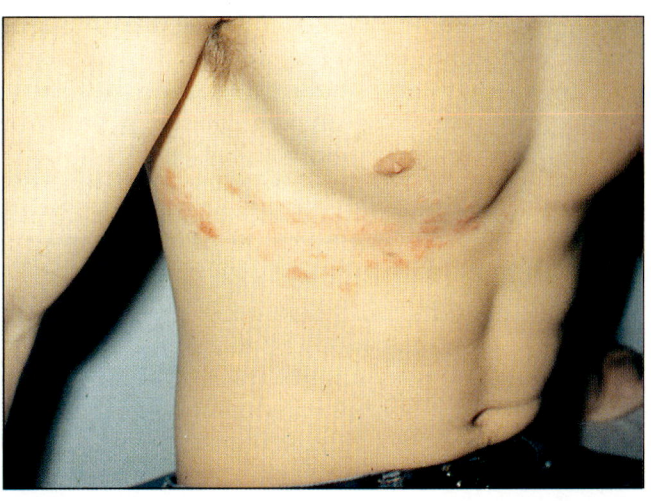

FIGURE 3-11 Zoster: vesicles in a dermatomal pattern.

TABLE 3-4 TREATMENT OF VARICELLA-ZOSTER INFECTION
Varicella Children: acyclovir 20 mg/kg daily orally in 4 divided doses for 7 d Adults: acyclovir 800 mg 5 times daily orally for 7–10 d
Zoster Localized: acyclovir 800 mg orally 5 times daily for 7–10 d or, famciclover orally 500 mg 3 times daily Burroughs solution compresses 3 to 4 times daily Topical antibiotic ointment after compresses Disseminated: acyclovir 10 mg/kg i.v. every 8h for 7 d
Post-zoster neuralgia Topical capsaicin cream 0.075% 6 times daily Amitriptyline 50 mg orally every h Oral analgesics Local nerve block by anesthesiologist

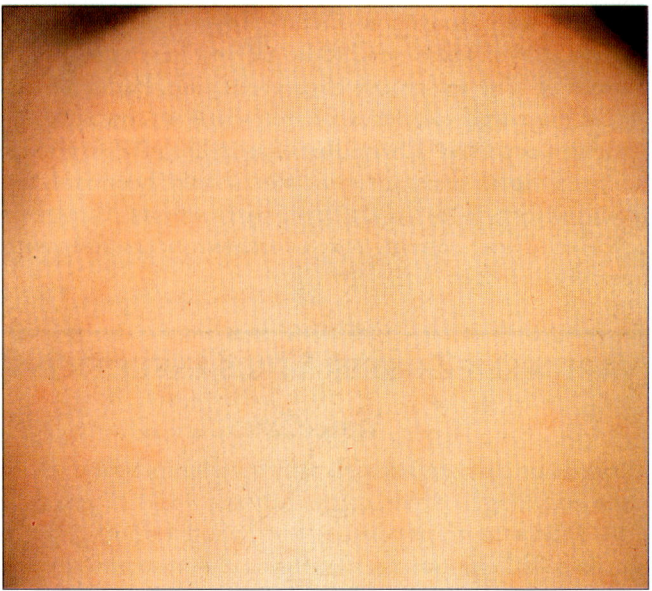

FIGURE 3-12 Roseola infantum. (*From* Flowers and Krusinski [24]; with permission.)

use of acyclovir [15]. Systemic corticosteroids have not been proven to be helpful in large, placebo-controlled studies [16].

Zoster requires larger doses of acyclovir than herpes simplex and acyclovir should be administered 800 mg orally five times per day for 7 to 10 days (Table 3-4). Severely immunocompromised patients who are at high risk for developing dissemination should be treated with intravenous acyclovir 10 mg per kg three times daily [17]. Institution of this therapy early in their disease decreases dissemination and visceral involvement.

Famciclovir is also available for the treatment of zoster in immunocompetent patients. Because of its greater bioavailability than acyclovir (77% absorption versus 20–30%) and its longer intracellular half-life, its recommended dosage is 500 mg orally three times daily. It has been shown to decrease viral shedding and shorten healing time in a similar manner to acyclovir. Some studies have shown that it may decrease zoster-associated pain perhaps even sooner than acyclovir. Famciclovir's safety profile appears to be similar to acyclovir. BVaraU (another nucleoside analogue) and valaciclovir are also being developed for their antizoster effect.

POST-HERPETIC NEURALGIA

Persistent pain greater than 3 to 6 months after resolution of the cutaneous symptoms of zoster is more frequently seen in elderly patients. At times, it is so severe as to be debilitating. Treatment with 0.075% capsaicin cream [18] topically four to six times daily or oral tricyclic antidepressants [19] has been shown to be helpful in 50% or more of patients. Many other therapies have also been suggested for postzoster neuralgia, but they have not been studied in a systematic

fashion. Use of nerve blocks performed by anesthesiologists may sometimes prove to be very helpful when all else fails.

The International Antiviral Consortium [20] has agreed that there is no universal definition for post-herpetic neuralgia. They suggest all pain during and after the eruption be called "zoster-associated pain." Studies of newer antivirals will use this terminology when assessing efficacy of zoster pain relief.

HERPESVIRUS TYPE 6

Exanthem subitum or roseola occurs in children between 6 months and 4 years of age and has been linked to human herpesvirus-6 (HH6) [21]. Characteristically, high fever remains constant for 3 to 5 days, developing with no other positive physical findings. Febrile seizures may occur in some of these patients. The rash appears at the time of defervescence and consists of discreet to confluent pink macules, primarily on the trunk (Fig. 3-12). Most infections due to HH6 in children present as a febrile illness with nonspecific findings, and therefore roseola is not diagnosed. Reactivation of HH6 later in life during periods of immunosuppression has recently been described.

HUMAN PARVOVIRUS

Erythema infectiosum or Fifth disease has now been linked to human parovirus B-19 [22]. Mild fever may accompany the distinctive eruption in this disease that consists of striking erythema of the cheeks with circumoral pallor or a slapped-cheek appearance (Fig. 3-13) and a reticulate erythematous, asymptomatic eruption on the extremities (Fig. 3-14). Some patients may have arthralgias associated

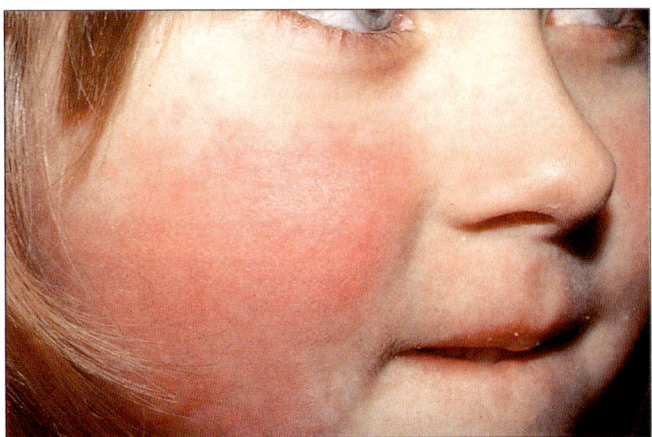

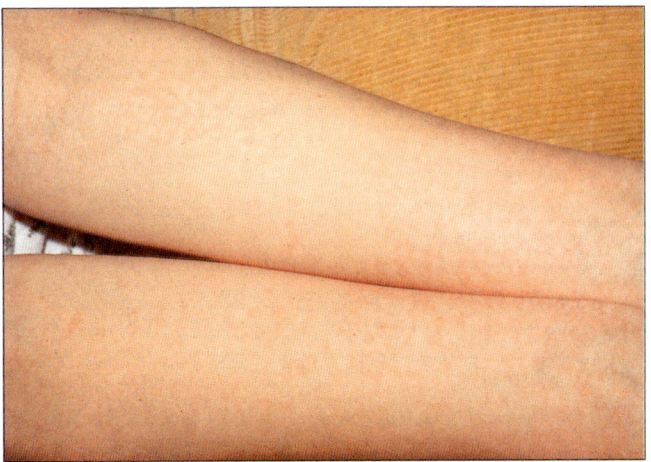

FIGURE 3-13 "Slapped cheek" facial erythema of Fifth disease. (*From* Flowers and Krusinski [24]; with permission.)

FIGURE 3-14 Reticulate eruption of Fifth disease.

with this distinctive eruption. Erythema infectiosum is self-limited and no treatment is necessary. However, epidemiologic studies have linked this virus to an increase in spontaneous abortion in women who are exposed early in pregnancy, and to aplastic crisis in patients with hemoglobinopathies and hematologic disorders [23]. Unfortunately, once the rash appears the patient is no longer infectious, and diagnosis is frequently made too late to prevent exposure to the above individuals, who are susceptible to serious complications.

MOLLUSCUM CONTAGIOSUM

Molluscum contagiosum are small, 2 to 6 mm flesh-colored or pink papules with a central umbilication. They are caused by a member of the poxvirus family and most frequently infect children, with lesions occurring on the trunk and face. In sexually active adults, the same clinical lesions will occur on the genitals and inner thighs as a sexually transmissible disease (Fig. 3-15). In patients with AIDS, molluscum contagiosum is quite common. These patients characteristically may develop hundreds of lesions which may grow to be quite large and become cosmetically disfiguring. The disease is self-limited and many children will observe spontaneous resolution within 6 to 18 months. However, patients with AIDS may have persistent lesions which require aggressive treatment. In adults, the papules may be curetted, nicked with a scalpel blade, or treated with liquid nitrogen cryocautery. The differential diagnosis in this group of patients includes condyloma acuminata and folliculitis. Sexual transmission of these lesions occurs during unprotected sexual exposure and questions regarding the symptoms and testing for syphilis, hepatitis B, and HIV must be raised in this group of patients.

HAND, FOOT, AND MOUTH DISEASE

A few strains of coxsackie virus (coxsackie A5,10,15, and 16) will cause this relatively mild disease. After a 7 to 10 day incubation period, patients develop a small number of 2 to 4 mm, flat-topped, gray pustules on their palms and soles with concomitant development of similar pustules involving the oral mucosa. These quickly rupture and may present as small, tender erosions. Only mild constitutional symptoms and low-grade fever accompany the cutaneous findings. The disease is self-limited and resolves spontaneously after 5 to 7 days. Infrequently, pneumonitis may complicate the illness. No treatment is available and usually none is necessary.

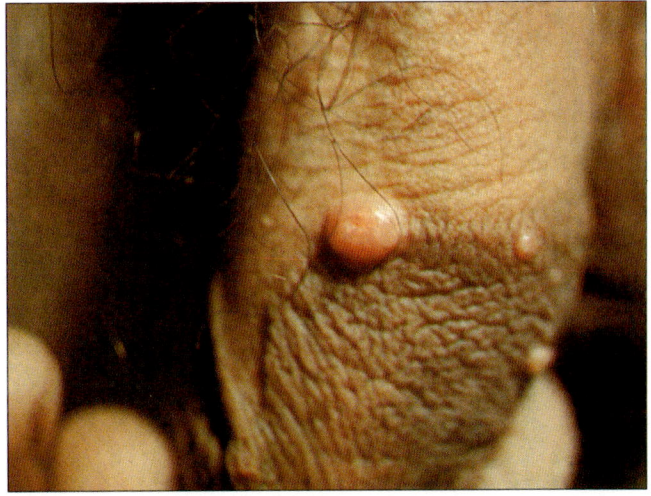

FIGURE 3-15 Molluscum contagiosum. (*From* Flowers and Krusinski [24]; with permission.)

References and Recommended Reading

Recently published papers of particular interest have been highlighted as:
• Of interest
•• Of outstanding interest

1.• Ramsey ML: Plantar warts: choosing treatment for active patients. *Physician and Sportsmed* 1992, 20:69–88.

2. Koutsky LA, Holmes KK, Critchlow CW, *et al.*: A cohort study of the risk of cervical intraepithelial neoplasia grade 2 or 3 in relation to papillomavirus infection. *N Engl J Med* 1992, 326:1272–1278.

3. Franco EL: Human papillomavirus and the natural history of cervical cancer. *Infect Med* 1993, 10:57–64.

4. Raimer SS, Raimer BG: Family violence, child abuse, and anogenital warts. *Arch Dermatol* 1992, 128:842–843.

5. Beutner KR, Friedman-Kien AE, Artman NN, *et al.*: Patient-applied podofilox for treatment of genital warts. *Lancet* 1989, i:831–834.

6.• Prober CG, Corey L, Brown ZA, *et al.*: The management of pregnancies complicated by genital infections with herpes simplex virus. *Clin Infect Dis* 1992, 15:1031–1038.

7. Gill MJ, Arlette J, Buchan KA: Herpes simplex virus infection of the hand. *J Am Acad Dermatol* 1990, 22:111–116.

8. Belongia EA, Goodman JL, Holland EJ, *et al.*: An outbreak of herpes gladiatorum at a high-school wrestling camp. *N Engl J Med* 1991, 324:906–910.

9. DeTorres O: Focus on foscarnet: a pyrophosphate analog for use in CMV retinitis and other viral infections. *Hosp Formul* 1991, 26:929–947.

10. Krusinski PA: Varicella (chickenpox). In *Clinical Dermatology*. Edited by Demis DJ. Philadelphia: JB Lippincott; 1988:1–7.

11. Weller TH: Varicella and herpes zoster: changing concepts of the natural history, control, and importance of a not-so-benign virus. *N Engl J Med* 1983, 308:1362–1367; *continues* 1434–1440.

12.• Dunkle LM, Arvin AM, Whitley RJ, *et al.*: A controlled trial of acyclovir for chickenpox in normal children. *N Engl J Med* 1991, 325:1539–1544.

13. Weibel RE, Neff BJ, Kuter BJ, *et al.*: Live attenuated varicella virus vaccine. *N Engl J Med* 1984, 310:1409–1415.

14. Krusinski PA: Herpes zoster. In *Clinical Dermatology*. Edited by Demis DJ. Philadelphia: JB Lippincott; 1988: 1–7.

15. Huff JC, *et al.*: Therapy of herpes zoster with oral acyclovir. *Am J Med* 1988, 85(suppl 2A):84–89.

16. Esmann V, Kroon S, Peterslund NA, *et al.*: Prednisolone does not prevent post-herpetic neuralgia. *Lancet* 1987, ii:126–129.

17. Shepp DH: Treatment of varicella-zoster virus infections in severely immunocompromised patients. *N Engl J Med* 1986, 314:208–212.

18. Bernstein JE, Bickers DR, Dahl MV, *et al.*: Treatment of chronic postherpetic neuralgia with topical capsaicin. *J Am Acad Dermatol* 1987, 17:93–96.

19. Watson CT, Evans RJ, Reed K, *et al.*: Amitriptyline versus placebo in postherpetic neuralgia. *Neurology* 1982, 32:671–673.

20. Wood M: How can the burden of zoster-associated pain be reduced? *International Herpes Management Forum*, Worthing: PPS Europe; 1993.

21. Yamanishi K, Shiraki K, Kondo T, *et al.*: Identification of human herpesvirus-6 as a causal agent for exanthem subitum. *Lancet* 1988, i:1065–1067.

22. Bell LM, Naides SJ, Stoffman P, *et al.*: Human parvovirus B19 infection among hospital staff members after contact with infected patients. *N Engl J Med* 1989, 321:485–491.

23. Ware R: Human parvovirus infection. *J Pediatr* 1989, 114:343–348.

24. Flowers FP, Krusinski PA: Dermatology in ambulatory and emergency medicine: a clinical guide with algorithms. Chicago: Year Book Medical Publishers; 1984.

Common Fungal Infections of the Skin 4

Boni E. Elewski

Key Points

- The dermatophyte fungi are the largest group of mycotic pathogens causing cutaneous diseases.

- Predisposing factors for the dermatophytoses include contact with infected animals, crowded living conditions, participation in contact sports, and use of gymnasiums.

- Not all annular or ringlike dermatoses are caused by dermatophytes. Similarly, only approximately 50% of dystrophic nails are caused by fungal organisms.

- There is an epidemic of *Trichophyton tonsurans* in urban areas of the United States. Prominent cervical lymphadenopathy, scale, and patches of alopecia are typical of the clinical presentation.

- Newer topical and systemic antifungals have significantly improved therapy. Oral antifungals are generally required when treating tinea capitis, onychomycosis, and extensive disease, and in those patients immunocompromised by disease or by therapy.

Cutaneous infections by the dermatophytes *Candida* and *Malassezia furfur* (*Pityrosporum*) are discussed in this chapter. Diagnosis and therapeutic options as well as common presentations of clinical disease are reviewed.

DERMATOPHYTOSES

Dermatophytoses are caused by a closely related group of organisms that are similar in morphology, pathogenicity, and physiology and have a special affinity for the keratinized tissues of the hair, skin, and nails [1•,2]. The dermatophytes encompass only three genera—*Epidermophyton*, *Microsporum*, and *Trichophyton*—but are collectively the largest group of fungi causing cutaneous diseases [2]. They are also referred to as ringworms because of the characteristic ring that develops on the infected skin. Diseases produced by these organisms are prefaced by the adjective *tinea*, and are named according to the body part infected (*eg*, tinea capitis refers to dermatophytosis of scalp hair, and tinea pedis to dermatophytosis of the plantar surface; Table 4-1). Although the causative organisms are closely related, the various dermatophytoses produce protean manifestations and can resemble numerous cutaneous diseases (Table 4-2).

Clinical Manifestations

Dermatophytoses have various presentations dependent upon the body site infected and the infecting fungus. For example, in a hair-bearing area, follicular invasion can result in folliculitis or alopecia. Disease in the nail unit can result in dystrophy, onycholysis, or loss of nail. Infection on the palm and sole can be particularly chronic owing to the lack of sebaceous glands, which contain fungistatic material [1•]. In addition, disease produced by some organisms, especially that acquired from animal sources, can be quite inflammatory and may

TABLE 4-1 SPECIFIC DERMATOPHYTOSES AND AREAS OF INFECTION	
Disease	**Area**
Tinea barbae	Beard region
Tinea corporis	Glabrous skin
Tinea cruris	Groin
Tinea pedis	Plantar surface or toe webs
Tinea manuum	Palmar surface
Tinea capitis	Scalp hair
Tinea unguium	Nails

resemble bacterial pyoderma [2]. In this chapter, presentations of common tineas are discussed.

Tinea corporis

Tinea corporis is dermatophytosis of the glabrous skin of the trunk, extremities, and face and occurs in all ages, ethnic backgrounds, and nationalities. It is most common in warm, humid climates. Predisposing factors include contact with animals (especially kittens, cattle, and horses), crowded living conditions, participation in contact sports and use of gymnasiums, and a variety of systemic disorders including diabetes mellitus and HIV infection. Contact with infected animals is a common cause as certain animals can harbor the organisms, resulting in disease in exposed persons. Kittens are particularly a problem, and large epidemics have resulted from a single infected animal.

Typical lesions of tinea corporis are pruritic, oval, annular (ringlike), erythematous, scaly patches that may have a slightly elevated border (Fig. 4-1). However, the presentation of tinea corporis is quite variable and can mimic many other dermatoses. It should be stressed that not all annular or ringlike dermatoses are tinea corporis. The diagnosis is especially challenging if blistering or pustular lesions occur

TABLE 4-2 DIFFERENTIAL DIAGNOSIS OF DERMATOPHYTOSIS
Tinea corporis, cruris, and pedis
Psoriasis, eczematous dermatitis, pityriasis rosea, granuloma annulare, bacterial pyoderma, subacute cutaneous lupus erythematosus
Tinea pedis
Psoriasis, eczema, candidiasis, eczematous dermatitis, erythrasma
Tinea cruris
Candidiasis, erythrasma, eczematous dermatitis, neurodermatitis
Tinea unguium or onychomycosis
Nail psoriasis, lichen planus
Tinea capitis
Inflammatory variety—bacterial pyoderma Noninflammatory variety—alopecia areata trichotillomania, discoid lupus, seborrheic dermatitis, psoriasis

(Fig. 4-2). The use of topical steroids may change the clinical appearance and produce tinea incognito (Fig. 4-3). Scratching may lead to lichenification and the appearance of a neurodermatitis or eczematous response. Occasionally, this lichenified presentation may mimic psoriasis. The diagnosis can be confirmed by potassium hydroxide preparation and by fungal culture.

Tinea pedis

Tinea pedis refers to dermatophytosis of the plantar surface or toe webs. There are three common recognized patterns: 1) moccasin or chronic hyperkeratotic; 2) interdigital; and 3)

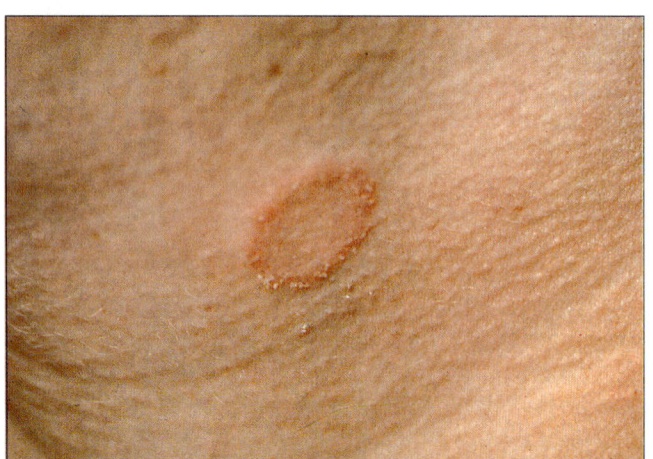

FIGURE 4-1 Tinea corporis. Annular scaly patch typical of dermatophytosis.

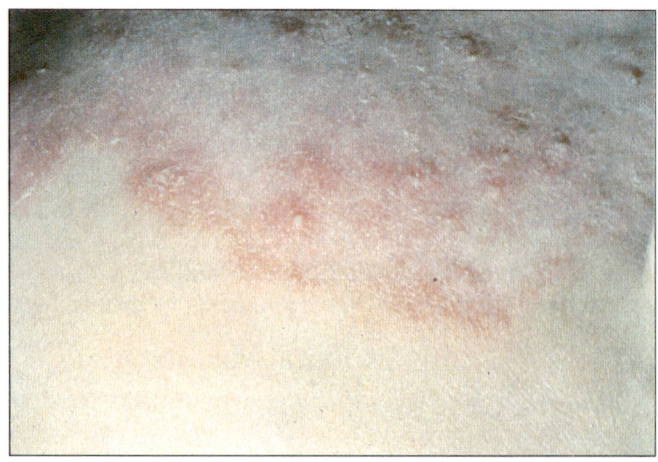

FIGURE 4-2 Tinea corporis with pustular lesions. This rash mimicked bacterial folliculitis.

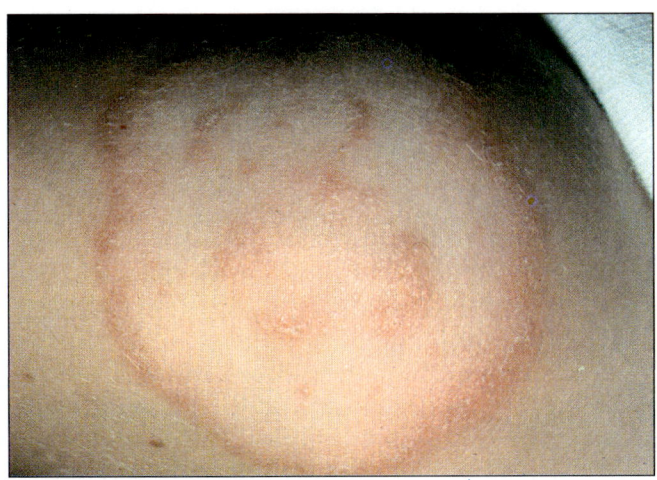

FIGURE 4-3 Tinea corporis. Use of topical steroids spread a small annular patch but reduced scale and itching. The rash progressed in size, but became less inflammatory.

inflammatory or vesicular [1•,2,3]. The interdigital variety is the most common, and the patient typically presents with macerated, fissured, scaling, interdigital lesions usually involving the web space of the fourth and fifth toes. Bacterial infections and cutaneous candidiasis can be differentiated by culture. Wood's light examination revealing bright coral red fluorescence is typical of infection by *Corynebacterium minutissimum* or erythrasma. In the vesicular variety of tinea pedis, the patient presents with painful pruritic vesicles or bullous lesions on the instep of one or both feet. Infection may be disabling, and this variety has historically been a particular problem in the military. The dermatophytid reaction can be associated with the vesicular variety. When this reaction occurs, the patient may have an eczematous-appearing rash on one or both hands that may resemble dishidrotic eczema on the palms or sides of

fingers. This rash is considered a hypersensitivity reaction to the fungal foot infection, and both cultures and potassium hydroxide (KOH) preparation taken from the hand produce negative results. The hyperkeratotic variety of tinea pedis or moccasin foot is characterized by dry, scaly, hyperkeratotic changes on the plantar surface of one or both feet (Fig. 4-4). Fungal nail disease is generally present, and the patient may also have palmar infection (tinea manuum). Chronic infections that are recalcitrant to therapy typically occur.

Tinea cruris

Tinea cruris refers to dermatophytosis of the inguinal region, including the gluteal folds, the crural folds, and proximal medial thighs. Intense pruritus is common and has led to the lay term "jock itch." Adult men are more commonly infected than women. Risk factors include maceration and occlusion. The scrotal skin appears immune to infection by dermatophytes, although candidiasis and erythrasma occur in this region (Fig. 4-5). Women are more likely to present with cutaneous candidiasis in the genital and inguinal areas than with dermatophytosis.

Tinea unguium

The terms *tinea unguium* and *onychomycosis* are often used interchangeably; however, the former specifies dermatophytic infection of the nail unit, whereas onychomycosis encompasses all forms of fungal infection causing nail disease. Onychomycosis is responsible for approximately 50% of dystrophic nails and occurs in an estimated 15% to 20% of people 40 to 60 years old [1•].

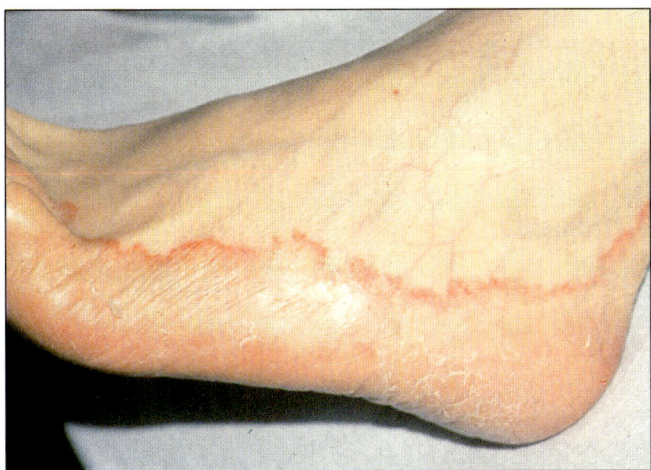

FIGURE 4-4 Moccasin tinea pedis. Entire plantar surface extending to lateral and medial borders of foot is red and scaly. (*From* Elewski [1•]; with permission.)

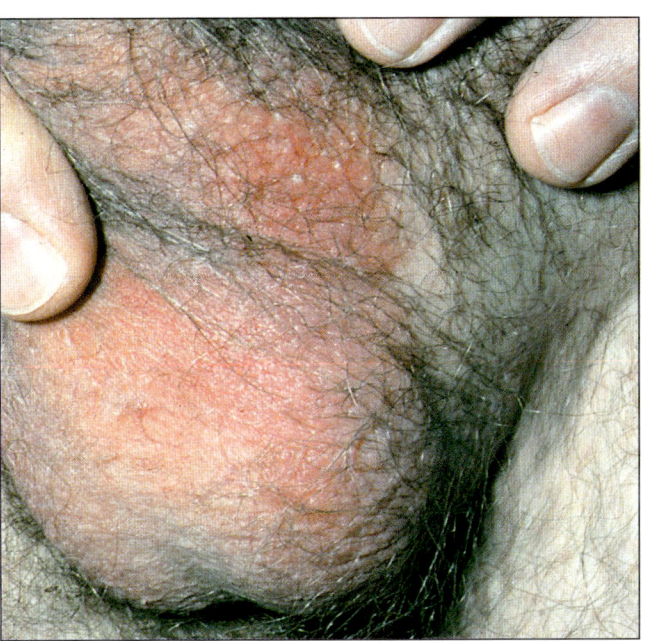

FIGURE 4-5 Tinea cruris. Note scrotal involvement—patient has cutaneous candidiasis, not dermatophytosis. The treatment would therefore be different than for dermatophytosis as griseofulvin would be ineffective.

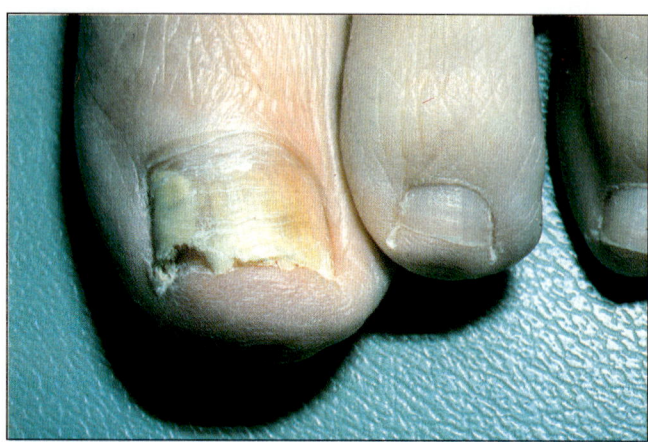

FIGURE 4-6 Tinea unguium or oncyomycosis. Note thickened nail bed with hyperkeratosis and onycholysis.

Toenails are more often involved than fingernails. The most common presentation is distal subungual variety manifested by subungual debris and thickening with associated onycholysis and thickening of the nail plate (Fig. 4-6) [4]. However, there are other presentations of fungal nail disease, including white superficial onychomycosis and candidiasis in nails [1•]. It is important to stress that not all patients with dystrophic nails have fungal disease. For example, psoriasis and lichen planus can mimic onychomycosis and can be differentiated by a culture.

Tinea capitis

Tinea capitis refers to dermatophytosis of the scalp hair follicle and occurs mostly in children [5]. Currently, there is an epidemic of *Trichophyton tonsurans* infection in urban areas of the United States [6–10]. Many infected children are black or Hispanic, and infection is often recalcitrant to griseofulvin therapy. The clinician must be suspicious of infection as this organism does not cause hair fluorescence [11], and therefore the diagnosis must made on clinical signs and by culture.

There are inflammatory and noninflammatory varieties of tinea capitis. With the inflammatory variety, the clinical picture varies from a few pustules in the scalp to widespread abscesses or kerions [5]. Alopecia and tender cervical lymphadenopathy are generally associated (Fig. 4-7). If untreated, a permanent scarring alopecia may result. The noninflammatory type may resemble alopecia areata and present with oval, generally scaly patches of alopecia. Prominent cervical adenopathy, presence of scale, and lack of exclamation point hairs in patches of alopecia point to a diagnosis of tinea capitis. As only a few species of dermatophytes are able to yield hair fluorescence under Wood's light examination, the diagnosis should be based upon culturing a dermatophyte, not on the presence or absence of scalp fluorescence [11]. It should be stressed that the presence of fluorescence is dependent upon the infecting dermatophyte rather than the clinical presentation.

Diagnosis

The clinical diagnosis of dermatophyte infection can be confirmed by direct microscopy of skin scrapings (KOH) and by fungal culture [2]. Methods of specimen collection vary depending on the body site infected. In nail disease, the specimen is best collected by cutting back diseased nails and curetting or scraping the hyperkeratotic and thickened nail bed in the area proximal to the cuticle area or proximal nail fold. With scalp infection, 10 to 12 hairs in the diseased area or at the border of alopecia should be epilated, and scale in the area can also be included in the specimen. With infections on the foot, hand, or elsewhere, the active raised border is the best site for collection of specimens. A glass slide or scalpel blade can be used to scrape off sufficient scale. In blistering conditions, the roof of the blister would be the best specimen. Once the specimen is obtained, a portion can be used for a KOH preparation and the remainder for culture. A KOH preparation is a simple, easy office procedure. Potassium hydroxide is a keratin-clearing agent and will dissolve the keratin in the specimen, permitting visualization of the fungal hyphae. As the KOH of all dermatophytes are indistinguishable, specific identification of the organism requires a culture (Fig. 4-8). Because dermatophytes can be acquired from animal, human, and soil sources, knowing the causative pathogen will help determine the pattern of spread [2]. Fungal cultures take considerable experience to correctly identify the genus and species. For this reason, many clinicians use a screening media, such as dermatophyte test media, that contains a phenol red indicator. With dermatophyte growth, the medium changes from yellow to red. Although a useful screen for dermatophytes, false-positive and false-negative results are common. In addition, *Candida albicans* will not change the color of the dermatophyte test media and therefore may lead to incorrect diagnoses [2]. Many reference laboratories are available for precise identification of fungal organisms.

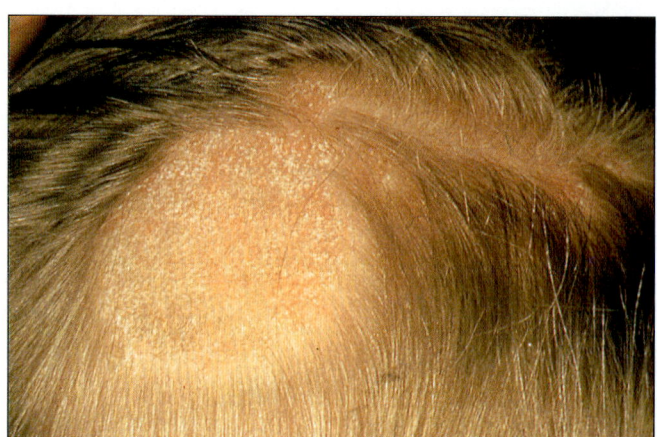

FIGURE 4-7 Tinea capitis. Patch of alopecia in a child's scalp. Note that not all patients with tinea capitis will fluoresce under Wood's light examination.

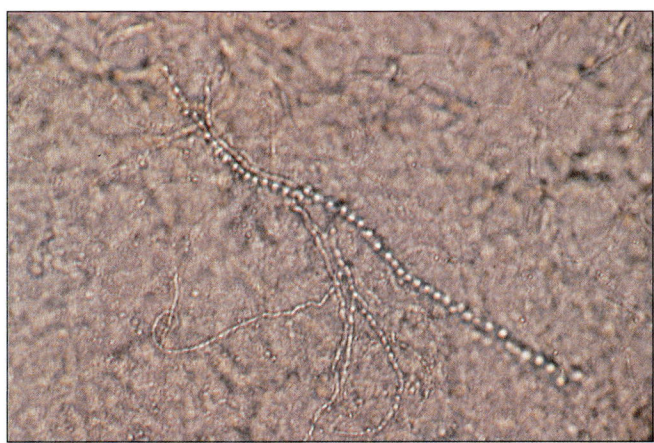

FIGURE 4-8 Positive potassium hydroxide preparation. Note branching hyphae typical of dermatophyte infection. The exact organism must be determined by culture.

Therapy

Newer topical and systemic antifungals have significantly improved the therapy for dermatophyte infections [12•, 13–17]. Oral antifungals available for therapy include grise-ofulvin, ketoconazole, itraconazole, fluconazole, and terbinafine (Table 4-3) [18]. Topical agents include the imidazoles, allylamines, ciclopiroxolamine, and a variety of miscellaneous agents (Table 4-4).

An oral therapeutic agent is necessary when treating tinea capitis and onychomycosis. Tinea capitis is generally treated until the patient is culture-negative and new hair is regrowing, and with griseofulvin, the duration of therapy is generally 2 to 3 months. Patients and their families should also use an antifungal shampoo—ketoconazole or selenium sulfide—on a daily basis [19]. In patients with *Microsporum canis* infections, the infected cat or dog should be appropriately treated. Onychomycosis has been historically treated with griseofulvin, which is administered until the new fungal-free nail has regrown [18]. Because of the slow growth of nails, this progress can take up to 2 years for toenails and 6 to 9 months for fingernails. Upon cessation of therapy, recurrence is common. However, newer agents appear promising using short-term or pulse courses (Table 4-5) and may prevent some relapses [14,17]. Further stud-

TABLE 4-3 ACTIVITY SPECTRUM OF ORAL ANTIFUNGALS

	Dermato-phytes	Candida	Malassezia furfur
Griseofulvin	+	–	–
Ketoconazole	+	+	+
Fluconazole	+	+	+
Itraconazole	+	+	+
Terbinafine	+	+/±	–

+, effective; –, ineffective; +/±. probably effective.

TABLE 4-4 ACTIVITY SPECTRUM OF TOPICAL ANTIFUNGALS

	Dermato-phytes	Candida	Malassezia furfur
Imidazoles	+	+	+
Clotrimazole			
Ketoconazole			
Miconazole			
Oxiconazole			
Sulconazole			
Allylamines	+	+	+
Naftifine			
Terbinafine			
Ciclopiroxolamine	+	+	+
Miscellaneous			
Tolnaftate	+	–	+
Nystatin	–	+	+
Selenium sulfide, 2.5%	–	–	+

+, effective; –, ineffective.

TABLE 4-5 THERAPY FOR DERMATOPHYTOSIS

Tinea corporis, cruris, and pedis

Topical imidazole, allylamine, or other effective agent twice daily for 4 wk or until clinically and mycologically resolved

Tinea capitis

Griseofulvin 5–15 mg/kg until mycologic cure obtained and normal hair is regrowing

*Itraconazole 100 mg/d for 30 d (dosage may vary according to body weight; duration may vary according to severity and clinical response)

Tinea unguium (toenails)

Griseofulvin (ultramicrosize strength) until nail has regrown and is culture-negative (generally 1–2 y toenail, 6–9 mo fingernail)

*Itraconazole 200 mg qd for 12 wk toenail, for 6 wk fingernail

*Itraconazole 400 mg qd for 1 wk–1 wk/mo 3–4 mo, toenail; 2 mo, fingernail

*Terbinafine 250 mg qd for 12 wk, toenail; for 6 wk, fingernail

*Fluconazole 100 mg qd or pulse dose† 300 mg/wk until nail has regrown and is culture negative

*Currently investigational in United States; dosage and duration may vary according to response. †With pulse dosage, nail is often not clinically normal when drug is discontinued.

ies are necessary to prove their effectiveness and dosage schedules.

Topical agents will generally suffice for tinea pedis, cruris, and corporis. The patient should be instructed to apply the topical agent twice a day to the involved skin and approximately 2 cm around the diseased area for 4 to 8 weeks. However, topical terbinafine has been shown effective for interdigital tinea pedis after a single 1-week course [20•]. In patients with extensive disease and patients immunocompromised by disease or therapy, an oral agent is justified as adjuvant therapy [21•]. Two weeks of ketoconazole 200 mg every day, or griseofulvin 250 mg twice daily (ultramicrosize) or 1 week of itraconazole 200 mg to 400 mg every day can be used adjunctively with appropriate topical therapy [18].

CUTANEOUS CANDIDIASIS

Both cutaneous and oral candidiasis are commonly encountered fungal infections. *Candida albicans* is the most frequently isolated species of *Candida* and is part of the normal flora of the alimentary tract and mucocutaneous areas, but is not ordinarily found on normal intact skin. Predisposing factors for clinical disease include: 1) underlying systemic disease; 2) impaired host immunity; 3) treatment with systemic antibiotics (>7 d) or immunosuppressive agents; 4) extremes of age; and 5) disrupted epithelial barrier (moisture, occlusion) [1•].

Clinical Presentation

Candida produces protean manifestations of the skin and mucous membranes. In many instances, disease may resemble dermatophyte or bacterial infection. The presence of risk factors should alert the clinician to Candida infection.

Candida intertrigo
With maceration, heat, occlusion, and friction, Candida overgrowth can occur. Areas predisposed include the groin, axillary vault, gluteal region, and under the pannus or pendulous breasts. The typical presentation is a bright red, moist skin surface with scaling borders and satellite papules or pustules (Fig. 4-9).

Candida paronychia
With prolonged exposure to water or manipulation of the cuticle, *Candida* can infect the proximal nail fold, developing erythema and edema with a purulent discharge. In chronic disease, the nail becomes dystrophic.

Candida diaper dermatitis
The occlusive nature of diapers promotes Candida overgrowth. The diaper area, including the folds of the groin, becomes red with satellite pustules (Fig. 4-10) [22].

Acute pseudomembranous candidiasis or thrush
White-gray curdlike patches develop in the buccal mucosa, tongue, gingiva, and pharynx. Risk factors include use of dentures, diabetes mellitus, systemic antibiotics (>7 d), HIV infection, and other immunocompromised states.

Angular cheilitis or perleche
Infection of the oral commisures is commonly caused by *Candida*, resulting in maceration, erythema, and scaling (Fig. 4-11).

Diagnosis

The diagnosis of all forms of cutaneous and mucosal candidiasis can be made by the potassium hydroxide wet mount, which reveals yeast and pseudohyphae. A fungal culture confirms the diagnosis [1•,2].

Therapy

Most cutaneous and oral candidiasis can be treated by topical agents. Topical agents such as ketoconazole or econazole creams are generally used twice daily for 2 to 4 weeks. In oral candidiasis, clotrimazole troches are very effective. Whenever possible, risk factors such as dentures should also

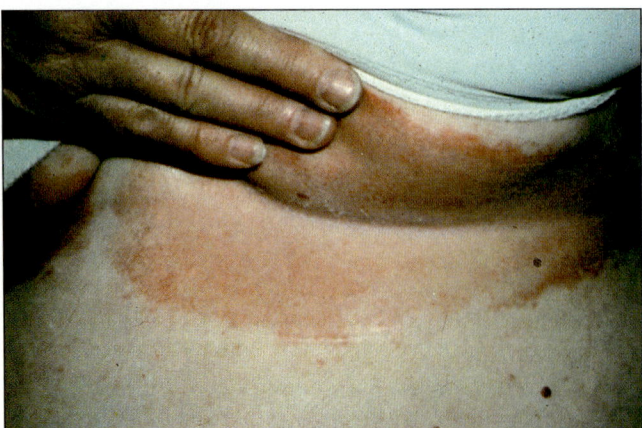

FIGURE 4-9 Red macerated rash under pendulous breasts is a common presentation of cutaneous candidiasis.

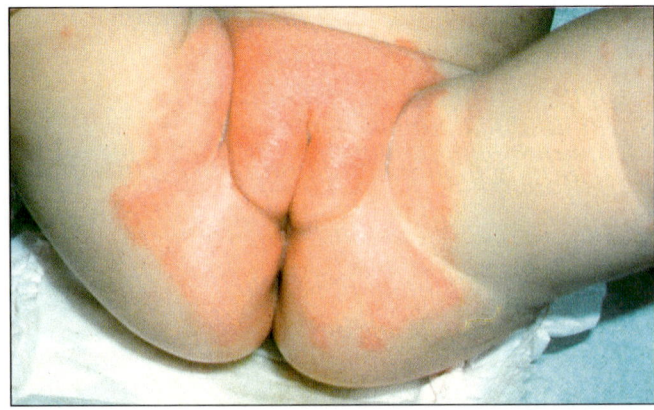

FIGURE 4-10 *Candida* diaper dermatitis. Note involvement of the folds of the groin that serve as a differentiating point from diaper dermatitis.

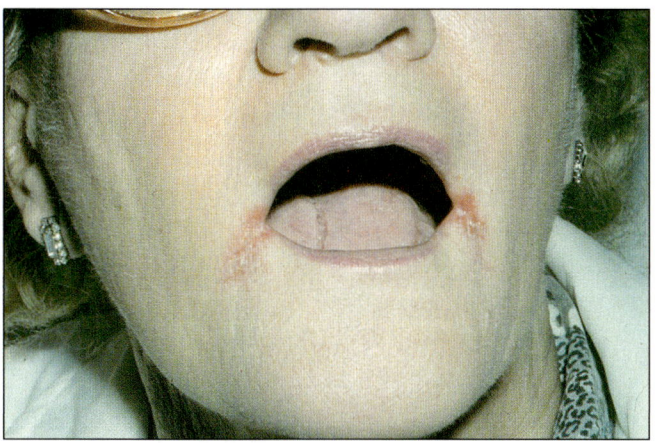

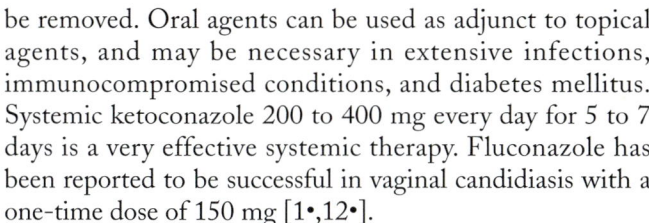

FIGURE 4-11 Perleche in an edentulous woman is a common presentation of cutaneous candidiasis.

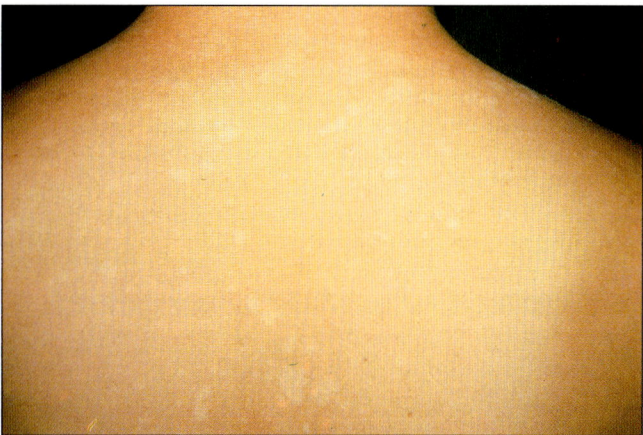

FIGURE 4-12 Pityriasis or tinea versicolor. Note hypopigmented and scaly patches on trunk and proximal extremities.

be removed. Oral agents can be used as adjunct to topical agents, and may be necessary in extensive infections, immunocompromised conditions, and diabetes mellitus. Systemic ketoconazole 200 to 400 mg every day for 5 to 7 days is a very effective systemic therapy. Fluconazole has been reported to be successful in vaginal candidiasis with a one-time dose of 150 mg [1•,12•].

TINEA VERSICOLOR OR PITYRIASIS VERSICOLOR

Pityriasis or tinea versicolor is caused by the yeast *M. furfur* [1•,2]. The typical presentation is asymptomatic, slightly scaly, hypopigmented or hyperpigmented, or even erythematous to salmon-colored patches on the trunk and upper arms (Fig. 4-12). Disease is most common during the summer months, and chronic infections are common.

The diagnosis is made by a KOH preparation showing short hyphae and yeast cells. Culture is not routinely done.

The treatment of pityriasis or tinea versicolor is topical application of an antifungal agent twice daily for up to 4 weeks (Table 4-4). Oral agents may occasionally be indicated (Table 4-3) [23,24,25•]. Ketoconazole 200 mg every day for 5 to 10 days is very effective, as is a single 400-mg dose of fluconazole. To avoid recurrence, prophylactic oral or topical treatment regimens may be important. Patients should also be instructed to avoid heavy oils on affected areas that may promote the growth of *M. furfur*.

REFERENCES AND RECOMMENDED READING

Recently published papers of particular interest have been highlighted as:
• Of interest
•• Of outstanding interest

1.• Elewski BE, ed. *Cutaneous Fungal Infections*. New York: Igaku-Shoin Medical Publishers; 1992.

2. Elewski BE, Hazen PG: The superficial mycoses and the dermatophytes. *J Am Acad Dermatol* 1989, 21:655–673.

3. Kearse HL, Miller OF: Tinea pedis in prepubertal children: does it occur? *J Am Acad Dermatol* 1988, 19:619–622.

4. Daniel CR III, Lawson LA: Tinea unguium. *Cutis* 1987, 40:326–327.

5. Herbert A: Tinea capitis. *Arch Dermatol* 1988, 124:1554–1557.

6. Bronson RM, Desai DR, Barsky S, *et al.*: An epidemic of infection with Trichophyton tonsurans revealed in a 20-year survey of fungal infections in Chicago. *J Am Acad Dermatol* 1983, 8:322–330.

7. Rasmussen JE, Ahmed R: Trichophyton reactions in children with tinea capitis. *Arch Dermatol* 1978, 114:371–372.

8. Babel DE, Baughman SA: Evaluation of the adult carrier state in juvenile tinea capitis caused by Trichophyton tonsurans. *J Am Acad Dermatol* 1989, 21:1209–1212.

9. Sharma V, Hall JC, Knapp JF, *et al.*: Scalp colonization by Trichophyton tonsurans in an urban pediatric clinic. *Arch Dermatol* 1988, 124:1511–1513.

10. Hebert AA, Head ES, MacDonald EM: Tinea capitis caused by Trichophyton tonsurans. *Pediatr Dermatol* 1985, 2:219–223.

11. Prevost E: The rise and fall of fluorescent tinea capitis. *Pediatr Dermatol* 1983, 1:127–133.

12.• Elewski BE: Mechanisms of action of antifungal drugs. *J Am Acad Dermatol* 1993, 28:S28–S34.

13. Lambert DR, Siegle RJ, Camisa C: Griseofulvin and ketoconazole in the treatment of dermatophyte infections. *Int J Dermatol* 1989, 28:300–304.

14. Hay RJ, Clayton YM, Moore MK, *et al.*: An evaluation of itraconazole in the management of onychomycosis. *Br J Dermatol* 1988, 119:359–366.

15. Lesher JL Jr, Smith JG Jr: Antifungal agents in dermatology. *J Am Acad Dermatol* 1987, 173:383–396.

16. Zaias N, Serrano L: The successful treatment of fingernail Trichophyton rubrum onychomycosis with oral terbinafine. *Clin Exp Dermatol* 1989, 14:120–124.

17. Goodfield MJD, Rowell NR, Forster RA, *et al.*: Treatment of dermatophyte infection of the finger and toenails with terbinafine (SF86-327, Lamisil), an orally active fungicidal agent. *Br J Dermatol* 1989, 12:1753–1757.

18. Gupta AK, Sauder DN, Shear NH: Antifungal agents: an overview, part II. *J Am Acad Dermatol* 1994, 30:911–933.

19. Allen HB, Honig RJ, Leyden JJ, *et al.*: Selenium sulfide: adjunctive therapy for tinea capitis. *Pediatr* 1982, 69:81–83.

20.• Bergstresser P, Elewski B, Hanifin J, *et al.*: Comparison of cure and relapse rates with 1- and 4-week regimens of terbinafine and clotrimazole 1% cream in patients with interdigital tinea pedis: results of a double blind, multicenter study. *J Am Acad Dermatol* 1993, 28:648–651.

21.• Elewski BE, Sullivan J: Dermatophytes as opportunistic pathogens. *J Am Acad Dermatol* 1994, 30:1021–1022.

22. Honig P, Gribetz B, Leyden JJ, *et al.* Amoxicillin and diaper dermatitis. *J Am Acad Dermatol* 1988, 19:275–279.

23. Lopez-Lopez JR, Gonzalez-Benavides JD: Pityriasis versicolor in children. *Med Cutan Ibero Lat Am* 1985, 13:381–383.

24. Ford GP, Ive FA, Midgley G: Pityrosporum folliculitis and ketoconazole. *Br J Dermatol* 1982, 107:691–695.

25.• Delescluse RCJ: Itraconazole in tinea versicolor: a review. *J Am Acad Dermatol* 1990, 23:551–554.

Premalignant and Malignant Epithelial Tumors

Lisa M. Seung
Daniel Rivlin
Ronald L. Moy

5

Key Points

- Epithelial malignant neoplasms have many potential etiologies, but the most common one and the one that can be protected against easily is actinic damage from the sun.

- Actinic keratosis is the most common precancerous lesion, and can be treated effectively with a variety of methods.

- Basal cell carcinoma is the most common epithelial malignancy and rarely if ever metastasizes, but can cause local destruction.

- Squamous cell carcinoma is the second most common epithelial malignancy and can metastasize.

- There are many methods for treating basal cell carcinoma and squamous cell carcinoma effectively, but Mohs micrographic surgery has the highest cure rate.

Although not all skin tumors are sun-related, ultraviolet radiation is the single most important cause of both premalignant and malignant epithelial tumors. Prevention plays a pivotal role in reducing the incidence of skin cancer. Thus, the risks of sun exposure and benefits of high-potency sun screens, with a sun protection factor of greater than 15, should be made common knowledge to all patients. In addition, generalists should learn to recognize premalignant lesions as early diagnosis and treatment of such lesions will decrease the morbidity rate of patients as well as the cost of treatment. When in doubt, a suspicious lesion should be biopsied rather than observed and allowed to develop into a malignant tumor.

PREMALIGNANT LESIONS

Actinic Keratoses

Actinic keratoses, also known as solar keratoses, are scaly, red papules of about 3 to 6 mm in diameter that develop on sun-exposed skin surfaces [1]. They are usually rough, keratotic lesions that are best detected by palpation (Fig. 5-1).

Actinic keratoses are most often induced by ultraviolet radiation and are thus more likely to develop in individuals who have had extensive sun exposure and are fair in complexion. The elderly, who have experienced the most cumulative sun exposure, are at the highest risk for development of actinic keratoses. The lesions are often multiple and most commonly appear on the face, dorsal surfaces of the hands and forearms, and the bald scalp.

If left untreated actinic keratoses have the potential to transform into squamous cell carcinoma. It is estimated that 12% to 25% of patients with actinic keratoses will develop invasive squamous cell carcinoma [2]; however, metastasis

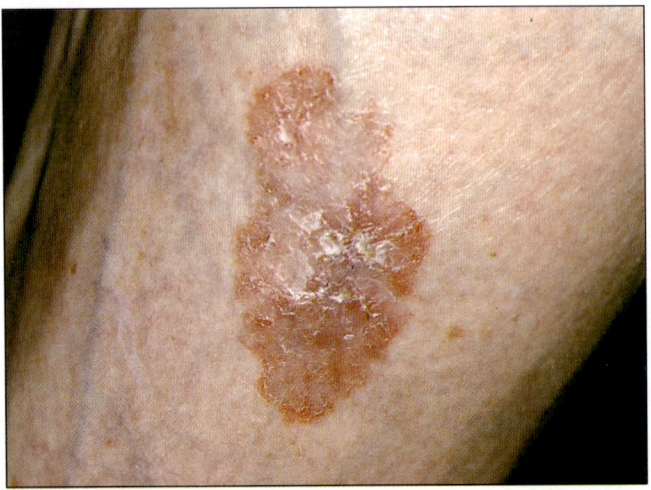

FIGURE 5-1 Red, scaly, erythematous plaque typical of both superficial basal cell carcinoma and Bowen's disease. This particular case represents superficial basal cell carcinoma.

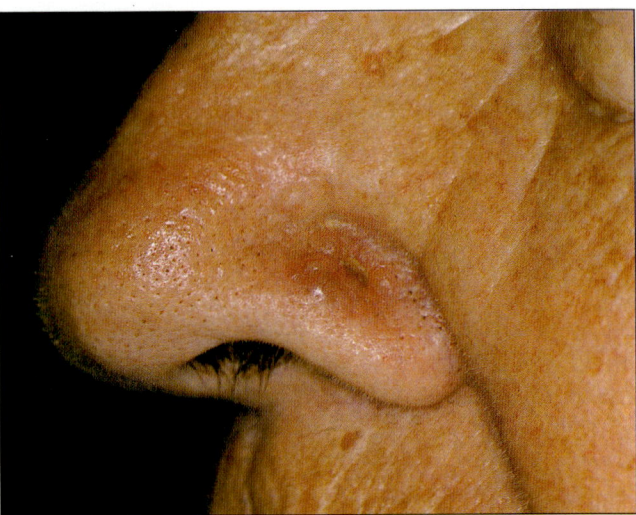

FIGURE 5-2 Typical nodular basal cell carcinoma with a pearly telangiectatic border and central erosion.

is rare in this type of squamous cell carcinoma [3•]. Although there have been controversies regarding whether treatment of actinic keratoses actually reduces morbidity in patients [4,5], it is generally accepted that the risks involved are too great to forgo therapy.

Treatment

Treatment of actinic keratoses in patients with a few lesions is best accomplished by cryosurgery or curettage. In cryosurgery, liquid nitrogen is sprayed onto the affected lesion or applied with a cotton-tipped swab. With curettage, an instrument (curette) is used to scrape out the lesions. A success rate of 99% has been shown for treatment with each of these procedures [1,3•]. In addition, both cryosurgery and curettage are quick procedures, and healing is usually prompt. However, with both procedures there may be some residual hypopigmentation.

In patients with numerous lesions, topical application of 5-fluorouracil (Efudex; Roche Dermatologics, Nutley, NJ, and Fluoroplex; Allergan Herbert, Irvine, CA) is extremely effective. One to five percent 5-fluorouracil is available in a cream or solution form and can be applied topically once or twice a day for about 4 to 6 weeks. A newer topical agent, masoprocol cream (Actinex; Reed & Carnrick, Jersey City, NJ), has also demonstrated effectiveness in treating multiple actinic keratoses. Masoprocol and 5-fluorouracil are especially useful, as they can destroy subclinical lesions as well as fully developed actinic keratoses. Unfortunately, they have uncomfortable side effects such as inflammation, erythema and irritation. In addition, patients should be warned that complications such as persistent redness may infrequently occur. Any lesion resistant to 5-fluorouracil or masoprocol can be further treated with cryosurgery or curettage.

Even after treatment, patients with actinic keratoses should be closely monitored at regular intervals for the development of further lesions. Also, proper precautions (*ie*, protection from the sun) should always be advised. The use of sunscreens and photoprotective clothing has been associated with spontaneous resolution of existing lesions, as well as reduction of new lesions.

Bowen's Disease

Bowen's disease is an in situ squamous cell carcinoma that has the potential to become invasive. It has been described as a well-demarcated, scaly, indurated red plaque that is often confused with benign dermatoses, such as chronic eczema or psoriasis (Fig. 5-2) [6••]. As a result of the confusion over its initial diagnosis, Bowen's disease is usually not properly diagnosed until a biopsy is performed. More often than not, the biopsy is taken after the presumed "dermatitis" has been present for several years and has been resistant to corticosteroid treatment.

Bowen's disease most frequently occurs in middle-aged to older white adults and can arise on both sun-exposed as well as nonexposed skin surfaces. A variety of agents have been implicated in the pathogenesis of Bowen's disease: 1) actinic damage (which accounts for the development of lesions on sun-exposed areas such as the face), 2) inorganic arsenic (a chemical formerly present in certain "bromide" medications and in fungicides and pesticides), 3) a viral factor (several human papillomavirus types have been linked to Bowen's disease), and 4) radiation exposure [7••]. In addition, a connection between Bowen's disease and internal cancer has been a topic of debate in the past. However, recent consensus is that there is no real increased risk of concurrent or subsequent visceral malignancy associated with Bowen's disease [8•].

Treatment options for Bowen's disease include surgical excision, curettage with electrodesiccation, topical 5-fluorouracil, cryosurgical destruction, radiation therapy, and laser surgery. For recurrent lesions Mohs micrographic surgery can be performed (*see* section on Squamous cell carcinoma).

MALIGNANT LESIONS

Squamous Cell Carcinoma

Squamous cell carcinoma is the second most frequent malignancy of the skin, second only to basal cell carcinoma. The lesions of squamous cell carcinoma arise from the keratin-producing squamous cells of the epithelium. Squamous cell carcinoma tends to occur on the sun-exposed skin regions of the elderly, such as the face, hands, and forearms. Also, it is often seen in conjunction with weathered and actinically damaged skin. In comparison with basal cell carcinoma, squamous cell carcinoma has the potential to metastasize and is able to develop from skin that has been chronically inflamed or irritated. In most instances, squamous cell carcinoma appears as a erythematous plaque, nodule, or ulceration (Table 5-1).

Etiology

The most common cause of squamous cell carcinoma is ultraviolet radiation and, in particular, ultraviolet-B exposure. Thus, fair-skinned individuals are the most likely victims of cutaneous squamous cell carcinoma. Other known causes of squamous cell carcinoma include certain chronic dermatoses, polycyclic aromatic hydrocarbons (seen in tars and petroleum), arsenic (which often causes lesions to appear on the palms and soles), human papillomavirus (especially types 16 and 18), genetic predisposition, and immunosuppression [9••]. Of special note is the well-documented incidence of squamous cell carcinoma arising in previously irradiated or burned skin, as well as its development from scars. Squamous cell carcinoma arising in such areas of skin injury is referred to as Marjolin's ulcer, and is usually located on the extremities [10]. Although Marjolin's ulcer is a rare entity, it is known to be an especially aggressive form of squamous cell carcinoma. Therefore, any chronic, intractable ulcer should be biopsied.

Keratoacanthoma, although originally believed to be a separate disorder, is now considered to be one form of squamous cell carcinoma. Keratoacanthomas tend to follow a course in which the lesions spontaneously involute. Nevertheless, they should be treated as other types of squamous cell carcinomas and excised or destroyed when discovered, as lesions have been known to metastasize.

Appearance

Squamous cell carcinoma may present with a variety of features. The lesions range in color from red to tan. In comparison with basal cell carcinoma, squamous cell carcinoma usually appears more scaly and may have some degree of ulceration, crusting, or erosion [11] (Fig. 5-3). In addition, the lesions usually lack the pearly hue and telangiec-

TABLE 5-1 METASTATIC RATES FOR SQUAMOUS CELL CARCINOMA	
Location of primary lesion	**Recurrence, %**
Sun-damaged skin	5.2
External ear	8.8
Lower lip	13.7
Osteomyelitic sinus	31.0
Scar	37.9
Data from **Rowe and coworkers [18].**	

tasias commonly associated with basal cell carcinoma. Because the appearance of squamous cell carcinoma may be variable, a biopsy should always be performed to establish diagnosis.

Local invasion and metastasis

Squamous cell carcinoma is known to grow more rapidly than basal cell carcinoma. However, it can penetrate through the subcutaneous and muscle layers and travel along nerve routes or through the lymphatics or the bloodstream. If allowed to grow indefinitely, the lesions may result in pain, necrosis of involved tissues, and functional impairment, including the loss of vision.

In metastasis, the regional lymph nodes are the most frequent targets of regional invasion. Distant organs such as bone, lung, and brain may also become sites of metastasis, but this is unusual. Once metastasis has taken place, (usually within 2 years of diagnosis of squamous cell carcinoma), prognosis tends to be poor. Tumors associated with ulcers, chronic irritation, or radiation exposure are more likely to metastasize, as are higher grade tumors. In addition, tumors of greater depth and size and those located on mucosal regions are more likely to metastasize as well as

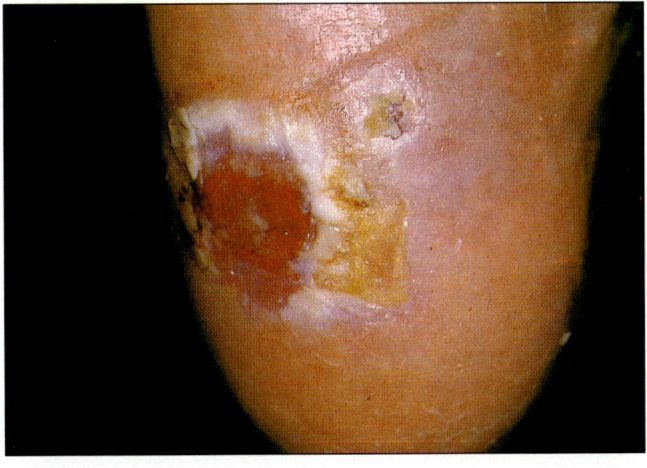

FIGURE 5-3 This ulcerated nodule with hyperkeratatic borders represents a deeply invasive squamous cell carcinoma.

recur. The incidence of metastasis is about 11% for patients with squamous cell carcinoma located on mucosal regions, 10% to 40% in patients with Marjolin's ulcer, and about 3% in patients with cutaneous squamous cell carcinoma [12].

Treatment

A number of different therapeutic options are available for squamous cell carcinoma, depending upon the location of the tumor, its size and depth of invasion, the age of the patient, and whether the tumor is a primary or recurrent lesion. Regardless of the choice of treatment, adequate follow-up is essential as recurrences tend to occur within the first 2 years after treatment of the primary lesion (Table 5-2).

Surgical excision

The conventional method for treating squamous cell carcinoma involves conservative surgical excision. This method achieves high success rates with rapid healing and good cosmetic results. After excision, margins should be examined histologically. The disadvantage of this form of treatment is that it may not be able to completely eradicate the tumor, especially if there is significant subclinical extension.

Cryosurgery and curettage

Options for small, primary lesions derived from sun damage (ie, actinically derived lesions) include destructive methods such as cryosurgery or curettage with electrodesiccation. These two modalities of treatment should only be performed on small lesions with distinct borders. In addition, they do not always achieve acceptable cosmetic results, and should be used with caution for lesions appearing on the face. When used for appropriate, small lesions, cryosurgery or curettage with electrodesiccation can achieve success rates equivalent to surgical excision. In addition, both are quick and economical modes of treatment.

Radiation treatment

Radiation treatment is especially useful for treating elderly or debilitated patients who are poor surgical candidates. Treatment requires multiple office visits and is costly. Other disadvantages to radiation therapy include lower success rates compared with other treatment modalities, and the often significant side effects with treatment.

Mohs micrographic surgery

To achieve the greatest amount of tissue preservation with the highest success rates, Mohs micrographic surgery is an important treatment. This procedure allows the physician to serially remove thin pieces of the specimen and microscopically examine 100% of the borders with frozen horizontal sections. Orientation is preserved and the edges of each slice are color-coded with dyes so that a map can be drawn, indicating any residual tumor [13]. The procedure is repeated but only in regions where, according to the map, the tumor is still remaining. Mohs surgery is the best treatment for large tumors, recurrent tumors, and for those

TABLE 5-2 RECURRENCE RATES IN PATIENTS TREATED FOR SQUAMOUS CELL CARCINOMA	
Therapeutic modality	**5-Year recurrence, %**
Cryotherapy	3.2
Curettage and electrodessication	3.7
Surgical excision	8.1
Radiation therapy	10.0
Mohs micrographic surgery	3.1

Data from Rowe and coworkers [18••].

regions where tissue preservation is deemed paramount (ie, for lesions on the face).

Metastatic disease

Treatment options for metastatic disease are limited. If there is invasion into regional lymph nodes, the options include lymph node dissection or radiation therapy [14••]. However, both lymph node dissection and radiation therapy can be used concomitantly. Once there are distant metastases (eg, metastases to the bones or lungs), prognosis is dismal. Combination chemotherapy for distant metastasis has been employed but has had limited effectiveness.

Basal Cell Carcinoma

Basal cell carcinoma is the most common cutaneous malignancy in the white population. Like squamous cell carcinoma, it has a tendency to occur in fair-skinned, elderly individuals who have been exposed to the harmful effects of the sun. Basal cell carcinoma appears most frequently on the face and neck as a small, pink, crusted, pearly lesion, often with rolled borders and telangiectasias. Of all the cutaneous malignancies, basal cell carcinoma is the slowest growing and is the least likely to metastasize. On initial presentation to a physician, patients often complain of a sore that tends to bleed or crust over, but which fails to heal.

Etiology

Many of the causes of basal cell carcinoma overlap with those of squamous cell carcinoma. For example, exposure to ultraviolet-B radiation, arsenic, and immunosuppressive states are known to predispose individuals to basal cell tumors. Occasionally, basal cell carcinoma may develop from trauma and scars including smallpox scars. However, unlike Marjolin's ulcers, they usually appear on the face and neck regions [15].

Appearance

Whenever basal cell carcinoma is suspected, the first step is to confirm the diagnosis with a biopsy. Nodular or nodular-ulcerative basal cell carcinoma is the most common basal cell carcinoma and presents as a small, pearly papule or nodule with a rolled border. Overlying telangiectasias are

TABLE 5-3 RECURRENCE RATES IN PATIENTS TREATED FOR BASAL CELL CARCINOMA

Therapeutic modality	5-Year recurrence, %
Surgical excision	10.1
Curettage and electrodessication	7.7
Radiation therapy	8.7
Cryotherapy	7.5
Mohs micrographic surgery	1.0

Data from Rowe and coworkers [19•].

frequently visible in these lesions. As they grow a central ulceration may develop along with crusting.

Superficial basal cell carcinoma is another common basal cell carcinoma that may present as multiple, red, scaly patches. The lesion commonly appears as a red plaque or patch with well-defined borders that may be pearly and scaly in appearance [16]. If allowed to develop for some time, these lesions tend to become nodular and may ulcerate.

Sclerosing or morpheaform basal cell carcinoma is a less common form of basal cell carcinoma that has the resemblance of a scar. It is yellowish-white in color and usually appears as a firm, indurated plaque with indistinct borders. Sclerosing basal cell carcinoma is a more aggressive form of basal cell carcinoma, as it often has subclinical extensions. These subclinical extensions make complete removal difficult and result in higher rates of recurrence.

Two other variants of basal cell carcinoma deserve mention. Pigmented basal cell carcinoma is a tumor that often resembles malignant melanoma but has the biologic behavior of common basal cell carcinoma. The other variant, infiltrating basal cell carcinoma, is a more aggressive tumor that, like sclerosing basal cell carcinoma, may have significant subclinical spread and high recurrence rates. The lesions of infiltrating basal cell carcinoma are ill-defined plaques that can resemble sclerosing basal cell carcinoma.

Local invasion and metastasis

Basal cell carcinoma tends to invade locally and rarely metastasizes. Like squamous cell carcinoma, local invasion can lead to infection, necrosis, and eventually pain and impairment of vital organs. The tumor can spread along nerves and bones. Basal cell carcinoma has an especially slow growth rate due to its dependence upon the stroma and an adequate blood supply for growth. Also, it may enter phases of regression alternating with periods of more aggressive growth.

Although recurrence rates for basal cell carcinoma vary greatly, two-thirds of recurrent lesions are known to develop within 3 years of diagnosis of the primary tumor [14••]. Tumors more likely to recur include those located on the nose, ear, or periorbital region (in descending order of

likelihood of recurrence). Also, tumors greater than 2 cm in diameter are more likely to recur [17] as are those with poor margins, such as sclerosing or infiltrating basal cell carcinoma. In general, any tumor with significant subclinical extension has a higher chance of recurring.

Treatment

As with squamous cell carcinoma, there are a number of methods to treat basal cell carcinoma. For small primary tumors of the nodular or superficial type, curettage with electrodesiccation is the most common mode of treatment. Cryosurgery is also a useful method for treating superficial basal cell carcinoma.

For larger tumors, conventional surgical excision or Mohs micrographic surgery is recommended. The margins for surgical excision should range from 2 to 4 mm for nodular basal cell carcinoma. However, for ill-defined lesions, lesions of the sclerosing or infiltrating type, or areas where a 2- to 4-mm surgical margin would not be cosmetically acceptable, it is recommended that Mohs surgery be performed. Mohs surgery has been shown to achieve success rates close to 99% for basal cell carcinoma, and should be the first-choice therapy for recurrent lesions (Table 5-3). Also, it is advocated that Mohs surgery be used for removing lesions located in regions with higher chances for recurrence, such as the nose, ear, and periorbital regions.

REFERENCES AND RECOMMENDED READING

Recently published papers of particular interest have been highlighted as:
• Of interest
•• Of outstanding interest

1. Balin AK, Lin AN, Pratt L: Actinic keratoses. *J Cutan Aging Cosmetic Dermatol* 1988, 1:77–86.

2. Kwa RE, Campana K, Moy RL: Biology of cutaneous squamous cell carcinoma. *J Am Acad Dermatol* 1992, 26:1–26.

3.• Callen JP: Possible precursors to epidermal malignancies. In *Cancer of the Skin.* Edited by Friedman RJ, Rigel DS, Kopf AW, Harris MN, Baker D. Philadelphia: WB Saunders; 1991:27–34.

4. Dodson JM, DeSpain J, Hewitt JE, Clark DP: Malignant potential of actinic keratoses and the controversy over treatment. *Arch Dermatol* 1991, 127:1029–1031.

5. Mostow EN, Johnson TM: Malignant transformation from actinic keratoses to squamous cell carcinomas. *Arch Dermatol* 1992, 128:560–561.

6.•• Beacham BE: Common skin tumors in the elderly. *Am Fam Physician* 1992, 46:163–168.

7.•• Cohen PR: Bowen's disease: squamous cell carcinoma in situ. *Am Fam Physician* 1991, 44:1325–1329.

8.• Chute CG, Chuang T-Y, Bergstralh EJ, Su WD: The subsequent risk of internal cancer with Bowen's disease. *JAMA* 1991, 266:816–819.

9.•• Johnson TM, Rowe DE, Nelson BR, Swanson NA: Squamous cell carcinoma of the skin (excluding lip and oral mucosa). *J Am Acad Dermatol* 1992, 26:467–484.

10. Edwards MJ, Hirsch RM, Broadwater JR, Netscher DT, Ames FC: Squamous cell carcinoma arising in previously burned or irradiated skin. *Arch Surg* 1989, 124:115–117.

11. Smoller J, Smoller BR: Skin malignancies in the elderly. Diagnosable, treatable, and potentially curable. *J Gerontol Nurs* 1992, 18:19–24.

12. Moller R, Reymann F, Hou-Jensen K: Metastases in dermatological patients with squamous cell carcinoma. *Arch Dermatol* 1979, 115:703–705.

13. Moy RL, Zitelli JA: Mohs micrographic surgery for treatment of skin cancer in the elderly. *Ger Med Today* 1989, 8:98–107.

14.•• Preston DS, Stern RS: Nonmelanoma cancers of the skin. *N Engl J Med,I>* 1992, 327:1649–1662.

15. Lang PG, Maize JC: Basal cell carcinoma. In *Cancer of the Skin.* Edited by Friedman RJ, Riegel DS, Kopf AW, Harris MN, Baker D. Philadelphia: WB Saunders; 1991:35–73.

16. Goldberg LH, Rubin HA: Management of basal cell carcinoma. *Postgrad Med* 1989, 85:57–63.

17. Roenigk RK, Ratz JL, Bailin PL, Wheeland RG: Trends in the presentation of basal cell carcinoma. *J Dermatol Surg Oncol* 1986, 12:860–865.

18.•• Rowe DE, Carroll RJ, Day CL: Prognostic factors for local recurrence, metastasis and survival rates in squamous cell carcinoma of the skin, ear and lip. *J Am Acad Dermatol* 1992, 26:976–990.

19.• Rowe DE, Carroll RJ, Day CL: Long-term recurrence rates in previously untreated (primary) basal cell carcinoma: implications for patient follow-up. *J Dermatol Surg Oncol* 1990, 15:315–328.

Benign and Malignant Pigmented Lesions

Arthur J. Sober
Raymond L. Barnhill

Key Points

- The incidence rate of cutaneous melanoma is increasing dramatically.

- Early diagnosis usually results in cure of the patient.

- Routine physical examination should include inspection of the skin, especially of the torso in men and the back and lower legs in women.

- Individuals at increased risk of developing melanoma are those with large numbers of nevi, clinical atypical moles, a personal or family history of melanoma, skin that tans poorly, and freckles.

- Most melanomas can be detected using the *ABCDE* rule: *A*ssymetry, *B*order irregularity, *C*olor variation, *D*iameter >6mm, and *E*nlargement.

Cutaneous melanoma is the most common cause of death from diseases developing initially in the skin [1•]. Because the frequency of cutaneous melanoma is increasing among white populations, it is imperative that the general physician be able to examine the skin in a discerning manner. The primary goal is to distinguish suspicious pigmented lesions from the myriad of other pigmented lesions on the skin.

Although a high proportion of melanomas are thought to be related to excessive sun exposure during childhood and adolescence, approximately 10% of cutaneous melanomas seem to have a genetic basis. Cutaneous melanomas that appear to follow a dominant inheritance pattern have been recognized for many years, and a linkage to chromosome 9 has recently been proposed.

NATURAL HISTORY

There are four distinct types of cutaneous melanoma which differ in clinical appearance, histologic appearance, and biologic behavior (Figs. 6-1 through 6-4). Three of these tend to exhibit horizontal growth in the superficial skin for extended periods of time (radial growth phase), during which surgical removal is usually curative. These types are the superficial spreading, lentigo maligna, and acral lentiginous melanoma [2] (Table 6-1).

These have relatively prolonged periods of evolution, during which they are either entirely intraepidermal or micro-invasive into the dermis with a negligible capacity for metastasis. Approximately 1 to 30 years may elapse before deeper invasion occurs with the attendant increased risk for metastasis via the lymphatics or the blood stream [2]. The fourth type, nodular melanoma, has no apparent radial growth phase and tends to rapidly invade the dermis from onset (Fig. 6-4; Table 6-1). Nodular melanoma appears to have capacity to metastasize from early in its development.

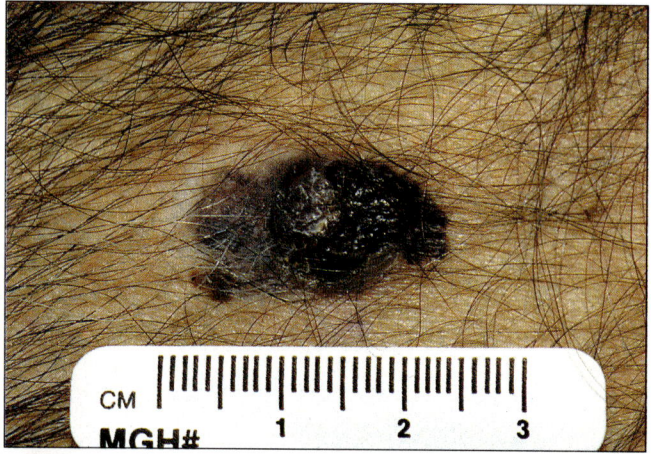

FIGURE 6-1 Superficial spreading melanoma is characterized by irregular borders and variation in color (blue color on left side).

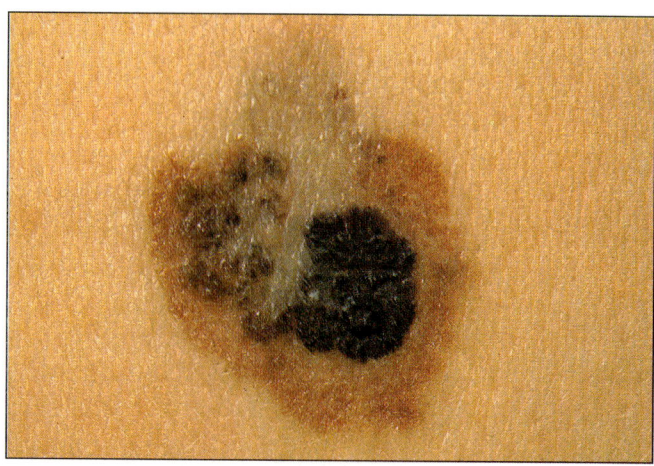

FIGURE 6-2 Superficial spreading melanoma shows irregular borders, variation in pigment pattern, and partial regression (whitish areas at 12 o'clock position).

The proportion of melanomas that arise *de novo* in apparently normal skin has been estimated to be anywhere from 30% to 70%. Conversely, the number of melanomas arising in pre-existing nevi also has been estimated to vary from 30% to 70%. Most authors believe that between 30% and 40% of melanomas arise in pre-existing nevi and the rest *de novo*.

Cutaneous melanoma spreads in three ways: within the adjacent skin, via the lymphatics to regional nodes, and via the blood stream to many visceral organs. In general, nodal presentation with metastatic disease occurs earlier than visceral presentation. The internal organs most frequently involved with metastatic disease are liver, lung, bone, and brain. Long disease-free intervals are not unusual with cutaneous melanoma so that 5 years disease-free survival does not necessarily represent cure. Thirteen percent of recurrences occur between 5 and 10 years and occasional

recurrences occur thereafter, especially with thinner tumors. Approximately 6% of patients with cutaneous melanoma will develop a second primary tumor during their lifetime. This figure is considerably higher in patients with familial melanoma, 30% of whom may develop a second primary tumor.

DIAGNOSIS

Clinical suspicion of cutaneous melanoma may be enhanced by applying the pneumonic *ABCDE: A*, asymmetry which refers to the lack of mirror image symmetry when the two halves of the lesion are compared; *B*, border irregularity; *C*, color variation; *D*, diameter >6 mm; and *E*, enlargement [3•]. Although certain melanomas may lack one or more of these features, or uncommonly all, their presence, especially in combination, should raise suspicion

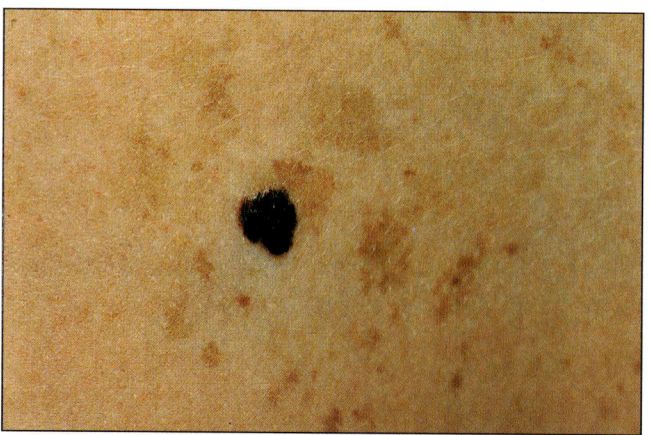

FIGURE 6-3 Early melanoma arising in markedly sun-damaged skin shows raised, dark-brown plaque with irregular border arising adjacent to a flat brown lesion.

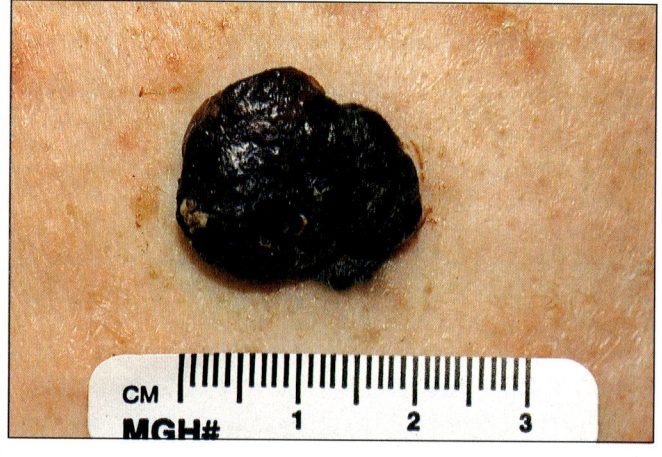

FIGURE 6-4 Nodular melanoma seen here is a brown-black nodule with no flat surrounding pigmentation.

TABLE 6-1 CLINICAL FEATURES OF MALIGNANT MELANOMA

Type	Site	Average age at diagnosis, y	Duration of known existence, y	Color
Lentigo maligna melanoma	Sun-exposed surfaces, particularly malar region of cheek and temple	70	5–20* or longer	In flat portions, shades of brown and tan predominant, but whitish gray occasionally present; in nodules, shades of reddish brown, bluish gray, bluish black
Superficial spreading melanoma	Any site (more common on upper back in men and on lower leg in women)	40–50	1–7	Shades of brown mixed with bluish red (violaceous), bluish black, reddish brown, and often whitish pink, and the border of lesion is at least in part visibly and/or palpably elevated
Nodular melanoma	Any site	40–50	Months to less than 5	Reddish blue (purple) or bluish black; either uniform in color or mixed with brown or black
Acral lentiginous melanoma	Palm, sole, nail bed, mucous membrane	60	1–10	In flat portions, dark brown predominantly; in raised lesions (plaques) brown-black or blue-black predominantly

*For much of this time (the precursor stage) active growth is confined to the epidermis.
Adapted from Sober and Koh [2]; with permission.

for melanoma [4]. Benign pigmented lesions may at times have one or more of these features, but by becoming aware of the clinical characteristics of the common benign pigmented lesions, most can be distinguished (Figs. 6-5 through 6-12 and Table 6-2). Those features most frequently present in early melanoma are increase in size and change in color. Increase in height correlates with deeper penetration within the skin and is a sign of more advanced disease, as are bleeding, pain, and ulceration. Itching in a pigmented lesion may raise suspicions because this symptom is present in approximately one quarter of patients with early melanomas.

Not everyone is at equal risk for developing melanoma. Those at greatest risk tan poorly, burn easily, freckle, have blonde or red hair, and blue or gray eyes, and have increased numbers of nevi [5,6]. Also at risk are those with a prior cutaneous melanoma, a positive family history of melanoma, and those who are immunosuppressed. Individuals who have had severe sunburns in childhood and adolescence also appear to have increased risk for development of melanoma later in life. Table 6-3 lists the factors associated with increased risk for development of melanoma. Increased regular surveillance would be appropriate for individuals with an elevated risk.

The best time to diagnose cutaneous melanoma is during the general physical examination. A complete skin examination of the patient should be performed in a room with bright lighting. A 5 to 10 power hand lens is also helpful in appreciating the differences noted in Figures 6-1 through 6-3 and Tables 6-1 and 6-2. Patients with a suspicious lesion should be considered for biopsy to establish the diagnosis [7], referred to a dermatologist for an additional opinion, or if suspicion is low-grade, given a follow-up appointment for reevaluation.

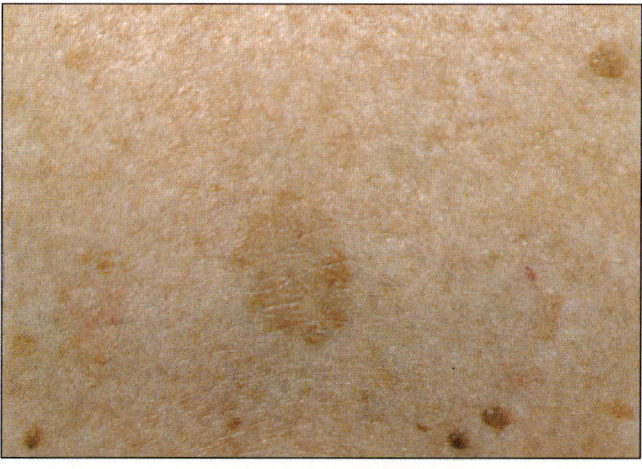

FIGURE 6-5 Solar lentigo (lentigines) results from chronic solar exposure. The face and back of the hands are the most common sites. Pigmentation is reticulate when magnified.

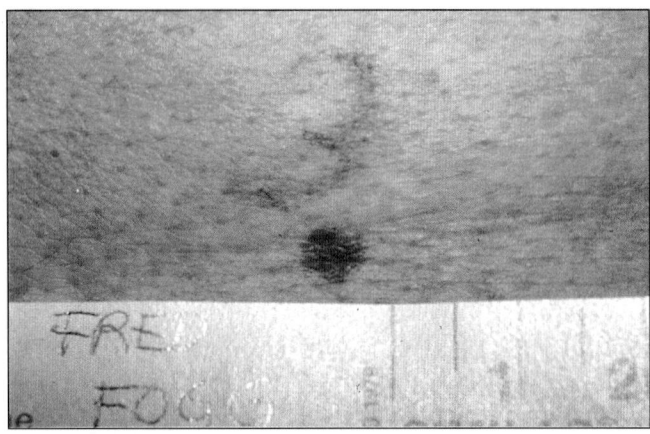

FIGURE 6-6 Lentigo is a flat (macular), sharply bordered medium- to dark-brown lesion that can vary in size from 2 mm to greater than 1 cm.

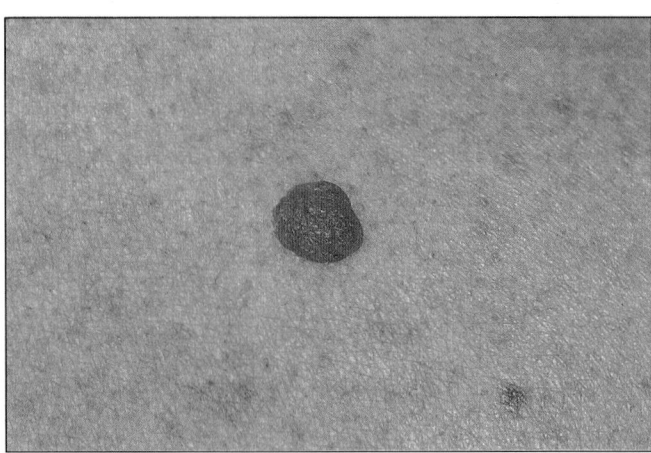

FIGURE 6-7 Dermal nevus is a flesh-colored papule or nodule usually with regular borders.

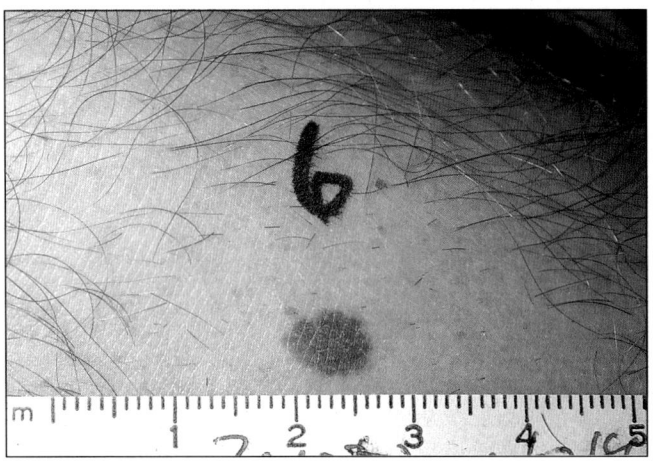

FIGURE 6-8 Compound nevus can be papillomatous or dome-shaped with smooth, well-demarcated borders. Colors may vary from light to very dark brown to flesh colored.

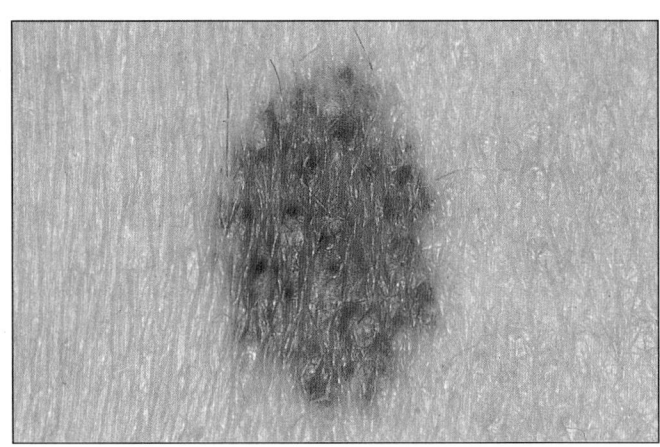

FIGURE 6-9 Congenital, melanocytic nevi are compound nevi present from birth. The size may range from less than 1 cm to greater than 144 in^2. Many will also have prominent dark hairs emerging from the nevus.

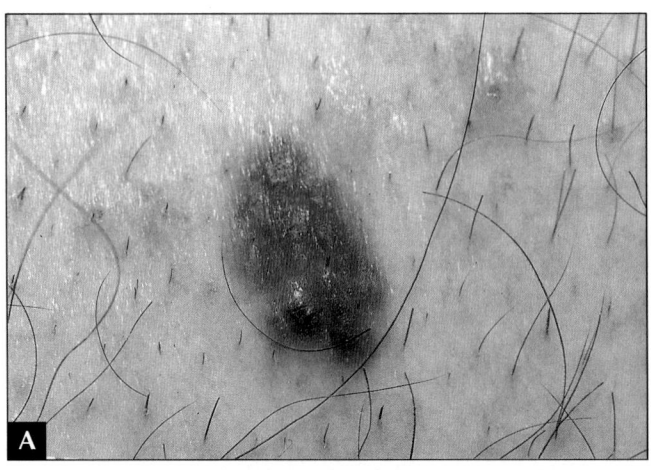

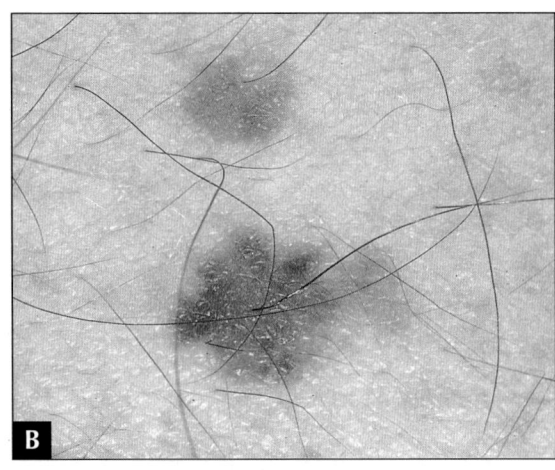

FIGURE 6-10 A, B, Dysplastic nevi, in contrast to benign acquired nevi, show more variable mixtures of tan, brown, and red or pink coloration, have irregular and sometimes hazy borders, are often 6 mm or larger, and may be present in great numbers.

Assessment

The most important evaluation in establishing the diagnosis of cutaneous melanoma is a biopsy of the lesion itself. Numerous studies have shown that a punch or incisional biopsy does not adversely affect outcome [7]. Total excisional biopsy with narrow margins is the procedure of choice, however, and can usually be performed under local anesthesia on an outpatient basis. This procedure provides the pathologist with the entire specimen for both diagnostic and prognostic purposes.

The prognosis of the patient with localized disease is directly related to the primary tumor thickness measured in millimeters from the granular cell layer of the epidermis to the deepest tumor cell. A second prognostic system depends on determining the anatomic level within the skin of the primary tumor, using Clark's levels of invasion: level I, intraepidermal (in situ); level II, into papillary dermis; level III, filling papillary dermis; level IV, into reticular dermis; and level V, into subcutaneous fat. Survival based

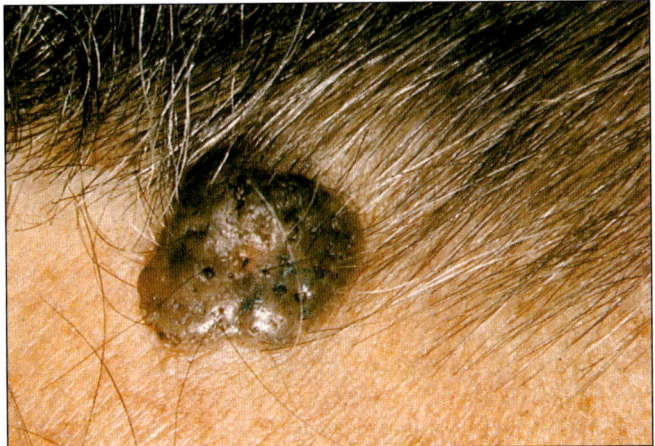

FIGURE 6-11 Seborrheic keratosis is a very common benign lesion which typically appears as a waxy "stuck-on" plaque. When highly pigmented or inflamed, differentiation from melanoma may be difficult. These lesions are typically multiple.

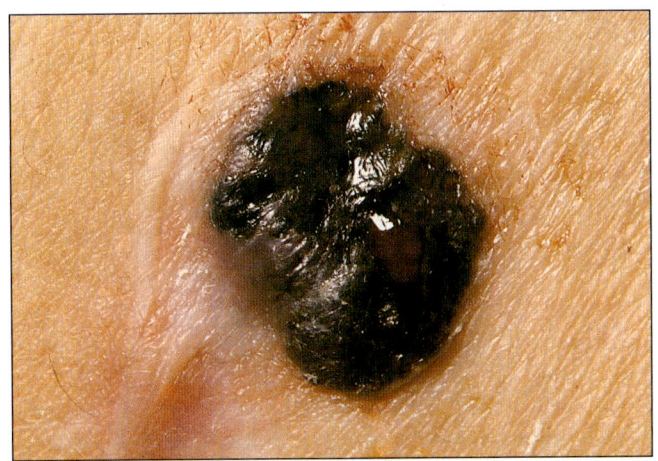

FIGURE 6-12 Pigmented basal cell carcinomas may appear as nodules such as this one or as barely raised plaques. In contrast to melanoma, which occurs more in fair-complexioned individuals with blue or gray eyes and lighter-colored hair, the pigmented basal cell carcinoma typically occurs in dark-complexioned individuals with dark brown or black hair and brown eyes.

TABLE 6-2 PIGMENTED LESIONS TO BE DISTINGUISHED FROM MELANOMA

Hemangioma

Reddish-brown or purple nodule. May blanch with compression (glass microscope slide), indicating its vascular nature

Subungual hematoma

Traumatic bleeding below the nail typically has maroon discoloration. A curved clear area is seen as the nail grows out

Tattoo

May be of medical origin (blue or green dots in a geometric pattern) or traumatic (pigmentation is irregularly dispersed and may appear black)

Blue nevus

Blue-gray, well-demarcated, stable 2–3 mm to 1 cm lesion. Occurs most often on hands, feet, and buttocks. The pigment is brown melanin, which appears blue because of the location in the mid-dermis

Pigmented dermatofibroma

Usually not pigmented, this firm, button-like fibrous response to injury may occasionally present with increased pigmentation. Dermatofibromas will ``dimple'' downward with lateral compression

TABLE 6-3 FACTORS THAT INCREASE RISK OF MELANOMA DEVELOPMENT

Greatly increase

Large numbers of nevi (>50 nevi ≥2 mm)

Clinically atypical moles in individuals with 2 family members with melanoma

Persistently changing pigmented lesion

Moderately increase

History of prior melanoma

Family history of melanoma

Clinically atypical nevi, nonfamilial melanoma

Light-complexioned whites versus blacks, Asians, or dark-complexioned whites

Modestly increase

Easily sunburned, poor at tanning

Freckles

Transplant suppression

on Clark's level is also shown in Table 6-4. Favorable prognostic factors are as follows:

Female sex
Patient age under 50 years
Clinically localized disease
Primary tumor located on arms and legs (other than hands and feet)
Thin primary tumor ≤ 0.75 mm)
Clark level II

Factors considered to be unfavorable are as follows:
Male sex
Patient age over 50 years
Evidence of metastases
Primary tumor located on head and neck, torso, or hands and feet
Thick primary tumor (> 1.70 mm)
Clark level IV or V
Ulcerated primary tumor
High mitotic rate of primary tumor
Presence of microscopic satellites

A variety of multifactorial models exist to further refine prediction of outcome, but these are beyond the scope of this chapter [8].

In the absence of positive signs or symptoms, patients with localized disease do not warrant extensive "high-tech" diagnostic investigations. A baseline chest radiograph is sufficient for individuals with low-risk disease, and for those at higher risk for recurrent disease, annual chest radiographs are recommended.

TREATMENT

Table 6-5 summarizes the treatment for primary melanoma [9•,10•]. In some centers, patients with localized disease who have primary tumors thicker than 1.50 mm undergo elective lymph nodal dissection if a single defined drainage pathway can be determined. The value of elective nodal dissection versus close observation followed by delayed dissection if nodes become clinically palpable is currently undergoing investigation by randomized clinical trial [11].

At present, there are no adjuvant therapies of proven value to lower risk of recurrence in patients with high-risk disease. Many agents are currently under investigation, including α-interferon, various tumor vaccines, and various types of monoclonal antibody therapy [12••].

The treatment for isolated metastatic disease is surgical excision, if possible. Some patients, especially those with lymph nodal and soft tissue disease, may have long disease-free intervals following surgery [13]. Such patients should be staged carefully before surgical treatment. Patients in whom metastatic disease cannot be surgically eliminated are candidates for palliative forms of therapy. At the present time, there is no highly successful form of chemotherapy or radiation therapy for metastatic cutaneous melanoma. Current treatment protocols usually involve multiple drugs, and referral to a medical oncologist is appropriate. Radiation therapy is palliative for metastasis to brain or bone.

ROLE OF THE GENERALIST

Most melanomas are detected either by the patient, patient's family members, or the family physician. As cutaneous melanoma can occur in relatively young individuals (mean age of melanoma is between 40 and 50 years), the early detection and subsequent cure of the patient translates into a gain of many years of productive life. In addition to early diagnosis, the generalist has an important role to play in primary and secondary prevention.

TABLE 6-4 FIVE-YEAR SURVIVAL RATES FOR LOCALIZED MELANOMA	
Thickness, *mm*	**5-Year Survival, %**
< 0.76	96
0.76–1.49	87
1.50–2.49	75
2.50–3.99	66
≥ 4.00	47
Clark level	
II (Into papillary dermis)	95
III (Filling papillary dermis)	82
IV (Into reticular dermis)	71
V (Into subcutaneous fat)	49

TABLE 6-5 SURGICAL GUIDELINES FOR PRIMARY TUMOR MANAGEMENT IN PATIENTS WITH LOCALIZED MELANOMA*		
Tumor thickness, *mm*	**Excision margin, *cm***	**Closure**
< 1.0	1.0	Primary
1.0–4.0	2.0	Primary
> 4.0	3.0†	Primary, flap, or graft

*These guidelines are arbitrary. They should be modified for individual patients, depending on overall assessment of prognosis. †Margins < 3 cm may be necessary to achieve primary closure.

PATIENT EDUCATION

Because there is no highly effective therapy for advanced melanoma, the cornerstone of decreasing melanoma mortality is based on a combination of early diagnosis and primary prevention. Primary prevention currently focuses on reducing the overall exposure of the population, especially those at increased risk, to sunlight from as early in life as possible. The three ways in which this is best done are avoidance of the most intense rays of the midday sun (10 a.m. to 2 p.m. eastern standard time or 11 a.m. to 3 p.m. daylight savings time), use of clothing cover-up such as a t-shirt with sleeves and a hat with a broad brim, and use of sunblocks with a high sun protection factor. Current recommendations suggest the use of a broad spectrum blocker so that both UVA (long wave) and UVB (sunburn) are reduced.

Identification of patients at increased risk is important so that they can be enrolled in a regular follow-up program and can be educated in self-examination. The American Cancer Society and the Skin Cancer Foundation have both published aids for patient education in learning self-examination. Every 6 to 8 weeks is a reasonable frequency for patients to check their own skin. The *ABCDE* warning signs should be part of the patient's health knowledge base. In addition, first-degree relatives of patients with melanoma or with clinically atypical moles should undergo skin examination (*see* Table 6-2 for features of clinically atypical moles).

REFERENCES AND RECOMMENDED READING

Recently published papers of particular interest have been highlighted as:
• Of interest
•• Of outstanding interest

1.• Koh HK: Cutaneous melanoma. *N Engl J Med* 1991, 325:171–182.

2. Sober AJ, Koh HK: Melanoma and other pigmented skin lesions. In *Harrison's Principles of Internal Medicine*, Edited by Isselbacher KJ, *et al.* New York: McGraw-Hill: 1994:1867–1871.

3.• Friedman RJ, Rigel DS, Kopf AW, *et al.*: *Cancer of the Skin.* Philadelphia: WB Saunders; 1991.

4. Sober AJ, Fitzpatrick TB, Mihm MC Jr, *et al.*: Early recognition of cutaneous melanoma. *JAMA* 1979, 242:2795–2799.

5. Rhodes AR, Weinstock MA, Fitzpatrick TB, *et al.*: Risk factors for cutaneous melanoma. *JAMA* 1987, 258:3146–3154.

6. MacKie RM, Aitchison TC, Freudenberger T: A personal risk factor chart for cutaneous melanoma. *Lancet* 1989, ii:487–490.

7. Lederman JS, Sober AJ: Does biopsy type influence survival in clinical stage I cutaneous melanoma? *J Am Acad Dermatol* 1985, 13:983–987.

8. Clark WH Jr, Elder DE, Guerry D IV, *et al.*: Model predicting survival in stage I melanoma based on tumor progression. *J Natl Cancer Inst* 1989, 81:1893–1904.

9.• Veronesi U, Cascinelli N: Narrow excision (1 cm-margin): a safe procedure for thin cutaneous melanoma. *Arch Surg* 1991, 126:438–441.

10.• Ho VC, Sober AJ: Therapy for cutaneous melanoma: an update. *J Am Acad Dermatol* 1990, 22:159–176.

11. Veronesi U, Adamus J, Bandiera DC, *et al.*: Delayed regional lymph node dissection in stage I melanoma of the skin of the lower extremities. *Cancer* 1982, 49:2420–2430.

12.•• Balch CM, Houghton AN, Milton GW, *et al.*: *Cutaneous Melanoma*, edn 2. Philadelphia: JB Lippincott; 1992.

13. Markowitz JS, Cosimi LA, Carey RW, *et al.*: Prognosis after initial recurrence of cutaneous melanoma. *Arch Surg* 1991, 126:703–708.

SELECT BIBLIOGRAPHY

Kelly JW, Rivers JK, MacLennan R, *et al.*: Sunlight: a major factor associated with development of melanocytic nevi in Australian school children. *J Am Acad Dermatol* 1994, 30:40–48.

Newton JA, Bataille V, Griffiths K, *et al.*: How common is the atypical mole syndrome phenotype in apparently sporadic melanoma? *J Am Acad Dermatol* 1993, 29:989–996.

7 Common Cutaneous Tumors

Tissa R. Hata
Kenneth A. Arndt

> ### Key Points
> - Common tumors of the skin are often difficult to recognize as "common," unless one can make an accurate diagnosis.
> - Treatment hinges on the pathology and natural history of the lesion.
> - Seborrheic keratosis is the most common benign tumor in adulthood.
> - Dermatofibromas are characterized by the "dimple" sign.
> - Sebaceous hyperplasia is often mistaken for basal cell carcinoma.
> - Fibrous papules of the nose and angiofibromas seen in tuberous sclerosis are similar both clinically and histologically.
> - Painful tumors are characterized by the acronym "*LEND AN EGG.*"

SEBORRHEIC KERATOSES

Seborrheic keratoses are benign lesions that are sometimes referred to as barnacles because of their "stuck on" appearance on the surface of the skin (Figs. 7-1 through 7-3). They are the most common benign tumor encountered in the older patient, and their number increases with age. Their onset is usually in patients aged in their late twenties to early thirties. These tumors are less common in native Americans and blacks.

Seborrheic keratoses may have several different appearances. Most typically they are raised brown waxy or greasy plaques with a verrucous surface, often containing small white inclusions which correspond to horn cysts seen on histopathologic examination. The second type is somewhat more difficult to recognize, and may be confused with lentigo maligna. These slightly raised waxy brown plaques often demonstrate variation in color, consisting of shades of brown or black. Even for dermatologists, this type of seborrheic keratosis is difficult to assess and may require biopsy for definitive diagnosis. Irritated seborrheic keratoses have a surrounding area of erythema, and may be associated with lesional swelling, bleeding, and oozing. Multiple seborrheic keratoses occurring in an eruptive manner may be a sign of internal malignancy, known as the sign of Leser-Trélat. The most common malignancy alleged to be associated with this is adenocarcinoma of the gastrointestinal tract [1].

Microscopically, these lesions display hyperkeratosis, acanthosis, and papillomatosis. Interspersed are multiple horn cysts or pseudo–horn cysts that show sudden and complete keratinization with only a very thin granular layer.

Seborrheic keratoses have a benign clinical course, but often the patient complains either of their unsightly appearance or of irritation of the lesion. Treatment by cryosurgery with liquid nitrogen is often sufficient to remove these lesions, but caution should be taken to ensure that the lesion is truly a seborrheic keratosis and not a lentigo maligna or melanoma. If the clinician is unsure of the

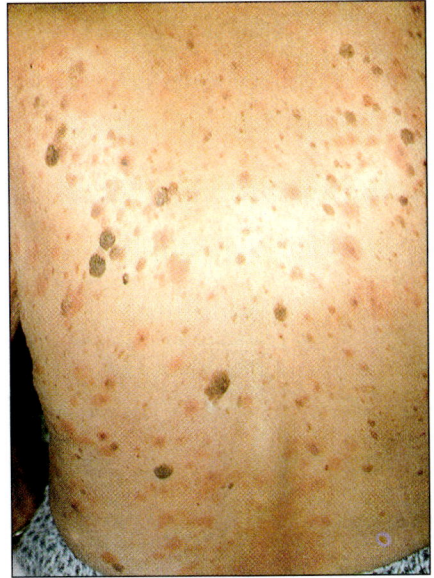

FIGURE 7-1 Seborrheic keratoses widely distributed on the trunk.

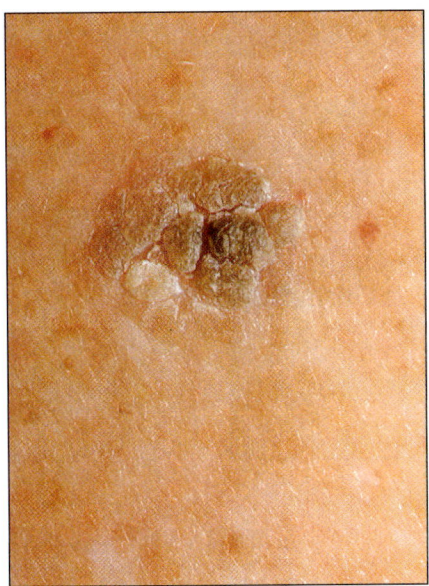

FIGURE 7-2 Seborrheic keratosis showing verrucous changes.

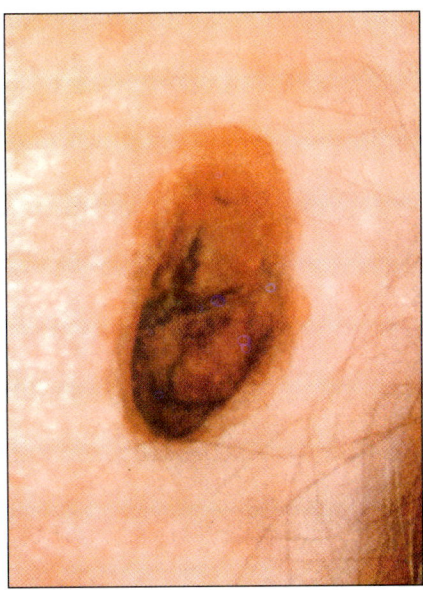

FIGURE 7-3 Seborrheic keratosis showing pigmentary variation.

diagnosis, treatment with gentle curettage and a hemostatic agent (Monsel's solution or aluminum chloride solution) applied to the base will provide a histologic specimen and effectively remove the keratosis. Surgical excision is strongly discouraged.

DERMATOSIS PAPULOSA NIGRA

Dermatosis papulosa nigra, which most often occurs on the faces of Hispanics and blacks, consists of 1- to 5-mm, stuck on–appearing, brown-black papules (Fig. 7-4). Histologically, these lesions are seborrheic keratoses, but they often have a different clinical presentation. The most typical areas of predilection are the malar regions and the forehead. They are of no medical consequence, but often the patient wishes to have them removed for cosmetic reasons.

Treatment is often limited to gentle curettage alone; electrodesiccation or freezing with a cotton-tipped swab is also effective but increases the risk of pigmentary sequelae. Vigorous treatment with liquid nitrogen or electrosurgery may cause postinflammatory hypopigmentation or hyperpigmentation of dark-skinned individuals, and should be avoided.

ACROCHORDONS

Acrochordons are soft, pedunculated, skin-colored polypoid papules, ranging from 1 to 5 mm in diameter, that are most commonly found on the neck, axillae, groin, and trunk (Fig. 7-5), although they can appear almost anywhere. They have a benign course, and removal is usually requested because of irritation in and around the lesion or for cosmesis.

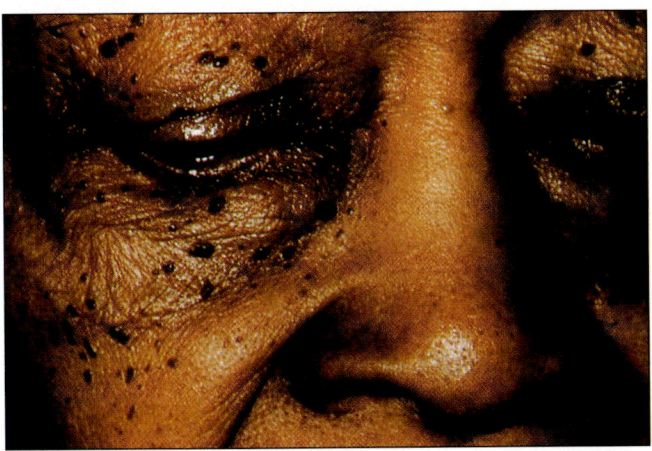

FIGURE 7-4 Dermatosis papulosa nigra.

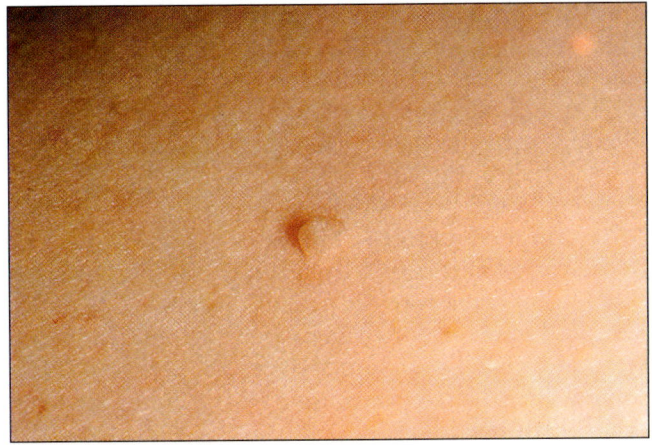

FIGURE 7-5 Skin tags.

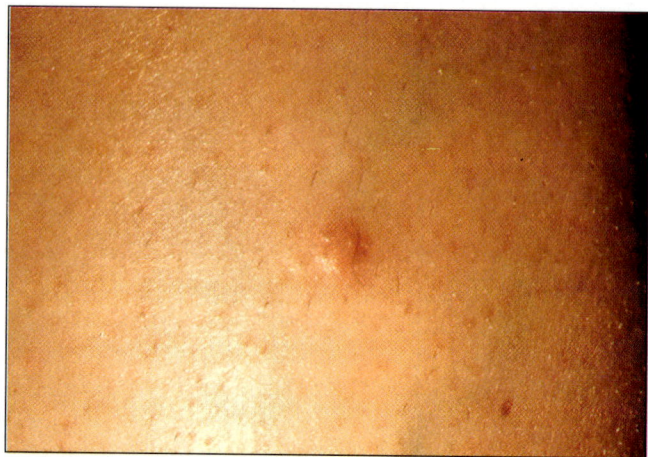

FIGURE 7-6 Dermatofibroma.

Histologically, these lesions have a connective tissue stalk composed of loose collagen fibers with numerous dilated capillaries, with overlying papillomatosis, hyperkeratosis, and acanthosis in the epidermis.

Treatment consists of removal with Gradle scissors, cryosurgery with liquid nitrogen, or gentle electrodesiccation. Most patients are able to tolerate these procedures without anesthesia. However, for large acrochordons, the use of local anesthesia is usually necessary.

DERMATOFIBROMAS

Dermatofibromas are usually pea-sized nodules that often occur on the lower legs or forearms and are associated with overlying hyperpigmentation (Fig. 7-6). These lesions are usually fixed within the skin but move freely over underlying tissues. They may be depressed or slightly elevated. A characteristic clinical sign is the "dimple" sign: on pinching, the dermatofibroma characteristically dimples into the skin. These lesions are very common. They may be noticed by the patient after minor trauma or an insect bite, but the relation of these incidents to the induction of lesions is unclear. Dermato fibromas are quite rare in children, and usually occur in adults. The etiology of these lesions is unknown.

Histologically, the dermatofibroma consists of spindle cells or histiocytes in association with collagen that is irregularly arranged in a storiform pattern. The overlying epidermis often shows elongation of the rete in a "dirty fingers" pattern. The best treatment for the dermatofibroma is usually none at all; the clinician should simply reassure the patient that these lesions are benign. However, for cosmetic reasons, surgical excision, tangential excision (shaving the lesion flat but leaving the base), or cryosurgery with liquid nitrogen can be performed.

Any dermatofibroma that is rapidly growing should be excised completely to rule out other causes, particularly dermatofibrosarcoma protuberans, which is a malignant soft tissue sarcoma. Primary excision of these tumors is usually inadequate, with a 40% recurrence rate with less than 1-cm margins [2], and excision by Mohs surgery is the treatment of choice [3].

SEBACEOUS HYPERPLASIA

Lesions of sebaceous hyperplasia often occur on the face as umbilicated or lobular yellow to orange-yellow papules of 2 to 5 mm in diameter (Fig. 7-7). They are often thought to be basal cell carcinomas because of their shared characteristics of translucency, telangiectasia, and central indentation. Sebaceous hyperplasia papules are most frequently located on the temples, cheeks, and forehead. They are usually first noted in patients who are aged over 40 years. Histologically, these lesions are composed of an enlarged sebaceous gland that consists of numerous lobules surrounding a centrally located wide sebaceous duct.

Sebaceous hyperplasia lesions do not require treatment unless the patient requests it for cosmetic purposes. They can be treated successfully with gentle electrodesiccation or electrofulguration if there is no doubt of the diagnosis. Alternative methods include the application of acids, cryosurgery, and carbon dioxide laser ablation. If there is any doubt, tangential excision or gentle curettage will also remove the lesion and provide a histologic specimen for examination.

HYPERTROPHIC SCARS AND KELOIDS

The hypertrophic scar is defined as a fibrous, thickened, firm reddish-brown plaque (Figs. 7-8 through 7-10) not overgrowing the boundaries of an original injury and often demonstrating partial resolution over 1 or several years. The keloid is an exuberant version of the hypertrophic scar that spreads well beyond the limits of the original scar and

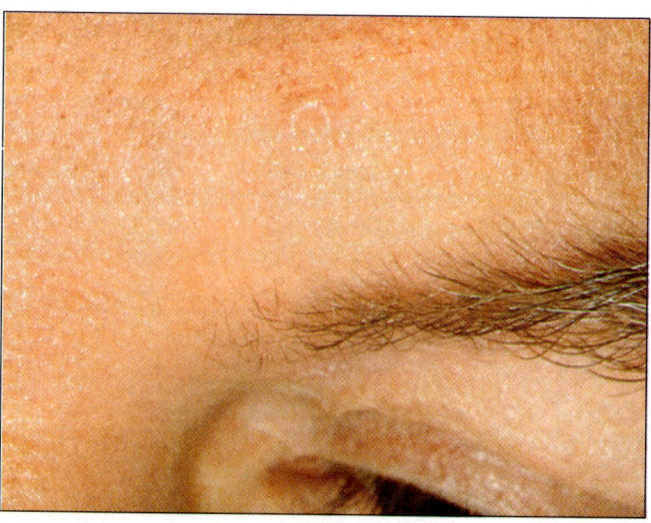

FIGURE 7-7 Sebaceous adenoma.

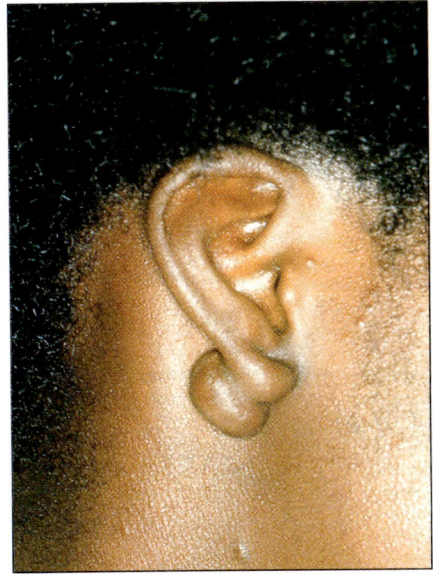

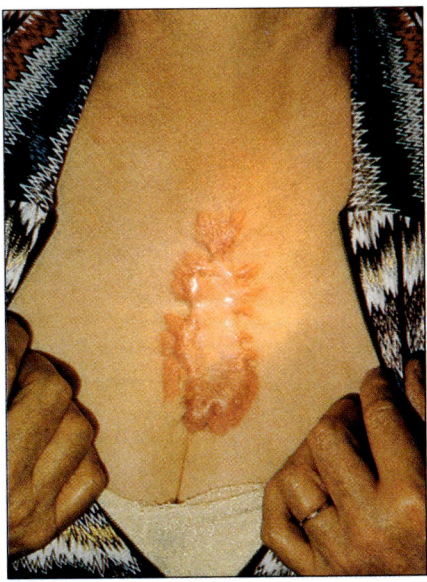

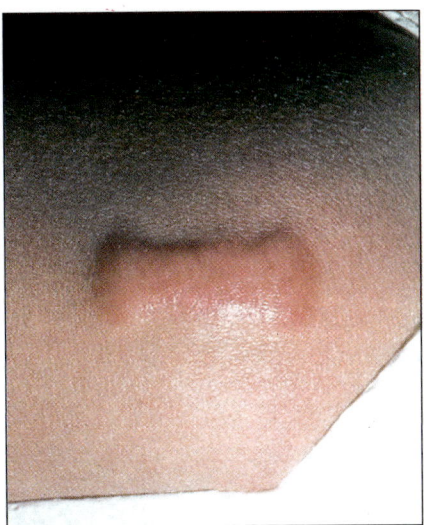

FIGURE 7-8 Ear keloid.

FIGURE 7-9 Presternal keloid.

shows no improvement with time. Keloids more often are accompanied by symptoms of itching or pain. Common sites for keloids are the sternal region, the neck and shoulders, the deltoid area, and the earlobes; a less common site is the trunk.

Histologically, the keloid or hypertrophic scar is composed of thick, highly compacted, hyalinized bands of collagen in a whirled or nodular pattern.

Effective treatment of keloids is quite difficult. The most effective therapy is prevention! First-line treatment is usually injection with an intralesional steroid such as triamcinalone acetonide, 10 to 40 mg/ml every 4 to 6 weeks, on one or several occasions, which flattens and softens the keloids. Other various treatment approaches are listed in Table 7-1.

TABLE 7-1 TREATMENT OF KELOIDS
Intralesional steroids
Cryosurgery with liquid nitrogen alone or in combination with intralesional steroids*†
Pressure dressings†
Silicone gel dressings‡
Excision and injection of intralesional steroids†
Excision and radiotherapy§
Ultrasound†
Laser surgery¶
Adhesive zinc tapes†
Topical retinoic acids**
Intralesional injection of interferon γ ††

Data from *Ceilley and Babin [4]; †Datubo-Brown [5•]; ‡Hirshowitz *et al.* [6]; §Darzi *et al.* [7•]; ¶Sherman and Rosenfeld [8]; **Haas and Arndt [9]; ††Granstein *et al.* [10•].

CHONDRODERMATITIS NODULARIS HELICIS

Chondrodermatitis lesions are typically small, very tender red nodules commonly occurring on the outer helix of the ear in older men (Fig. 7-11). They may be single or multiple, are typically 2 to 6 mm in diameter, and often present as erythematous red nodules firmly attached to the underlying cartilage. The surface may be covered with an adherent crust that on removal reveals a central ulceration.

The etiology is unclear; however, pressure or chronic trauma, particularly over skin altered by actinic exposure, is believed to be important in their evolution. Histologically, the epidermis of these lesions shows an ulcer filled with necrotic dermal debris and covered with a crust. The dermis in the center of the lesion shows degenerated collagen

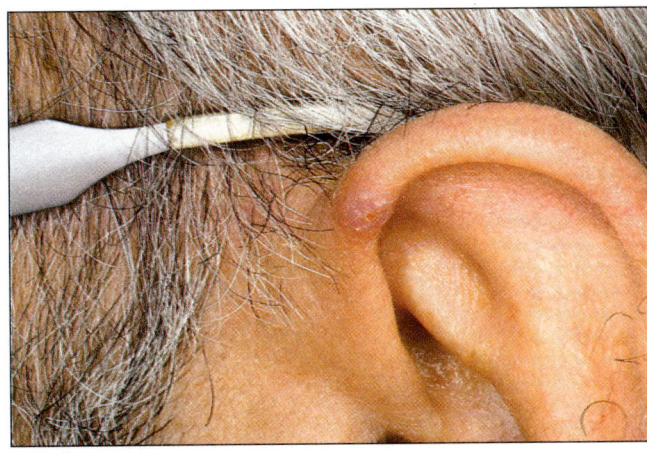

FIGURE 7-11 Chondrodermatitis nodularis helicis.

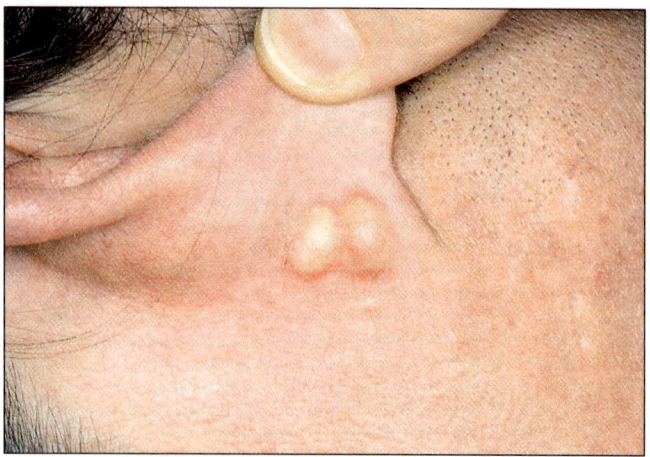

Figure 7-12 Epidermal inclusion cyst.

Table 7-2 Types of Cysts

Epidermoid	Branchial cleft cyst
Eruptive vellus hair cyst	Thyroglossal duct cyst
Dermoid cyst	Thymic cyst
Trichilemmal cyst	Cutaneous ciliated cyst
Steatocystoma	Digital mucous cyst
Median raphe cyst	Omphalomesenteric duct
Bronchogenic cyst	cyst

Data from Golitz and Poomeechaiwong [14].

surrounded by granulation tissue. The perichondrium is often thickened, and focal degeneration of the cartilage itself may occur.

Treatment options include injection of intralesional corticosteroids [11•], excision along with the underlying cartilage [11•], electrodesiccation and curettage [12], and carbon dioxide laser surgery [13].

EPIDERMAL INCLUSION CYSTS

Epidermal inclusion cysts are lesions that are typically 0.5 to 2 cm in size and are most commonly seen on the face, neck, and trunk (Fig. 7-12). These lesions are freely movable over underlying structures, but they are often connected to the overlying skin by a central punctum. The content of the cyst is usually a pasty, cheesy material that is formed of macerated keratin and cheesy, fatty material.

There are many different types of cysts (Table 7-2), but the ones most commonly confused with epidermal inclusion cysts are trichilemmal cysts, or pilar cysts (Table 7-3). It may be impossible to differentiate clinically between the appearance of epidermal inclusion cysts and that of trichilemmal cysts, however, clinical differentiation is often not important because the treatment regimens are identical.

Treatment of inflamed cysts is by intralesional injection of corticosteroids. Once the inflammation has subsided, the lesions can be excised. Drainage of a cyst may provide relief or cure; however, because the wall of the cyst remains, the lesion may recur.

LIPOMAS

Lipomas are soft subcutaneous nodules approximately 1 to 2 cm in diameter that commonly occur on the posterior trunk, abdomen, forearm, buttocks, and thighs. They usually arise as solitary lesions but may also be multiple. Frequently, lipomas are first noted between the fourth and fifth decades of life and are most common in women. The skin overlying these benign tumors is freely movable, and no textural or pigmentary changes are evident. Lipomas are usually asymptomatic, as opposed to a painful variant, the angiolipoma (Table 7-4). Painful tumors of the skin can be characterized using the acronym *LEND AN EGG* (Table 7-5).

Several syndromes are associated with multiple lipomas occurring in adult life. Madelung's disease refers to the occurrence of multiple large, painless, coalescent lipomas around the neck, shoulders, and upper arms, most commonly occurring in older men [16]. Dercum's disease, or adiposis dolorosa, occurs primarily in obese menopausal women and presents as symmetric, tender, circumscribed fatty deposits that are often associated with weakness and psychiatric disturbances [17].

Lipomas may be left untreated unless they are cosmetically bothersome or painful. The most effective treatment

Table 7-3 Epidermal Inclusion Cysts Versus Trichilemmal Cysts

	Inclusion cyst	Trichilemmal cyst
Clinical appearance	Identical	Identical
Location	Face, scalp, neck, trunk	90% on scalp
Histopathology	Cystic structure with wall of true epidermis containing a granular layer, filled with horny material arranged in laminated layers	Cystic structure derived from the middle portion of the hair follicle, with a wall of epidermis without a granular layer or visible intercellular bridging. Palisade arrangement of cells peripherally
Inheritance	Unknown	May be autosomal dominant

TABLE 7-4 LIPOMAS VERSUS ANGIOLIPOMAS

	Lipomas	Angiolipomas
Symptoms	Asymptomatic	Painful
Groups affected	Frequently first noted between the 4th and 5th decades; most common in women	Typically arise in young adults
Histologic findings	Surrounded by a connective tissue capsule; contains normal fat cells similar to those found in the subcutaneous tissue	Similar to those for lipoma, except for an increase in vascular tissue often containing fibrin within the capillaries
Appearance	Identical	Identical

TABLE 7-5 PAINFUL TUMORS

Leiomyoma	Angiolipoma
Eccrine spiradenoma	Neurilemmoma
Neuroma	Endometrioma
Dermatofibroma	Glomus tumor
	Granular cell tumor

Data from Naversen *et al.* [15•].

for lipomas is excision, although liposuction has also been reported to be effective [18].

FIBROUS PAPULES OF THE NOSE

The fibrous papule is a dome-shaped, often singly occurring skin-colored papule, 1 to 3 mm in diameter, that is most often located on the nose. Lesions can also occur on the forehead, cheeks, chin, and neck. These benign growths are of little but cosmetic consequence. However, they may be mistaken for dermal nevi or basal cell carcinoma. Table 7-6 compares fibrous papules with the angiofibromas of tuberous sclerosis.

No treatment is necessary for the isolated fibrous papule of the nose. However, if excision is indicated, tangential excision is usually the treatment of choice. It will remove the lesion with good results and will also provide tissue for histologic examination. Laser surgery with the carbon dioxide or argon laser has been shown as effective in treating angiofibromas of tuberous sclerosis.

MILIA

Milia are firm white papules 1 to 2 mm in diameter that often give the appearance of containing a grain of sand or a pearl immediately beneath the epidermis (Fig. 7-13). These lesions can occur either spontaneously, secondary to an associated disease state (*eg,* bullous pemphigoid, dystrophic epidermolysis bullosa, or porphyria cutanea tarda), or after trauma.

TABLE 7-6 FIBROUS PAPULES VERSUS ANGIOFIBROMAS

	Fibrous papule	Angiofibroma
Age group affected	Middle aged adults	Children
Inheritance	Acquired	Autosomal dominant
Clinical appearance	Usually singly occurring; most often located on the nose, but may also occur on the forehead, cheeks, chin, and neck	Multiple; often occur on the nasolabial folds, cheeks, and chin; associated cutaneous findings include periungual fibromas, shagreen patch, and ash leaf macules*
Histologic findings	Papular lesions with a localized area of fibrosis and vascular proliferation in the upper portion of the dermis	*Same as* fibrous papule
Internal associations	None	Mental retardation, seizures, retinal phakomas, renal angiomyolipomas, cardiac rhabdomyomas
Treatment of fibrous papule or angiofibroma	Tangential excision, argon or CO_2 laser	*Same as* fibrous papule

Data from Fitzpatrick *et al.* [19].

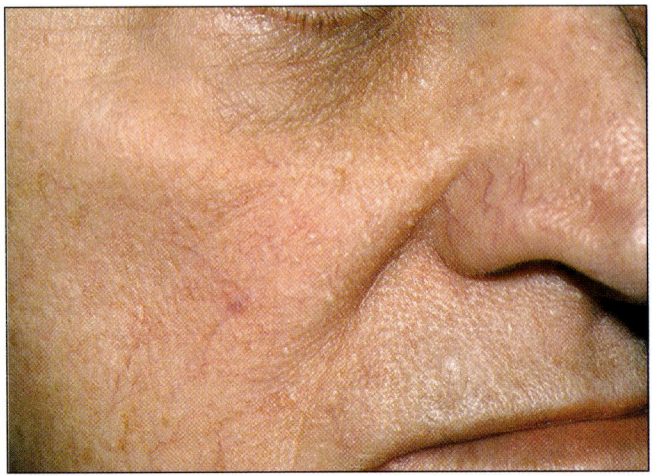

FIGURE 7-13 Milia.

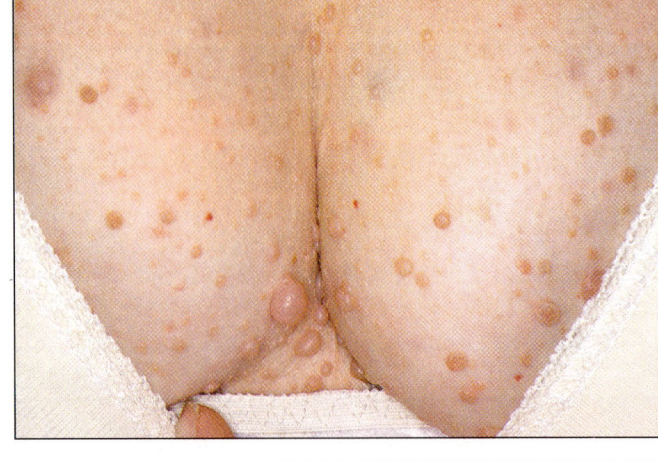

FIGURE 7-14 Neurofibroma.

Histologically, they represent miniature epidermal inclusion cysts and are derived from the lowest portion of the infundibulum of vellus hairs. Treatment is by incision with a no. 11 blade scalpel and expression of the cyst contents.

NEUROFIBROMAS

Neurofibromas may appear as soft, skin-colored pedunculated or sessile polyps (Fig. 7-14). They are often confused with acrochordons or as skin-colored lesions mistaken for nevi. Frequently, these tumors exhibit "buttonholing," which occurs when the soft tumor is invaginated into the skin by pressure with a finger. They can be solitary or multiple, and if they are multiple, the syndrome of neurofibromatosis must be considered.

Neurofibromas are benign nerve sheath tumors composed of thin wavy collagen fibers in association with spindle cells with slightly wavy nuclei and slender elongated cytoplasmic processes that extend in various directions. These lesions are usually well circumscribed but not encapsulated. Treatment is by either tangential excision or surgical excision. Superficial ablation procedures, such as defocused carbon dioxide laser surgery, may also be useful for flattening lesions.

SYRINGOMAS

Syringomas are multiple skin-colored to yellow papules usually occurring on the lower eyelids and cheeks (Fig. 7-15), although they may occur in any location. Their typical diameter is 2 to 3 mm, and they usually occur in women in the second or third decade of life. One association of syringomas has been made in patients with Down's syndrome: there is a 39% occurrence rate in these patients [20].

Histologically, these lesions represent adenomas of the intraepidermal eccrine ducts. They are embedded in a fibrous stroma and consist of small ducts whose walls are lined by two rows of epithelial cells. The ducts often possess small, comma-like tails, which give them the characteristic tadpole appearance. Treatment is usually by gentle electrolysis, laser ablation, or cautious cryotherapy.

CHERRY ANGIOMAS

Cherry angiomas are one of the most common benign skin tumors. Their onset is in early adult life, and they increase in number with age. Lesions can occur anywhere, but the trunk is the most common site (Fig. 7-16). They most often appear as nonblanching, bright red, smooth dome-shaped lesions one to several millimeters in diameter.

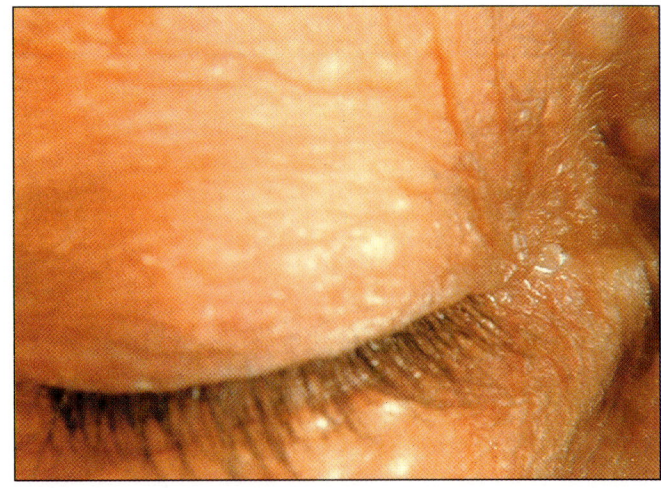

FIGURE 7-15 Periorbital syringoma.

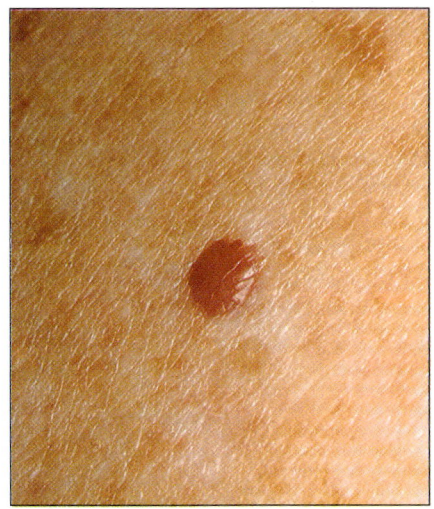

FIGURE 7-16 Cherry hemangioma.

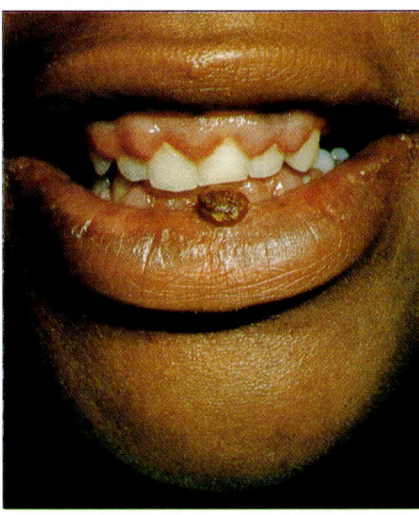

FIGURE 7-17 Pyogenic granuloma.

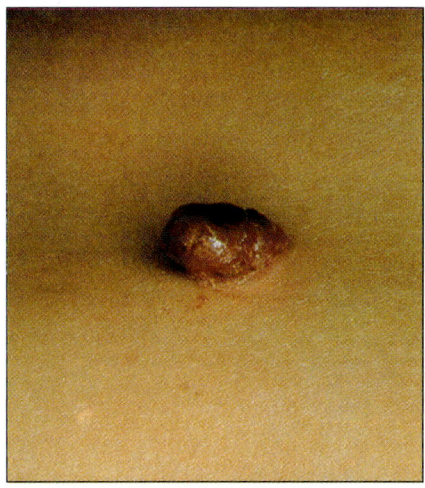

FIGURE 7-18 Pyogenic granuloma of pregnancy.

Histologically, they are composed of numerous moderately dilated capillaries lined by flattened endothelial cells. The epidermis is thinned and often surrounds most of the angioma in a collarette.

These lesions respond well to electrosurgery or laser surgery [21].

PYOGENIC GRANULOMAS

Pyogenic granulomas are small, solitary erythematous growths, either sessile or pedunculated, that are most commonly seen on an exposed surface such as the hands, forearms, face, or mouth (Figs. 7-17 and 7-18). Typically, these lesions begin as small erythematous papules that rapidly enlarge and become pedunculated. They are quite common in children, although all age groups are affected. There is often a history of trauma to the area preceding the appearance of the pyogenic granuloma. This lesion tends to be friable and bleeds easily, and it commonly recurs after treatment.

Histologically, pyogenic granulomas are composed of circumscribed lesions covered by a flattened epidermis that forms an epidermal collarette around the lesions, in association with a lobular capillary proliferation and an edematous stroma.

Treatment is usually most effective if the lesion is first curetted, and the base is then destroyed by electrofulguration. Laser ablation and excision also are effective.

WHEN TO REFER

Although each case is individually different, there are certain rules which one can apply to decide if referral is appropriate. In general, pigmented lesions should be referred unless one is 100% sure of the diagnosis. Differentiation from melanoma is difficult even for the best of dermatologists. If the lesion is behaving in an atypical manner, for example by continuing to enlarge, becoming multiple, bleeding, or becoming painful, this is a signal to refer. Also, referral is appropriate if the lesion is not responding to conventional treatment.

REFERENCES AND RECOMMENDED READING

Recently published papers of particular interest have been highlighted as:
• Of interest
•• Of outstanding interest

1. Sperry K, Wall J: Adenocarcinoma of the stomach with eruptive seborrheic keratosis: the sign of Leser-Trélat. *Cancer* 1980, 45:2434–2437.

2. Roses DF, Valensi Q, LaTrenta G, *et al.*: Surgical treatment of dermatofibrosarcoma protuberans. *Surg Gynecol Obstet* 1986, 162:449–452.

3. Robinson JK: Dermatofibrosarcoma protuberans resected by Mohs surgery. *J Am Acad Dermatol* 1985, 12:1093–1098.

4. Ceilley RI, Babin RWQ: The combined use of cryosurgery and intralesional injections of suspensions of fluorinated adrenocorticosteroids for reducing keloids and hypertrophic scars. *J Dermatol Surg Oncol* 1979, 5:54–56.

5.• Datubo-Brown DD: Keloids: a review of the literature. *Br J Plast Surg* 1990, 43:70–77.

6. Hirshowitz B, Ullmann Y, Har-Shai Y, *et al.*: Silicone occlusive sheeting (SOS) in the management of hypertrophic and keloid scarring, including the possible mode of action of silicone, by static electricity. *Eur J Plast Surg* 1993, 16:5–9.

7.• Darzi MA, Chowdri NA, Kaul SK, *et al.*: Evaluation of various methods of treating keloids and hypertrophic scars: a 10-year follow-up study. *Br J Plast Surg* 1992, 45:374–379.

8. Sherman R, Rosenfeld H: Experience with the Nd:YAG laser in the treatment of keloid scars. *Ann Plast Surg* 1988, 21:231–235.

9. Haas AA, Arndt KA: Selected therapeutic applications of topical tretinoin. *J Am Acad Dermatol* 1986, 15:870–877.

10.• Granstein RD, Rook A, Flotte TJ, *et al.*: A controlled trial of intralesional recombinant interferon-gamma in the treatment of keloidal scarring. *Arch Dermatol* 1990, 126:1295–1302.

11.• Coldiron BM: The surgical management of chondrodermatitis nodularis chronica helicis. *J Dermatol Surg Oncol* 1991, 17:902–904.

12. Kromann N, Hoyer H, Reymann F: Chondrodermatitis nodularis chronica helicis treated with curettage and electrocauterization. *Acta Derm Venereol (Stockh)* 1983, 63:85–87.

13. Taylor MB: Chondrodermatitis nodularis chronica helicis: successful treatment with the carbon dioxide laser. *J Dermatol Surg Oncol* 1991, 17:862–864.

14. Golitz L, Poomeechaiwong S: Cysts. In *Pathology of the Skin.* Edited by Farmer ER, Hood AF. Norwalk: Appleton & Lange; 1990:513–529.

15.• Naversen DN, Trask DM, Watson FH, *et al.*: Painful tumors of the skin: "LEND AN EGG." *J Am Acad Dermatol* 1993, 28:298–300.

16. Ruzicko T, Vieluf D, Landthaler M, *et al.*: Benign symmetric lipomatosis Launois-Bensaude. *J Am Acad Dermatol* 1987, 17:663–674.

17. Palmer ED: Dercum's disease: adiposis dolorosa. *Am Fam Physician* 1981, 24:155–157.

18. Coleman WP: Noncosmetic applications of liposuction. *J Dermatol Surg Oncol* 1988, 14:1085–1090.

19. Fitzpatrick TB, Szabo G, Hori Y, *et al.*: White leaf-shaped macules. *Arch Dermatol* 1968, 98:1–6.

20. Carter DM, Jegasothy BV: Alopecia areata and Down's syndrome. *Arch Dermatol* 1976, 112:1397–1399.

21. Arndt KA: Argon laser therapy of small vascular lesions. *Arch Dermatol* 1982, 118:220–224.

Psoriasis 8

Karen Simpson
Nicholas J. Lowe

Key Points
- Increased epidermal proliferation, aberrant keratinocyte differentiation, and inflammatory abnormalities characterize psoriasis.
- Clinical diagnosis can be made by careful examination of skin lesions in most patients. Skin biopsies are occasionally needed.
- Management should commence with topical therapy and patient education for those patients with localized disease. More severely affected patients should be referred to a dermatologist.
- Psoriasis is a chronic relapsing disease, and treatment toxicity should always be considered and monitored.

Psoriasis is a chronic skin disease usually characterized by discrete erythematous papules and plaques covered by a silvery white scale. Some patients develop sterile pustules, while others develop total body or erythrodermic psoriasis. Patients with psoriasis are concerned with cosmetic disfigurement and the resultant social isolation that the disease may cause. Associated itching and pain resulting from fissuring of the lesions may also be present.

Approximately 2% of the US population is affected. Psoriasis is an inherited disorder, and current investigations are attempting to localize the gene responsible for the disease. The onset is frequently in early adult life, but the disease may be seen first in childhood or old age. When psoriasis occurs earlier in life, there is often an associated family history of psoriasis. In contrast, psoriasis that appears for the first time later in life (*eg*, in the fifth decade) often lacks a family history [1]. Arthritis is seen in approximately 10% of patients with psoriasis, and it may occasionally occur before skin manifestations.

The primary physician should be able to treat mild and localized psoriasis. An understanding of the pathophysiology of the disease, and knowledge of the different treatment modalities available will facilitate collaboration with a dermatologist for those patients with moderate and severe psoriasis.

DIAGNOSIS

There are several forms of psoriasis: plaque, guttate, erythrodermic, and pustular. In addition, distinct manifestations of psoriasis may depend on body location (*eg*, the scalp, nails, palms, or soles).

Plaque Psoriasis

The most classic form is plaque psoriasis. Clinically, patients with plaque psoriasis present with well-marginated, erythematous, elevated papules that coalesce into plaques. If it has not previously been treated by the patient, thick, silvery scaling will be seen (Fig. 8-1). The differential diagnosis of plaque psoriasis includes

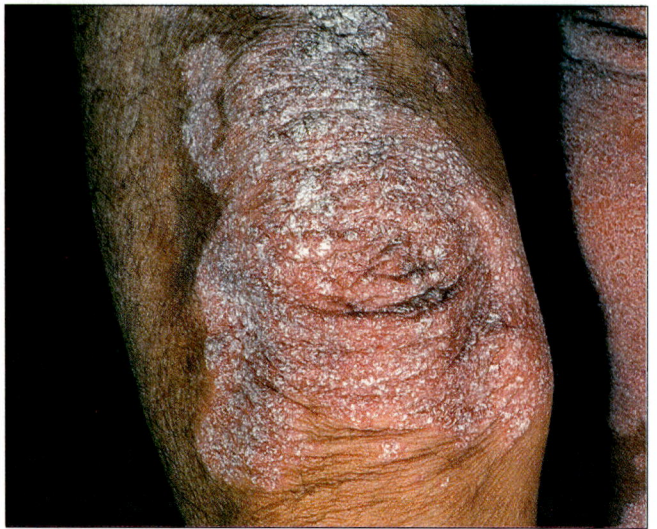

FIGURE 8-1 Plaque psoriasis.

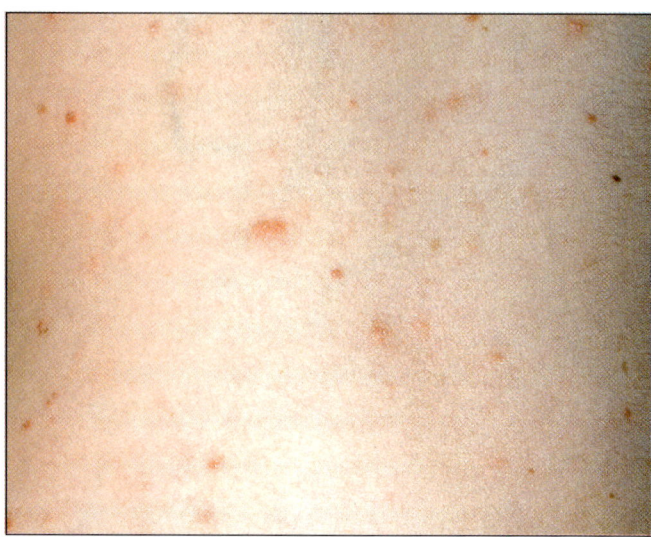

FIGURE 8-2 Guttate psoriasis.

nummular eczema and cutaneous T-cell lymphoma (Table 8-1). Removal of this scale reveals punctate bleeding points known as Auspitz's sign. Mucous membranes are rarely involved.

Histologically, the epidermis is thickened, and immature nucleated cells are seen in the horny layer. An accompanying dilation of the subepidermal blood vessels and infiltration with mononuclear cells accounts for erythema. Neutrophils are often seen within the stratum corneum, forming characteristic micropustules.

Guttate Psoriasis

Another clinical type is guttate psoriasis (Fig. 8-2), which presents with small, discrete, erythematous papular lesions that may appear suddenly after an upper respiratory tract infection. This form is often associated with *Streptococcus pyogenes* infection, but it is not serotype specific [2]. The differential diagnosis of guttate psoriasis includes pityriasis rosea, parapsoriasis guttata, and secondary syphilis. Table 8-2 lists some distinguishing characteristics.

Erythrodermic Psoriasis

An exfoliative or erythrodermic form of psoriasis shows generalized erythema without any characteristic lesions

(Fig. 8-3). This form must be differentiated from Sézary syndrome and pityriasis rubra pilaris (Table 8-3).

Pustular Psoriasis

An uncommon but serious variation is generalized pustular psoriasis (Fig. 8-4), which is often accompanied by systemic symptoms. The patient has sudden onset of fever and arthralgias, followed by the eruption of 2- to 3-mm sterile pustules on erythematous skin. The original pustules may resolve in a few days; however, the patient continues to experience new waves of fever followed by the formation of new pustules. Patients with this type of psoriasis usually require hospitalization and intensive treatment. At times, generalized pustular psoriasis is life threatening.

Localized pustular psoriasis of the palms and soles (Fig. 8-5) may also be seen without characteristic lesions of psoriasis elsewhere.

Scalp Psoriasis

Scalp psoriasis may accompany any form of psoriasis, or it may be the only visible sign of psoriasis. It may at times be difficult to distinguish from seborrheic dermatitis. Some distinguishing features of these conditions appear in Table 8-4.

	TABLE 8-1 DIFFERENTIAL DIAGNOSIS OF PLAQUE PSORIASIS		
	Plaque psoriasis	**Nummular eczema**	**Cutaneous T-cell lymphoma**
Lesion	Sharply marginated erythematous plaques; silvery scale	Erythematous, vesicular; scale present often	May be identical to plaque psoriasis; varying thickness; little or no scale
Location	Symmetric	May be asymmetric	Asymmetric
Diagnosis	Skin biopsy	Skin biopsy	Skin biopsy
Pruritus	Usually not pruritic	Yes	Yes

TABLE 8-2 DIFFERENTIAL DIAGNOSIS OF GUTTATE PSORIASIS

	Guttate psoriasis	Pityriasis rosea	Parapsoriasis guttata	Secondary syphilis
Lesion	Fine maculopapules; silvery scale	Small, thin oval plaques; fine scale at periphery of plaque	Fine maculopapules; silvery scale	Papules or small plaques; usually fine but may be marked
Location	Entire body	Trunk in "Christmas tree" pattern; initial single plaque (herald patch)	Mainly on trunk	Trunk, palms, soles, mouth
Pruritus	Yes	Usually mild	Uncommon	Usually none
Course	Abrupt onset; occasional spontaneous recovery in 6 wk	Spontaneous resolution, generally in 6–8 wk; may be longer	Chronic	Resolves with therapy
Diagnosis	Skin biopsy	Skin biopsy	Skin biopsy	Serologic tests for syphilis, skin biopsy

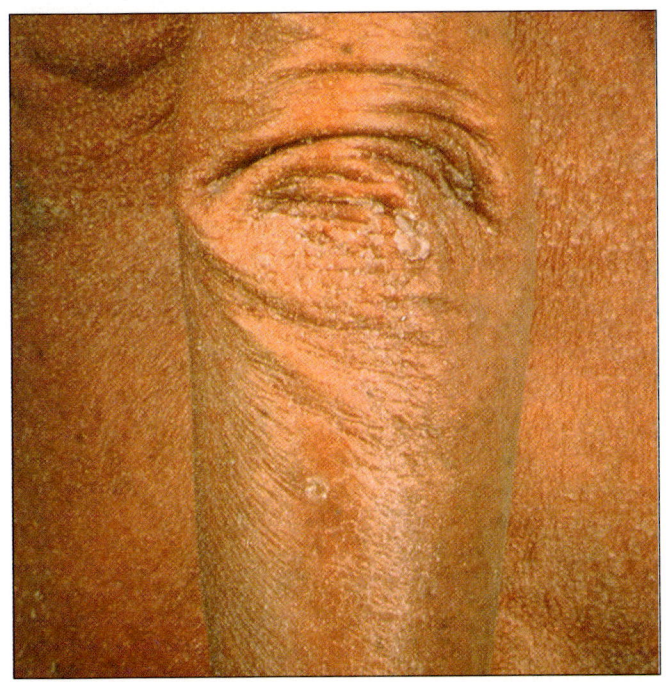

FIGURE 8-3 Erythrodermic psoriasis.

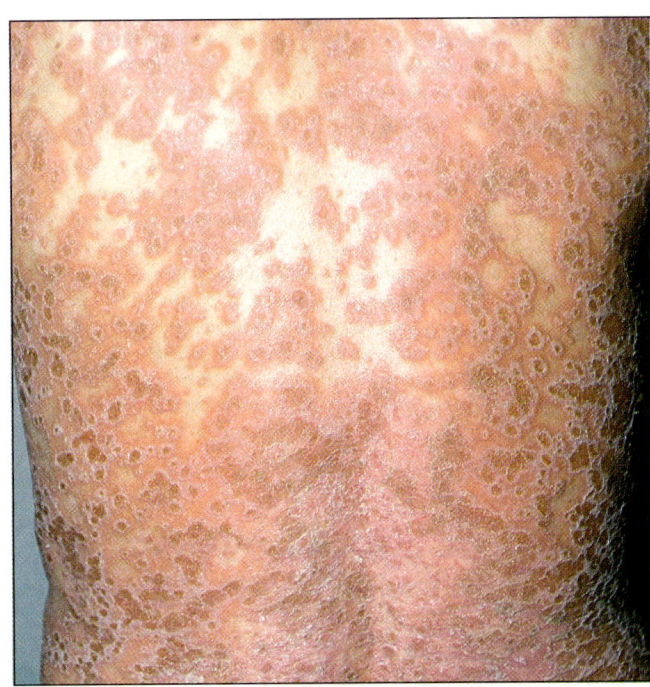

FIGURE 8-4 Generalized pustular psoriasis.

TABLE 8-3 DIFFERENTIAL DIAGNOSIS OF ERYTHRODERMIC PSORIASIS

	Erythrodermic psoriasis	Pityriasis rubra pilaris	Sézary syndrome
Lesion	Whole body erythema and scaling	Discrete papules; areas of generalized erythema; islands of normal skin; perifollicular lesions	Same as erythematous psoriasis
Location	Whole body	Whole body; thick, smooth yellow palms and soles	Whole body
Pruritus	Severe	Severe	Extreme
Diagnosis	Skin biopsy	Skin biopsy	Minimum 5% Sézary cells (abnormal lymphocytes)

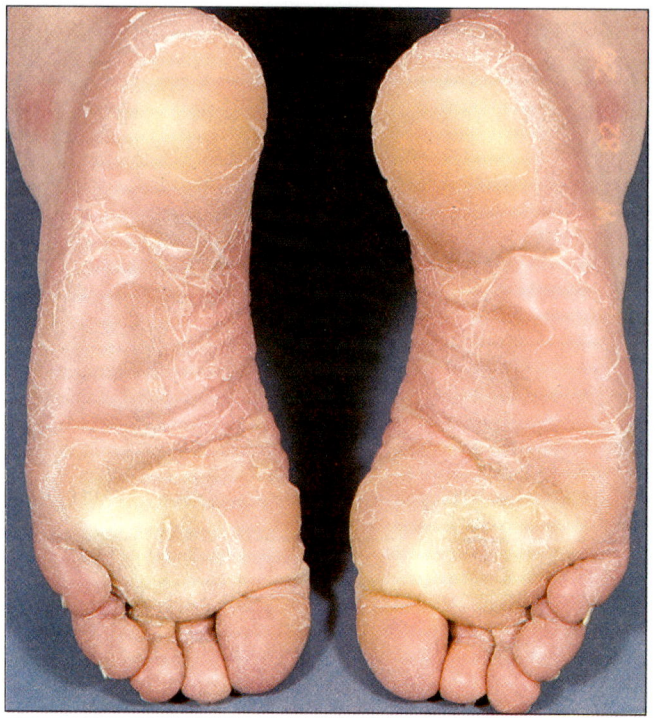

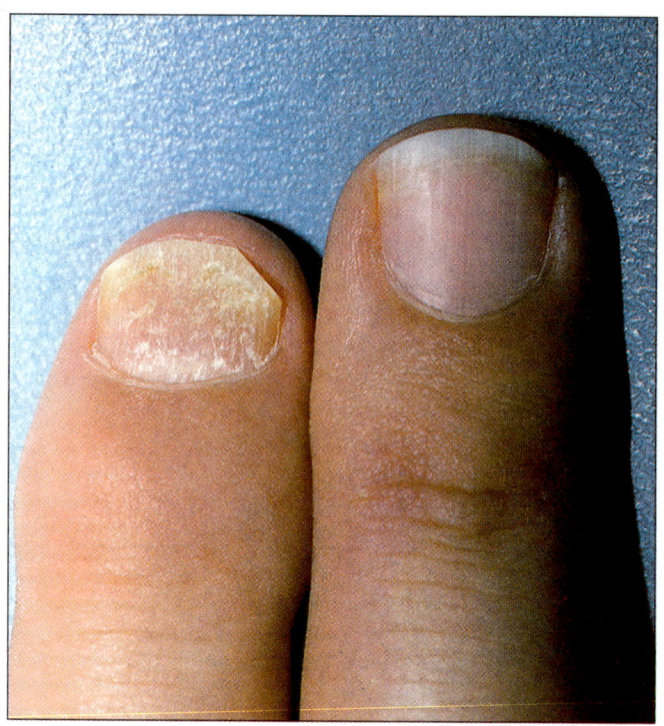

FIGURE 8-5 Pustular psoriasis of the soles.

FIGURE 8-6 Pitting and discoloration seen in psoriatic nails.

Nails often show punctate pitting and a characteristic discoloration of the nail surface that resembles an oil spot (Fig. 8-6). Subungual collections of keratotic material are also common and can be confused with tinea unguium. Fungal infections can be distinguished clinically by their usual lack of nail pitting. A scraping of the keratotic material placed in 10% potassium hydroxide may reveal fungal hyphae.

TOPICAL THERAPY

Topical Steroids

Topical corticosteroids are widely used, especially for ambulatory patients, because they are relatively easy to apply. The ability of topical steroids to produce vasoconstriction, with resultant pallor of the skin, has been used to rank them for anti-inflammatory potency. In most patients with psoriasis, the more potent steroids are usually required to produce a good response. Topical steroids are sometimes effective in clearing psoriasis and may be used in certain situations (*eg*, for exposed and unsightly areas of psoriasis and flexural psoriasis); however, caution is needed in their use. Table 8-5 lists some commonly used steroid preparations.

With the exception of the face, skin fold areas, and genitals, treatment begins with a superpotent corticosteroid preparation (group 1), followed by the use of a less potent preparation to maintain the improvement achieved. Some of the superpotent steroids may not be used for longer than 2 weeks or at dosages of greater than 50 g/wk.

Fluorinated steroids should be avoided on the face, genitals, and skin fold areas because they are more likely

	TABLE 8-4 DIFFERENTIAL DIAGNOSIS OF SCALP PSORIASIS	
	Scalp psoriasis	**Seborrheic dermatitis**
Lesion	Discrete patches; may be raised	Diffuse with fine scale; erythematous areas not raised
Location	Scalp; rarely on face; common on elbows, knees, and extremities	Scalp; common on face, chest, and upper back; rarely on elbows, knees, and extremities
Course	Waxing and waning; increased severity with stress; may respond to sunlight; winter flare-up common	Same

to cause skin atrophy. Group 6 steroids can be used on a short-term basis in these areas (no longer than 2 or 3 weeks). Group 7 steroids may be used for extended periods on the face and skin fold areas with little risk of atrophy. Most patients prefer creams; however, ointments are used when there is thick psoriatic scale. Solutions are used for scalp lesions. An example of patient instructions for the use of topical steroids is given in Table 8-6.

Maintenance therapy with pulse "weekend" steroids has proven to be clinically beneficial and well tolerated [3•]. Once plaques are clear or nearly clear, relapse rates may be kept to a minimum with the use of three consecutive applications 12 hours apart, once a week.

Side effects
Side effects seen with potent topical steroids include skin atrophy, rebound worsening of psoriasis after discontinuation

---

TABLE 8-5 POTENCY RANKING OF SOME COMMONLY USED BRAND-NAME CORTICOSTEROIDS*

Group 1

Ultravate cream 0.05% (*a*: Westwood-Squibb; Buffalo, NY)

Ultravate ointment 0.05% (*a*: Westwood-Squibb)

Temovate cream 0.05% (*b*: Glaxo Dermatology; Research Triangle Park, NC)

Temovate ointment 0.05% (*b*: Glaxo Dermatology)

Diprolene cream 0.05% (*c*: Schering-Plough; Kenilworth, NJ)

Diprolene ointment 0.05% (*c*: Schering-Plough)

Psorcon ointment 0.05% (*d*: Dermik Laboratories; Blue Bell, PA)

Group 2

Cyclocort ointment 0.1% (*e*: Lederle; Wayne, NJ)

Diprolene AF cream 0.05% (*c*: Schering-Plough)

Diprosone ointment 0.05% (*f*: Schering-Plough)

Elocon ointment 0.1% (*g*: Schering-Plough)

Florone ointment 0.05% (*h*: Dermik)

Halog cream 0.1% (*i*: Westwood-Squibb)

Lidex cream 0.05% (*j*: Syntex; Palo Alto, CA)

Lidex gel 0.05% (*j*: Syntex)

Lidex ointment 0.05% (*j*: Syntex)

Maxiflor ointment 0.05% (*h*: Herbert Laboratories; Irvine, CA)

Topicort cream 0.25% (*k*: Hoechst-Roussel; Sommerville, NJ)

Topicort gel 0.05% (*k*: Hoechst-Roussel)

Topicort ointment 0.25% (*k*: Hoechst-Roussel)

Group 3

Aristocort A ointment 0.1% (*l*: Fujisawa Pharmaceutical; Deerfield, IL)

Cyclocort cream 0.1% (*e*: Lederle)

Cyclocort lotion 0.1% (*e*: Lederle)

Diprosone cream 0.05% (*f*: Schering-Plough)

Florone cream 0.05% (*h*: Dermik)

Lidex E cream 0.05% (*j*: Syntex)

Halog ointment 0.1% (*i*: Westwood-Squibb)

Maxifor cream 0.05% (*h*: Herbert Laboratories)

Valisone ointment 0.1% (*m*: Cheesebrough Ponds; Research Triangle Park, NC)

Group 4

Cordran ointment 0.05% (*n*: Schering-Plough)

Elocon cream 0.1% (*g*: Schering-Plough)

Kenalog cream 0.1% (*l*: Westwood-Squibb)

Synalar ointment 0.025% (*o*: Syntex)

Westcort ointment 0.2% (*p*: Westwood-Squibb)

Group 5

Cordran cream 0.05% (*n*: Oclaussen Pharmaceutical; San Rafael, CA)

Diprosone lotion 0.05% (*f*: Schering-Plough)

Kenalog lotion 0.1% (*l*: Westwood-Squibb)

Locoid cream 0.1% (*q*: Ferndale; Ferndale, MI)

Synalar cream .025% (*m*: Syntex)

Valisone cream 0.1% (*n*: Ferndale)

Westcort cream 0.2% (*p*: Westwood-Squibb)

Group 6

Alcovate cream 0.05% (*r*: Glaxo Dermatology)

Alcovate ointment 0.05% (*r*: Glaxo Dermatology)

Aristocort cream 0.1% (*l*: Fujisawa)

Desowen cream 0.05% (*s*: Owen/Galderma; Fort Worth, TX)

Synalar solution 0.01% (*o*: Syntex)

Synalar cream 0.01% (*o*: Syntex)

Tridesilon cream 0.05% (*s*: Miles Pharmaceutical; Elkhart, IN)

Valisone lotion 0.05% (*m*: Ferndale)

Group 7

Topicals with hydrocortisone, dexamethasone, flumethalone, prednisolone, and methylprednisolone

*Group 1 is the superpotent category; potency descends with each group, to group 7, which is least potent (2 and 3, potent steroids; 4 and 5, midstrength steroids; 6 and 7, mild steroids). There is no significant difference between agents in groups 2 through 7; the compounds simply are arranged alphabetically. However, within group 1, Temovate cream or ointment is more potent than Diprolene cream or ointment and Psorcon ointment.

a—halobetasol; b—clobetasol propionate; c—betamethasone dipropionate (optimized vehicle); d—diflorasone diacetate (optimized vehicle); e—amcinonide; f—betamethasone dipropionate; g—mometasone furoate; h—diflorasone diacetate; i—halcinonide; j—fluocinonide; k—desoximetasone; l—triamcinolone acetonide; m—betamethasone valerate; n—flurandrenolide; o—fluocinolone acetonide; p—hydrocortisone valerate; q—hydrocortisone butyrate; r—alclometasone dipropionate; s—desonide.

TABLE 8-6 INSTRUCTIONS FOR PATIENTS UNDERGOING TOPICAL CORTICOSTEROID (STEROID) THERAPY FOR PSORIASIS

These are often very effective preparations, but they have to be used with care

Apply only small amounts twice daily to psoriatic skin, unless advised otherwise by your physician; rub them well into your psoriasis

Unless specified by your doctor, do not continue treatment after the psoriasis has cleared; this can lead to skin thinning

Do not apply any steroid to the face or skin folds unless you are specifically advised to do so by your physician

If any new skin irritation, skin bruising, ulcers, or skin infections occur, stop using the corticosteroid until you have checked with your physician

of steroid use, a tendency to convert "stable" psoriasis to "unstable" (erythrodermic or pustular) types, significant skin absorption, systemic steroid effects in patients with extensive psoriasis, and the possibility of rosacea-like syndrome after long-term use of potent steroids on the face.

After an initially good response, steroid resistance often occurs. The clinician should discontinue the steroid temporarily and switch to a different topical agent, such as anthralin or calcipotriene, if there are no contraindications. If a different topical agent is not effective or is contraindicated, the clinician should refer the patient to a dermatologist.

Sunlight

Many patients with milder psoriasis experience an improvement in their psoriasis with exposure to sunlight; however, they must take care not to get sunburned because this may cause a Koebner reaction with worsening of their psoriasis in the sunburned areas.

Coal Tar Preparations

Goeckerman described the combination of ultraviolet (UV) light and coal tar in 1925 [4]. Numerous modifications of this treatment have been proposed. Crude coal tar application may be no more effective than petrolatum when combined with aggressive erythemogenic UVB (290 to 320 nm) therapy for psoriasis. However, suberythemogenic UVB plus 1% crude coal tar or a coal tar extract in oil has proved to be more effective than suberythemogenic UVB plus petrolatum [5•]. Thus, coal tars themselves are probably therapeutic and enhance the effect of suberythemogenic UVB.

Although tar used alone has some beneficial effect in treating psoriasis, it is generally used as adjunctive therapy. Some commercial purified tar preparations available for body and scalp psoriasis are:

Aquatar gel (Herbert Laboratories; Irvine, CA)
Baker's P & S Plus gel (Baker Cummins; Miami, FL)

Estar tar gel (ICN Pharmaceuticals; Costa Mesa, CA)
Fototar tar cream (Westwood-Squibb; Buffalo, NY)
Psorigel (Owen/Galderma; Fort Worth, TX)
T-Derm tar oil (Neutrogena; Los Angeles, CA)
T-Derm tar and salicylic acid scalp lotion (Neutrogena)

Liquor carbonis detergens is available as an alternative to crude coal tar, usually in 5% to 20% concentrations in cream, ointment, or oil. Balnetar and Doak oil are available as additives for bathwater. One possible treatment for localized psoriasis is a combination of tar and topical steroids. The patient may apply a purified tar at night and allow it to dry for a minimum of 10 to 15 minutes before going to bed. This will minimize staining. Once or twice during the day, a steroid cream or ointment is then applied to the localized lesions.

Folliculitis is a possible side effect of the use of tar products. If folliculitis occurs, a less occlusive base or a lower concentration of crude coal tar can be used. The purified tar preparations listed in Table 8-7, provided with instructions for patients' use, present less risk of folliculitis.

Anthralin

Anthralin is trihydroxyanthracene, an aromatic compound with three benzene rings that has been used topically for psoriasis since the 19th century. It is available commercially in creams and ointments. The use of 0.1% anthralin for at least 8 hours daily improves psoriasis. The relapse rate is increased by the addition of topical corticosteroids to the regimen. Interestingly, the application of much higher concentrations (1% and above) of anthralin, which are washed off after 10 to 60 minutes, improves psoriasis and makes outpatient psoriasis treatment with anthralin practical. This is known as as short-contact anthralin therapy.

TABLE 8-7 INSTRUCTIONS FOR PATIENTS USING COAL TAR PRODUCTS FOR PSORIASIS

Many of these products can be messy and stain your clothing and furnishings

Apply small amounts and rub them well into the skin; use old or stained garments as clothing after applying the coal tars

Many purified tar gels, lotions, creams, and oils will cease staining your clothes after they have been on the skin for several minutes

Avoid any sun exposure of coal tar–treated skin unless advised by your physician; your physician may advise sun or ultraviolet treatments after you apply the coal tar, but these have to be done with your physician's advice to avoid skin burning

If skin infections, infections around hairs, increased redness of the skin, or stinging or smarting of the skin occurs, stop using the coal tar until you have checked with your physician

The patient gradually increases the time the anthralin is left on the skin, as long as no irritation occurred with the previous contact time. The patient starts using anthralin for 10 minutes and reaches a maximum contact time of 60 minutes. Caution is needed to avoid skin irritation. Anthralin may also stain adjacent skin reddish-brown, and clothing may be stained purple.

Anthralin is often very effective, but patients resent the staining of skin and clothing. Careful instruction and good physician–patient rapport are helpful when anthralin is prescribed (Table 8-8). Anthralin is best used by physicians familiar with its use.

Vitamin D Analogues

Calcipotriol (1,24-dihydroxyvitamin D_3), which will be known as calcipotriene in the United States, is a promising new topical treatment that has been recently approved by the Food and Drug Administration. Several studies with calcipotriol ointment have shown approximately 70% improvement after a 3-month course of therapy [6–8]. It is used extensively in several countries, including Denmark, New Zealand, the United Kingdom, and Canada.

Calcipotriol ointment has been shown to be significantly superior to betamethasone valerate and anthralin in recent clinical trials [9•]. Long-term use is not likely to cause skin atrophy.

This agent may cause skin irritation when applied to the face and skin fold areas, so these areas must be avoided. Patients should apply it sparingly to psoriatic lesions while avoiding surrounding normal skin. Side effects include local perilesional skin erythema and irritation, as well as facial dermatitis in approximately 5% of patients, even when the agent is not applied to the face [8]. This may have been caused by accidental transference of the drug from the hands to the face.

Scalp Treatment

Scalp psoriasis is often frustrating to treat, both from the clinician's and the patient's points of view. Different regimens may be used according to the severity of the psoriasis, and whether the hair is color treated, blond, or gray.

Mild, diffuse scalp psoriasis

Mild, diffuse scalp psoriasis may be easily confused with seborrheic dermatitis, especially if no other signs of psoriasis are present. Mild scalp psoriasis often responds well to regular shampooing with tar or salicylic acid preparations, which may be alternated with an antifungal shampoo if needed (ketoconazole). The use of tar must be avoided with color-treated, blond, or gray hair because it will cause discoloration of the hair. At night, phenol and saline solutions, for example, P & S liquid (Baker-Cummins) or Keralyt gel (Westwood-Squibb) or a steroid in an oil base such as Dermasmoothe (Hill Dermaceuticals, Orlando, FL), applied to the scalp, will help loosen scale. This effect is intensified with occlusion (eg, wearing a shower cap to bed). Application of midpotency steroid lotions or sprays during the day can be useful [10]. A high-powered shower nozzle may also be helpful in removing some of the scale when patients shampoo their hair.

Ketoconazole theoretically acts by depleting the surface yeast contaminants, which are thought to activate the complement cascade in psoriatic skin, leading to leukocyte chemotaxis [11].

Localized plaque scalp psoriasis

Local application of tar, anthralin, or salicylic acid compounds is often useful. Again, tar should not be used with light-colored hair or color-treated hair. Anthralin can also cause discoloration in these cases, although red hair tends to tolerate the anthralin without much discoloration.

TABLE 8-8 SOME AVAILABLE ANTHRALIN PREPARATIONS WITH USUAL CONCENTRATIONS

Form of preparation	Product	Concentrations, %
Paste	Formulated by pharmacist in Lassar's paste (best used under dermatologist's supervision)	0.1–5.0
Ointment	Anthra-Derm*; (Dermik Laboratories, Blue Bell, PA)	0.1, 0.25, 0.5, 1.0
Cream	Drithocream*†; (Dermik Laboratories)	0.1, 0.25, 0.5
	Drithocream*†; (Dermik Laboratories)	0.1, 0.25, 0.5, 1.0
	Drithoscalp; (Dermik Laboratories)	0.5
	Anthranol†; (Stiefel Laboratories, Coral Gables, FL)	0.1, 0.2, 0.4
	Psoradrate†; (Eaton, UK)	0.1, 0.2
Stick	Anthra-Derm†; (Brocades, UK)	0.5, 1.0
Future options: Solutions, Gels, Tapes, Possibility of effective anthralin analogues		

*Available in the United States and Canada; †available in the United Kingdom.

Ultrapotent corticosteroid lotions or aerosols may be used during the day. Occasional use of intralesional steroids may be useful; however, several precautions should be followed. Injections should not be given more frequently than every 4 to 6 weeks because skin atrophy, folliculitis, and systemic effects from the corticosteroid can result with repetitive use. At each treatment session, no more than 2 mL of triamcinolone at a concentration of 3 to 5 mg/mL should be used. Treatment regimens for mild psoriasis may be followed in between injections [10•].

Extensive, severe scalp psoriasis

Treatment of extensive, severe scalp psoriasis can be a particularly arduous task and often requires day care or hospitalization under a dermatologist's supervision. The first step should be a home treatment regimen. A tar or salicylic acid gel or lotion, or a combination may be applied by the patient at night.

Examples of available preparations are provided below:

•*Steroid preparations*
Aristocort lotion (Fujisawa Pharmaceutical; Deerfield, IL)
Cordran lotion (Oclaussen Pharmaceutical; San Rafael, CA)
Cyclocort lotion (Lederle; Wagner, NJ)
Dermasmoothe lotion (Hill Dermaceuticals)
Diprolene lotion (Schering-Plough, Kenilworth, NJ)
Diprosone lotion (Schering-Plough)
Diprolene gel aerosol (Schering-Plough)
Lidex gel (Syntex; Palo Alto, CA)
Temovate lotion (Glaxo Dermatology; Research Triangle Park, NC)
Valisone lotion (Cheesebrough Ponds; Research Triangle Park, NC)
•*Purified tar preparations*
Bakers P & S Plus gel (Baker-Cummins)
Estar tar gel (ICN Pharmaceuticals)
Fototar tar cream (Westwood-Squibb)
Psorigel (Owen/Galderma)
T-Derm tar and salicylic acid scalp lotion (Neutrogena)
•*Salicylic acid preparations*
Keralyt gel (Westwood-Squibb)
•*Other*
P & S liquid (Baker Cummins)

These formulations should be rubbed well into the scalp and then covered with a plastic or a paper shower cap. In the morning, the patient should wet the scalp and rub in a shampoo containing tar, salicylic acid, or ketoconazole, wrapping the scalp in a damp warm towel afterward. The towel should be left on for 15 to 30 minutes. The patient should shower off this initial shampoo and continue shampooing until the cream or gel preparations have been removed. The scalp may then be treated with a single application of a high-potency corticosteroid lotion such as Temovate lotion (Glaxo Dermatology), Lidex solution (Syntex), or Diprolene lotion (Schering-Plough) [10•].

If response to this therapy is slow, referral to a dermatologist is indicated. Short-contact anthralin may be added to the regimen for home treatment. If this fails, day care or hospital scalp treatment may be needed. For truly incapacitating scalp psoriasis that does not respond to topical treatment regimens, systemic treatment may be indicated. This should be done under a dermatologist's supervision.

SYSTEMIC TREATMENT

Systemic treatment is indicated only for severe or incapacitating psoriasis. This includes generalized pustular psoriasis, exfoliative psoriasis, severe psoriatic arthropathy, and extensive psoriasis (> 20% body surface area). Systemic treatments include psoralen photochemotherapy and the administration of methotrexate, retinoids, cyclosporine, or systemic corticosteroids. These systemic treatments are best used by dermatologists familiar with their effects.

PREVENTION

Although nothing can be done to decrease the chance of getting psoriasis, several things can be done to decrease the chance of exacerbating the disease. Stress (physical and emotional) in the patient's life should be minimized. Although this may be easier said than done, psychological support from the treating physician, the psychiatrist or psychologist, and support groups are important measures [12•]. Cautious sun exposure and careful topical therapy can prevent relapse in many patients for prolonged periods. An excellent resource for patients with psoriasis is the National Psoriasis Foundation, which provides information on the latest treatment modalities and educational materials (PO Box 9009, Portland, Oregon 97207).

REFERENCES AND RECOMMENDED READING

Recently published papers of particular interest have been highlighted as:
• Of interest
•• Of outstanding interest

1. Schmitt-Egenolf M, Boehncke W-H, Christophers E, *et al.*: Type I and type II psoriasis show a similar usage of T-cell receptor variable regions. *J Invest Dermatol* 1991, 97:1053–1056.

2. Funk J, Langeland T, Schrumpf E, *et al.*: Psoriasis induced by interferon alpha. *Br J Dermatol* 1991, 125:463–465.

3.• Katz H, Prawer S, Medansky R, *et al.*: Intermittent corticosteroid maintenance treatment of psoriasis: a double-blind multicenter trial of augmented betamethasone diproprionate ointment in a pulse dose treatment regimen. *Dermatologica* 1991, 183:269–274.

4. Goeckerman WH: The treatment of psoriasis. *Northwest Med* 1925, 24:2–9.

5.• Lowe N: Tars, keratolytics, and emollients. In *Practical Psoriasis Treatment*, edn 2. Edited by Lowe N. St. Louis: Mosby; 1993:45–57.

6. Kato T, Rokugo M, Terui T, *et al.*: Successful treatment of psoriasis with topical application of active vitamin D_3 analogue, 1,24-dihydroxycholecalciferol. *Br J Dermatol* 1986, 115:431–433. 1993:45–57.

7. Kragballe K: Treatment of psoriasis by the topical application of the novel cholecalciferol analogue calcipotriol. *Arch Dermatol* 1989, 125:1647–1652.

8. Morimoto S, Yoshikawa K, Kozuka T, *et al.*: An open study of vitamin D_3 treatment in psoriasis vulgaris. *Br J Dermatol* 1986, 115:421–429.

9.• Murdoch D, Clissold S: Calcipotriol: a review of its pharmacological properties and therapeutic use in psoriasis vulgaris. *Drugs* 1992, 43:415–429.

10.• Lowe N: Therapy of scalp psoriasis. In *Practical Psoriasis Treatment*, edn 2. Edited by Lowe N. St. Louis: Mosby; 1993: 207–217.

11. Rosenberg E, Belew P: Role of microbial factors in psoriasis. In *Proceedings: The Third International Symposium*. Edited by Katz SI. New York: Grune & Stratton; 1982:343–344.

12. •Koo J: Emotional and psychological aspects of psoriasis. In *Practical Psoriasis Treatment*, edn 2. Edited by Lowe N. St. Louis: Mosby; 1993:23–31.

SELECT BIBLIOGRAPHY

Baker H: Psoriasis. In *Textbook of Dermatology*, edn 4. Edited by Rook A, Wilkinson DS, Ebling FJG, *et al.* Oxford: Blackwell Scientific Publications; 1986:1469–1532.

Christopher E, Krueger GS: Psoriasis. In *Dermatology in General Medicine*, edn 3. Edited by Fitzpatrick TB, Eisen AZ, Wolff K, *et al.* New York: McGraw-Hill; 1987:461–491.

Lowe NJ, ed.: *Practical Psoriasis Therapy*, edn 2. St. Louis: Mosby; 1993.

Morison WL: Management of psoriasis vulgaris. In *Phototherapy and Photochemotherapy of Skin Disease*, edn 2. Edited by Morison WL. New York: Raven Press; 1991:53–93.

Roenigk HH, Maibach HI, eds: *Psoriasis*, edn 2. New York: Marcel Dekker; 1991.

9

The Eczemas

Terrence Hopkins
Richard A.F. Clark

Key Points

- Eczema is dermal inflammation. It is associated with epidermal edema that can sometimes appear as vesiculation.
- Acute, subacute, and chronic eczema do not refer to chronicity but rather to clinical and histologic manifestations of eczema.
- The eczemas are categorized by clinical appearance or location, etiologic cause, or associated conditions.
- Although management varies according to the type of eczema, certain basic principles apply, such as the need for topical steroids in acute eczema or hydration, moisturizers, and nonsteroidal topical medication in subacute and chronic eczema.

The terms *dermatosis*, *dermatitis*, and *eczema* are often loosely applied to inflammatory skin disorders; therefore, they should be clearly defined to limit confusion and enable classification of the eczemas. The term *dermatosis* refers to the entire spectrum of skin disorders, varying from inflammatory to neoplastic. Dermatitis relates to all inflammatory disorders of the skin, such as sunburn, contact dermatitis, and psoriasis. Finally, *eczema*, or *eczematous dermatitis* embraces only those dermatitis conditions that are associated with intraepidermal edema (spongiosis), which is often manifested clinically as vesiculation.

Eczema is defined by its clinical and histologic characteristics; however, the clinical manifestations of eczema can vary during the disease evolution. Often, the clinical characteristics of eczema are subdivided into three stages: acute, subacute, and chronic (Figs. 9-1 through 9-4). These stages frequently overlap within a given patient; nevertheless, general topical therapy can be tailored to the most prominent stage of eczema present (Fig. 9-1).

Six general histopathologic findings often occur in eczematous dermatitis: in the epidermis, spongiosis (intraepidermal edema), acanthosis (thickening of the epidermis), and parakeratosis (retention of nuclei within the cells of the stratum corneum); in the dermis, blood vessel dilatation, infiltration of lymphocytes and monocytes, and edema. The exact histopathologic pattern depends on the stage of clinical evolution.

A particular type of eczema can be classified by etiology, clinical pattern, or associated phenomena that distinguish it from the group.

CONTACT DERMATITIS

Contact reactions can be separated into three major categories: allergic contact dermatitis, irritant contact dermatitis, and contact urticaria. Each category is defined by its time of onset, specific immunologic mechanism or mechanisms, and inciting agents (Table 9-1).

Allergic Contact Dermatitis

Allergic contact dermatitis first requires sensitization to an antigen, which takes approximately 1 week. Eczema is usually not present at this time. On reexposure to the antigen, an eczematous reaction may become clinically apparent in 1 to 2 days. Allergic contact dermatitis can at times be difficult to discern from other eczematous reactions; however, specific patterns of distribution often suggest an exogenous etiology, as shown in Table 9-1. Linear, arcuate, or well-demarcated patches of eczema occur in the configuration of the contact with the inciting agent.

Diagnosis of this condition is often elicited either by history, anatomic location, or morphologic configuration. For example, a patient who worked in the garden 1 week ago presents with linear patches of eczema. Clearly, plant allergic contact dermatitis, such as from contact with poison ivy or poison oak, is likely. Often, cases are not so straightforward, and patch testing is required. Standardized chemical preparations are placed on the back under occlusion for 48 hours, and reactions at 72 hours are noted.

Allergic contact dermatitis may present as acute, subacute, or chronic eczema and must be treated accordingly

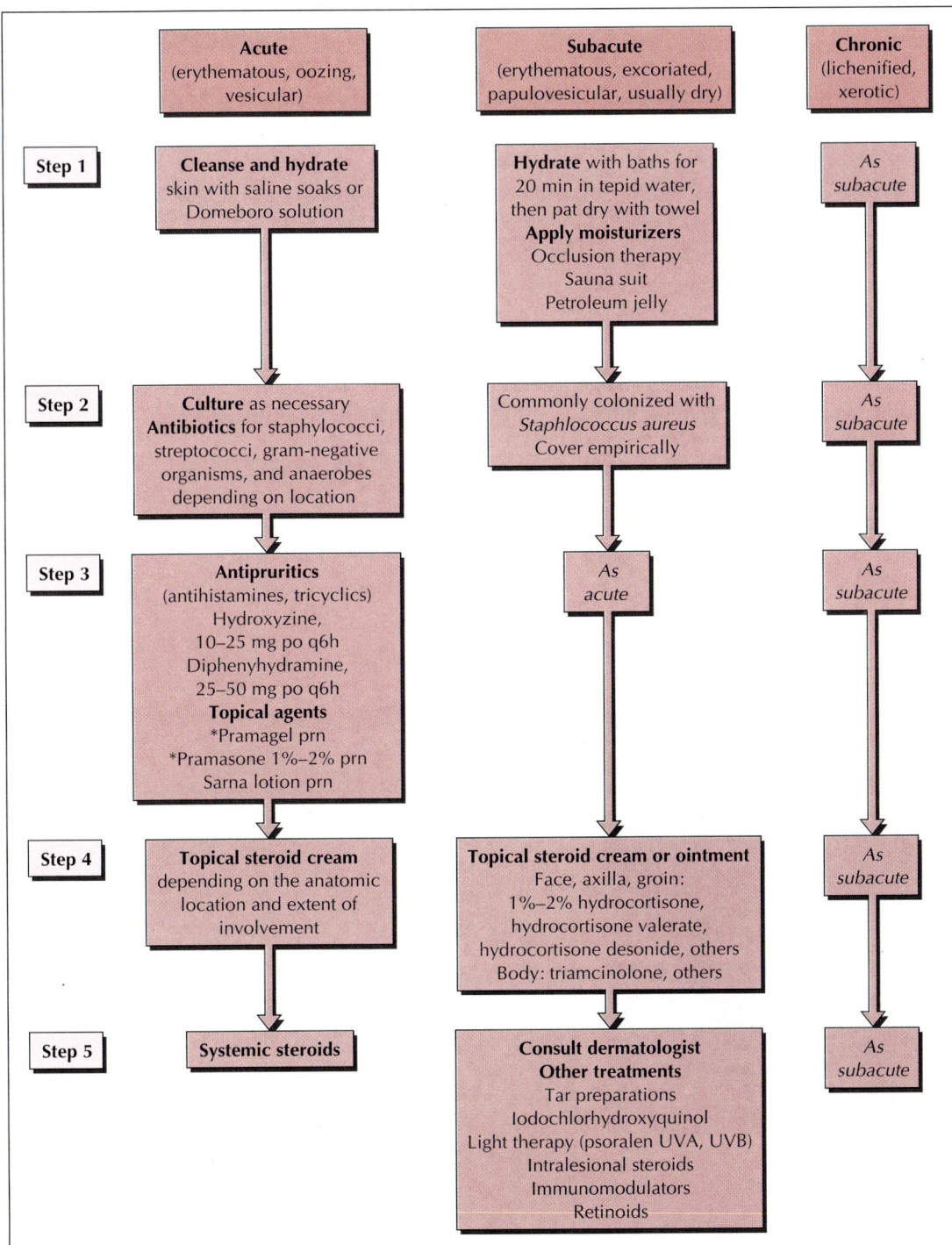

FIGURE 9-1 General principles of eczema treatment according to reaction stage. po—orally; prn—as needed; q6h—every 6 hours. *Ferndale Laboratories, Ferndale, MI.

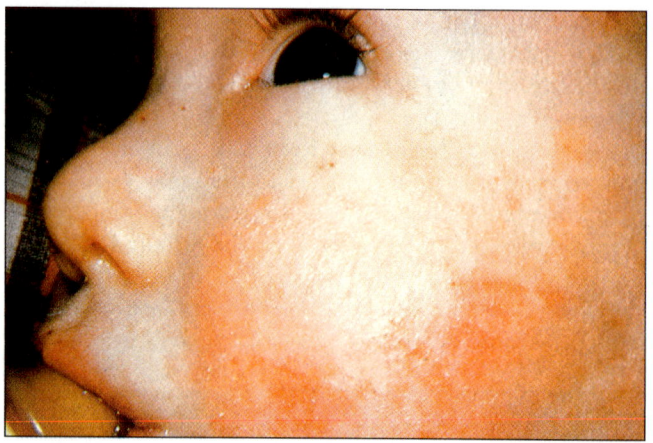

FIGURE 9-2 Acute eczema is manifest by erythema, epidermal edema, or vesiculation with oozing, crusting, or both.

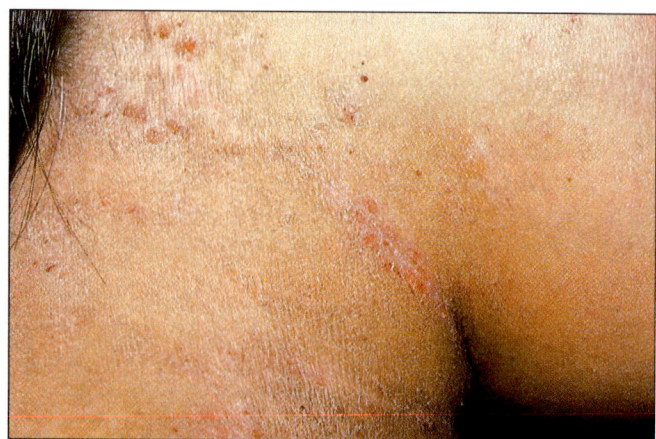

FIGURE 9-3 Subacute eczema is manifest by erythema, lichenification, scaling, and excoriations.

(Fig. 9-1). Recently, Grevelink and coworkers [1•] showed that the use of barrier preparations can be effective in the prevention or attenuation of poison ivy or poison oak dermatitis.

Irritant Contact Dermatitis

Irritant contact dermatitis is another extremely common eczema. Key to its recognition is the sharply demarcated morphologic configuration in the area of the applied irritant. Patient age; dry, cold, or windy environment; frictional trauma; and underlying skin disorders such as atopic dermatitis may predispose patients to irritant contact dermatitis. The epidermal permeability barrier is disrupted from reductions in stratum corneum lipids. The reaction can vary from mild to severe and can present as acute, subacute, or chronic eczema.

The diagnosis of this condition can usually be made by compiling information on morphologic characteristics, history, and anatomic location. The treatment options are shown in Figure 9-1. The patient's ability to avoid inciting agents greatly influences prognosis [2•].

Contact Urticaria

Contact urticaria is not eczema or even a dermatitis, but is an important contact dermatosis to recognize. A wheal-and-flare reaction occurs within minutes after exposure to certain agents and usually resolves within 24 hours. This reaction may be associated with anaphylaxis. Latex gloves have recently attracted much attention as an inciting agent of contact urticaria [3•]. Treatment principally relies on identification and avoidance of the inciting agent. Symptomatic relief can be obtained with antihistamine H_1 and H_2 blockers. Such patients should be observed for the development of hoarseness; shortness of breath; and tongue, lip, or throat swelling. If these signs are apparent, appropriate supportive and emergency measures must be employed.

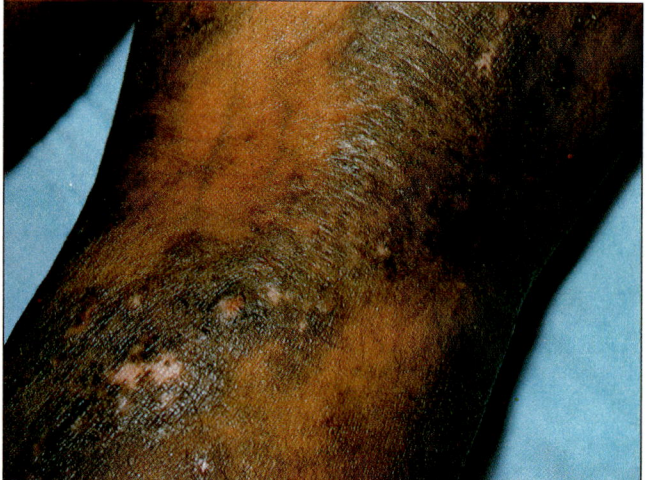

FIGURE 9-4 Chronic eczema is manifest by erythema, increased skin markings (lichenification); and hypopigmentation, hyperpigmentation, or both.

TABLE 9-1 DISTRIBUTION OF CONTACT DERMATITIS AND COMMON INCITING AGENTS

Distribution of eczema	Inciting agent
Allergic	
Hairline	Hair dye, hat band
Eyelids	Nail polish, cosmetics
Earlobes, neck, wrists	Nickel, cobalt
Sides of neck	Perfume
Hands	Gloves, chemicals
Feet	Shoe leather or dye
Exposed extremities	Plants (poison ivy)
Sites of topical application	Preservatives
Irritant	
Hands	Soaps, detergents, oils, greases, other chemicals

ATOPIC DERMATITIS

Atopic dermatitis is a chronic relapsing, pruritic dermatitis that usually occurs in individuals with a personal or family history of atopy (food allergy or allergic asthma, rhinitis, or conjunctivitis). The onset is usually in childhood, but the disease may persist in adults. In older patients in whom a diagnosis of atopic dermatitis is being entertained for the first time, a childhood history should be ascertained [4•]. If the patient does not have a childhood history of this condition, he or she may have another eczema or an eczematous reaction to a medication or an underlying malignancy.

Much evidence suggests that IgE-mediated immediate and late-phase reactions play a role in the development of atopic dermatitis. In addition, recent evidence has suggested that an immunologic dysregulation may cause overactivation of a variant delayed-type hypersensitivity reaction distinct from classic delayed-type hypersensitivity. House dust mite antigen, molds, pollens, animal dander, and other proteinaceous aeroallergens, as well as certain foods, may precipitate flares of eczema in these patients [5]. Important questions include those about the home environment, including the presence of pets, and those about disease variation with the season or with travel.

The distribution of eczema varies with age, but a characteristic distribution is usually seen by the age of 3 or 4 years (Fig. 9-5). Atopic dermatitis is usually associated with other manifestations of atopy and can be complicated by cutaneous infection as well as a variety of other problems (Table 9-2). Herpes simplex infection may begin as a cold sore and then become generalized and complicated by ocular involvement. Therefore, when pustules form on these patients, both a Gram stain and Tzanck preparation should be performed. In adult patients who give a history of no previous atopy, an itemization of medications and exposures and a thorough

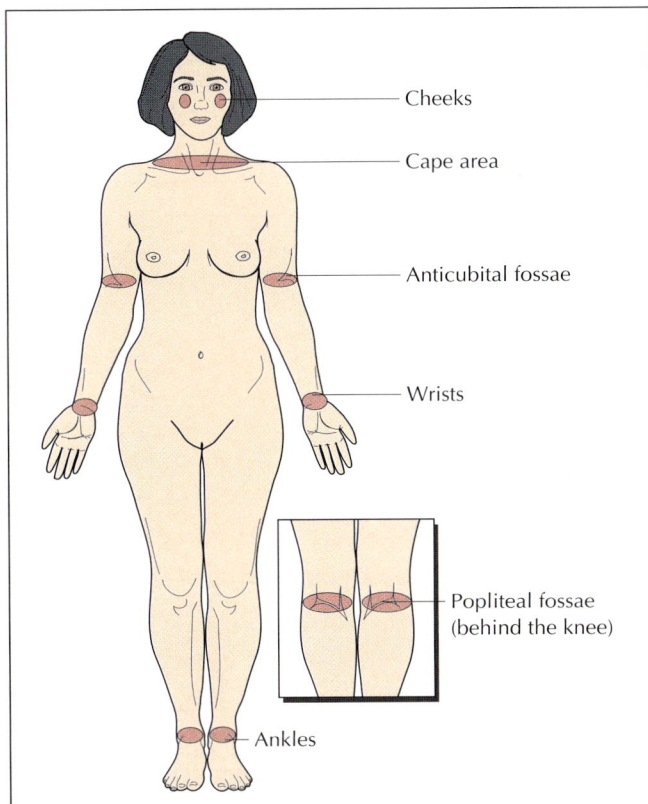

FIGURE 9-5 Characteristic distribution of eczema in older children and adults with atopic dermatitis.

Cheeks

Cape area

Anticubital fossae

Wrists

Popliteal fossae (behind the knee)

Ankles

TABLE 9-2 ATOPIC DERMATITIS

Variants
Infants
  Involves the face, scalp, extensor surfaces
Older children
  Tends to localize to flexural areas, especially antecubital
    and popliteal fossae
Adults
  Usually involves the flexural areas, but may be localized to
    the hands and feet only
Erythroderma (any age)
  Generalized flare
Neurodermatitis or prurigo nodularis (older children and
  adults)
  Excoriations or excoriated nodules on the extremities

Potential allergens
Dust mite antigen, animal dander, cockroach, molds
Pollens
Foods (especially in children younger than 5 y)

Associated conditions
Atopic diathesis (*ie*, allergic asthma, rhinitis, or dermatitis):
  familial inheritance
Xerosis, ichthyosis vulgaris, keratosis pilaris
Eye findings
  Periorbital dermatitis, allergic or vernal conjunctivitis
  Posterior cataracts, keratoconus, glaucoma
Postinflammatory hypo- or hyperpigmentation
White dermatographism

Complications
Cutaneous infections
  Viral: herpes simplex, vaccinia, molluscum contagiosum,
    papillomavirus infection
  Bacterial: *Staphylococcus aureus* infection
  Fungal: dermatophyte infection
Exoliferative erythroderma
Growth retardation and weight loss
Mental and emotional dysfunction

Laboratory findings
Blood eosinophilia
Increased serum IgE level
Positive reaction to immediate hypersensitivity testing

physical examination, including lymph node palpation and an abdominal examination, are appropriate.

IgE levels are not diagnostic but may help guide the diagnosis. Prick skin testing and patch testing may be indicated in patients with recalcitrant disease. The treatment is outlined in Figure 9-1; however, the use of systemic steroids should be avoided. Some success has been seen with psoralen-UVA photochemotherapy and immunomodulatory agents.

HAND AND FOOT DERMATITIS

Table 9-3 categorizes hand and foot eczema. Irritant hand and foot dermatitis usually appears on the palms and soles, respectively (Fig. 9-6), and often occurs in adults with a history of atopic dermatitis. Allergic contact dermatitis usually appears on the dorsal surfaces of the hands and feet (Fig. 9-6). Allergic contact dermatitis, however, can be superimposed on irritant contact dermatitis [6,7•]. Patch testing can be useful for documenting allergic contact. Nummular eczema appears as coin-shaped lesions in a mirror image distribution over the trunk and extremities, including the hands and feet, in middle-aged adults. There is no known pathogenesis. Asteatotic eczema is a form of eczema that is derived from dry skin and often has the appearance of "cracked porcelain" (eczema craquelé). Usually seen in elderly patients during the winter, it most commonly affects the hands, feet, and lower extremities. Stress can be associated with the development or the recurrence of hand and foot eczema, especially pompholyx, in which patients develop deep-seated vesicles bilaterally and symmetrically over the sides of the fingers, over the thenar and hypothenar eminences, or along the sides of the feet.

When confronted with a patient who has hand and foot eczema, the physician should ask about wet work (eg, cleaning, bartending, cooking, and nursing) and exposure to potential contact allergens [6,7•]. Bacterial infections are a common complication of hand dermatitis and should be excluded when vesiculopustular formation is present.

Dermatophyte infection should be considered when vesiculation occurs on the feet. Psoriasis can masquerade as recalcitrant hand and foot dermatitis associated with sterile pustules.

The treatment of hand dermatitis follows the outline in Figure 9-1. In addition, the patient should avoid wet work or any inciting chemical or chemicals. For difficult cases, tar soaks, followed by the application of a layer of diiodohydroxyquinone cream and a potent topical steroid ointment, can be tried. This treatment is aided by occlusion with

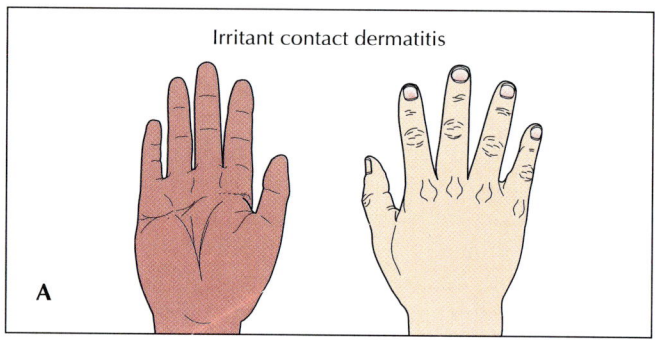

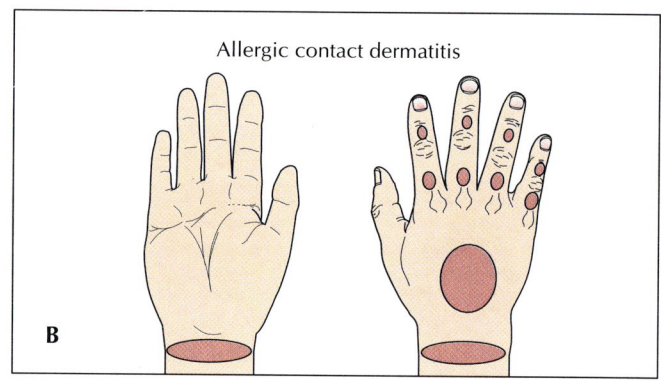

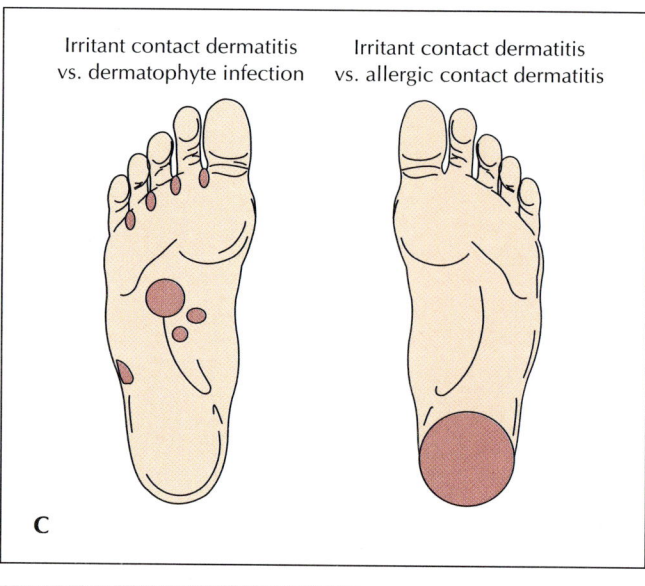

FIGURE 9-6 The location of eczema on the hands and feet may help distinguish irritant contact dermatitis from allergic contact dermatitis or dermatophyte infection.

TABLE 9-3 HAND AND FOOT ECZEMA	
Endogenous factors	**Exogenous factors**
Nummular eczema	Irritant contact
Xerosis (dry skin)	Soaps, detergents
Atopic dermatitis	Chemicals (especially solvents)
	Cold air
	Friction
	Allergic contact
	Chemicals
	Foods
	Plants
	Metals

cotton or vinyl gloves for several hours or overnight. Oral antibiotics are used for bacterial superinfection.

SEBORRHEIC DERMATITIS

Seborrheic dermatitis is a common waxy, scaling, superficial eczematous dermatitis showing a predilection for areas of increased sebaceous gland activity (ie, seborrheic areas) (Fig. 9-7 and Table 9-4). Seborrheic dermatitis affects approximately 3% of the general population. In AIDS or AIDS-related complex, the incidence of seborrheic dermatitis ranges from 20% to 80%. It is more common in men than in women and appears to be associated with an oily complexion (ie, the seborrheic diathesis). Seborrheic dermatitis was historically found in two major age groups: infants in the first 3 months of life and persons 40 to 70 years of age. However, in patients with AIDS, severe seborrheic dermatitis can be seen at any age.

Pityrosporum ovale, a saprophyte found in the seborrheic areas of normal adults, may be an important inciting factor. It grows exuberantly on patients with AIDS [8]. The disease also has a predilection for patients with neurologic disorders, such as mental retardation, parkinsonism, cerebrovascular trauma, facial nerve palsy, syringomyelia, and quadriplegia; patients with alcoholism; patients with endocrinologic disease; and patients receiving neuroleptic

drugs. Treatment of seborrheic dermatitis is outlined in Table 9-5.

NEURODERMATITIS

Neurodermatitis is characterized by skin changes that occur because of itching, scratching, and rubbing. It is associated with many conditions that predispose the patient to a habitual itch-scratch cycle, including insect bites, drug reactions, atopic dermatitis, contact dermatitis, photodermatitis, other chronic eczematous conditions, lichen planus, cutaneous T-cell lymphoma, other malignancies, AIDS, metabolic causes of pruritus, and stress or psychiatric disorders. Patients with this condition classically have pruritus out of proportion to the appearance of the lesion.

Clinically, neurodermatitis is characterized by excoriations, erythematous excoriated papules, plaques with increased skin markings (lichenification), or fibrous nodules. In addition, changes in pigmentation may be present. It is more commonly observed in middle-aged women than in men. The acute form is commonly associated with insect bites. The subacute form often presents as widespread excoriations (Fig. 9-8). The chronic forms, well

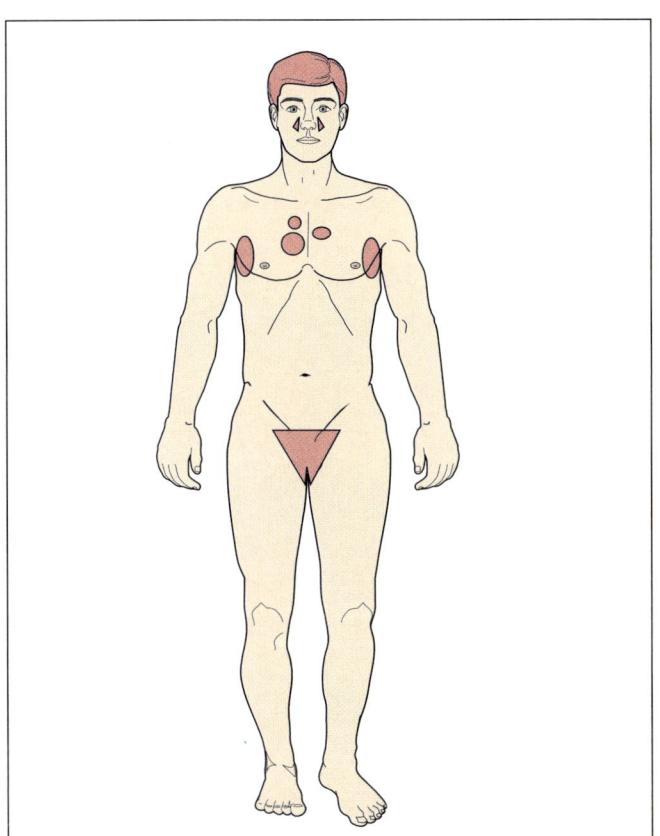

FIGURE 9-7 Seborrheic dermatitis has a predilection for the seborrheic areas of the body.

TABLE 9-4 CLINICAL VARIANTS OF SEBORRHEIC DERMATITIS	
Scalp Pityriasis sicca: dandruff without inflammation Inflammatory: often extends beyond the hairline onto the postauricular area **Facial** Eyebrows Marginal blepharitis Conjunctivitis Nasolabial fold Beard area: often follicular	Forehead, cheeks, chin: diffuse or plaques **Otitis externa** **Flexural** Axillary Inframammary Umbilical Intergluteal Groin **Generalized** Erythroderma

TABLE 9-5 TREATMENT OF SEBORRHEIC DERMATITIS
Scalp   Antidandruff shampoo (tar, selenium sulfide, zinc pyrithione, salicylic acid)   Glucocorticoid lotion   **Glaborous skin**   Topical steroids (1%–2% hydrocortisone) twice daily   Topical ketoconazole cream (2%) twice daily   Tar preparations (LCD 5% or 10% in Aquaphor [Biersdorf, Norwalk, CT]) at bed time

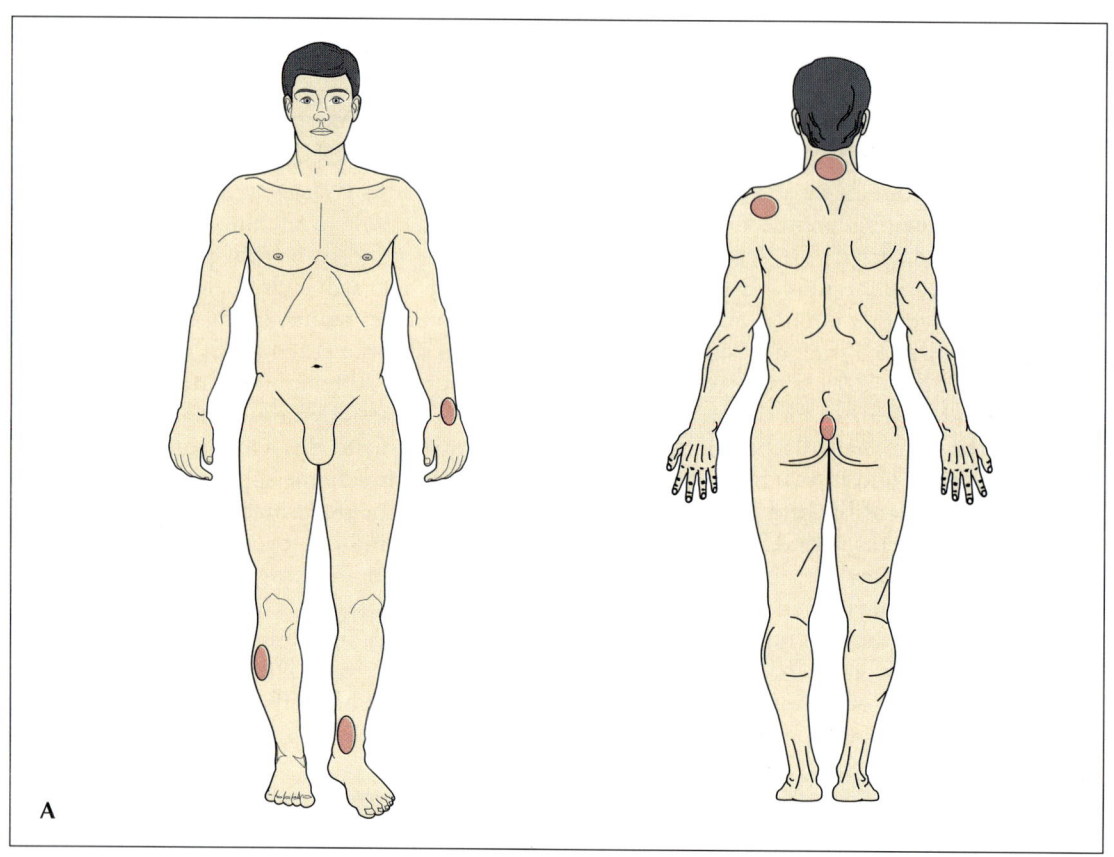

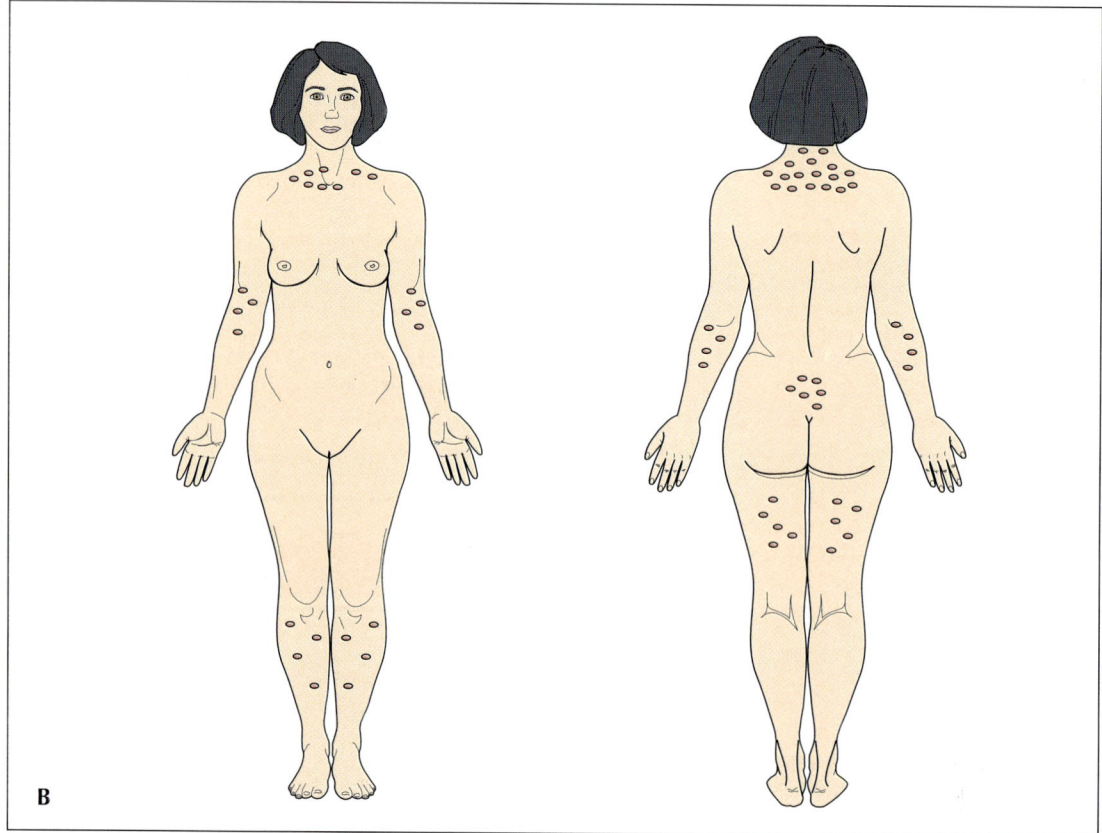

FIGURE 9-8 Neurodermatitis has characteristic locations when it presents as chronic eczema (*panel A*; lichen simplex chronicus) or subacute eczema (*panel B*; neurotic excoriations).

known as lichen simplex chronicus and prurigo nodularis, present as localized plaques or nodules (Fig. 9-8). If no etiology is obvious, a thorough history taking and physical examination for underlying illness are indicated [9].

The treatment of this condition is based initially on preventing patients from continuing to rub or scratch. This outcome can be achieved in a number of ways, among them cutting the patient's nails; administering antipruritics (topical and systemic) or topical and intralesional glucocorticoids; using tar products or barrier systems such as an occlusive dressing over a localized area; and having the patient undergo a psychiatric consultation. Alternative modalities have been tried; however, these methods are best handled by an experienced dermatologist.

ERYTHRODERMA

The terms *erythroderma* and *exfoliative dermatitis* are commonly used synonymously in the literature. Both terms imply the widespread dilation of cutaneous blood vessels associated with inflammation. When increased epidermal cell proliferation causes marked scaling, *exfoliative dermatitis* is the preferred term.

Clinically, patients have generalized erythema with or without scaling. Involvement of the hair and nails may result in alopecia and nail dystrophy. The condition may be acute or chronic. An underlying malignancy should be sought in chronic forms [10].

In adults, preexisting skin disease, (*eg*, psoriasis, atopic dermatosis, stasis dermatitis, contact dermatitis, and seborrheic dermatitis), drug allergy, and underlying malignancy (internal malignancy, leukemia, lymphoma, and cutaneous T-cell lymphoma) can lead to erythroderma. Therefore, close examination of the skin, as well as lymph node palpation and abdominal examination, is important. In a variable but substantial number of patients described, no cause was found [10]. Except when secondary to atopic dermatitis, seborrheic dermatitis, or ichthyosiform erythroderma, erythroderma will usually occur in individuals over 40 years old. Men appear to be affected about twice as often as women.

Metabolic complications of erythroderma are shown in Table 9-6. In acute erythroderma, patients usually need to be followed up closely and are usually hospitalized. These patients can become hypothermic very easily, as manifested by chills. A high-output cardiac failure state may occur. Thus, fluid and electrolyte levels should be monitored closely. Associated liver function abnormalities may indicate underlying drug hypersensitivity or internal malignancy.

The treatment is described in Figure 9-1. Underlying disease should be sought [11•], and any suspected medications should be discontinued. A dermatologic consultation is strongly suggested.

INTERTRIGO AND DIAPER DERMATITIS

Intertrigo is a superficial traumatic dermatitis that occurs in skin folds. Diaper dermatitis is an irritant contact secondary to urine and feces.

Intertrigo occurs in patients of all ages. Most adults who acquire intertrigo tend to be obese, diabetic, or both. Intertrigo also occurs more in hot and humid environments.

Clinically, intertrigo begins as well-marginated, diffuse erythema confined to areas within skin folds. When the rubbing between apposed skin surfaces continues, maceration and frank erosions compound the dermatitis. If the area is left untreated, it will become superinfected with bacteria or yeast. Candida superinfected intertrigo usually involves the inframammary area, the genitocrural area, or the scrotum and can extend to the buttock in the patient receiving long-term broad-spectrum antibiotics. Often, patients become sensitized to topical agents being used to treat the intertrigo.

Diaper dermatitis affects convex surfaces in closest contact with the wet diaper. Inadequate cleansing, frequent loose stools, high environmental temperature, and occlusive rubber or plastic pants are frequent contributing factors. With the use of disposable diapers, diaper dermatitis has markedly decreased in the United States [12]. Infants, however, still develop candida infection and nonspecific intertrigo.

The differential diagnosis of inguinal eruptions is vast (Table 9-7). However, the clinician should concentrate on the most common possibilities. Treatment is tailored to the underlying etiology. Concerted efforts should be made to preserve good hygiene and encourage weight loss. To reduce maceration, powders free of cornstarch can be used. Antibacterial and antifungal creams may also be helpful. A low-potency topical steroid cream may be used along with appropriate antimicrobial therapy until the acute inflammation has resolved. Gentian violet may be effective in patients with mixed superinfections in whom conventional therapy fails.

STASIS DERMATITIS

Stasis dermatitis is eczema secondary to venous hypertension of the lower extremity. This condition has a predilection for middle-aged to elderly women with venous incompetence or an inadequate calf pump. It is also seen in patients who have had deep venous thromboses.

The exact mechanism for the development of eczematous skin changes in patients with venous hypertension remains

TABLE 9-6 METABOLIC COMPLICATIONS OF ERYTHRODERMA	
Skin dysfunction	**Complication**
Loss of permeability barrier	Xerosis, water loss, dehydration
Marked scaling	Protein loss, hypoalbuminemia
Increased vasopermeability	Edema
Marked vasodilation	Chills, hypothermia, high-output cardiac failure

obscure; however, trauma, rubbing, scratching, and topical steroid use can perpetuate and exacerbate the condition.

Clinically, the dermatitis can begin rapidly or insidiously. A rapid onset of stasis dermatitis is usually associated with deep venous thrombosis. The lower leg becomes erythematous, warm, and eczematous. This process can progress proximally from the ankle. The skin can be seen in any of the classically described stages of eczema. Frequent flares of acute dermatitis are often precipitated by the application of topical medications and moisturizers. Recurrent inflammation in the dermis and subcutaneous tissue results in repeated erythrocyte extravasation, with hemosiderin deposition in the dermis and sclerosis of the subcutaneous tissue. Together, these changes give the skin a woody appearance called *liposclerosis* [13••]. As liposclerosis becomes established, edema no longer accumulates around the ankle and lower leg but rather proximal to the sclerosis. The skin of the lower leg is prone to ulceration; however, not all ulcerations are secondary to venous incompetence. Diagnosis and treatment of the ulcers are geared toward the potential etiology. However, basic principles of wound care must be kept in mind. The general treatment of stasis dermatitis consists of leg elevation, the use of support stockings, the administration of diuretics as necessary, the use of end-diastolic pneumatic compression boots, the administration of low- or intermediate-potency corticosteroids in a petrolatum base, the application of petrolatum after a bath or shower, and the use of systemic antibiotics for cellulitis.

TABLE 9-7 DIFFERENTIAL DIAGNOSIS OF INTERTRIGO IN ADULTS

Fungal
Candida (especially in obesity and diabetes)
Dermatophyte
Deep fungal (blastomycosis, actinomycosis, trichomycosis)

Bacterial
Staphylococcal or streptococcal (toxic shock syndrome)
Pseudomonas aeruginosa
Corynebacterium minutissimum (erythrasma)

Venereal diseases
Lymphogranuloma venereum
Granuloma inguinale

Skin diseases
Psoriasis or impetigo herpetiformis
Contact dermatitis
Acrodermatitis enteropathica
Migratory epidermal necrolysis (glucagonoma)
Short bowel syndrome
Darier's disease
Pemphigus foliaceus, subcorneal pustular dermatosis
Benign familial pemphigus (Hailey-Hailey disease)
Pemphigus vegetans

REFERENCES AND RECOMMENDED READING

Recently published papers of particular interest have been highlighted as:
• Of interest
•• Of outstanding interest

1.• Grevelink S, Dedee FM, Olsen EA: Effectiveness of various barrier preparations in preventing and/or ameliorating experimentally produced toxicodendron dermatitis. *J Am Acad Dermatol* 1992, 27:182–188.

2.• Hogan D, Dannaker C, Maibach H: The prognosis of contact dermatitis. *J Am Acad Dermatol* 1990, 23:300–307.

3.• Hamann C: Natural rubber latex protein sensitivity in review. *Am J Contact Dermatitis* 1993, 4:4–21.

4.• Larsen FS: Atopic dermatitis: a genetic-epidemiologic study in a population-based twin sample. *J Am Acad Dermatol* 1993, 28:719–723.

5. Adinoff AD, Tellez P, Clark RAF: Atopic dermatitis and aeroallergen contact sensitivity. *J Allergy Clin Immunol* 1988, 81:736–742.

6. Epstein E: Dermatitis: practical management and current concepts. *J Am Acad Dermatol* 1984, 10:395–424.

7.• Wall L, Gebauer KA: Occupational skin disease in Australia. *Contact Dermatitis* 1991, 24:101–109.

8. Wikler JR, Nieboer C, Willemze R: Quantitative skin cultures of pityrosporum yeasts in patients seropositive for the human immunodeficiency virus with and without seborrheic dermatitis. *J Am Acad Dermatol* 1992, 27:37–39.

9. Kantor GR, Lookingbill DP: Generalized pruritus and systemic disease. *J Am Acad Dermatol* 1983, 9:375–382.

10. Thestrup-Pederson K, Halkier-Sorenson L, Sogaard H, Zachariae H: The Red Man syndrome. *J Am Acad Dermatol* 1988, 18:1307–1312.

11.• Bakels V, van Oostveen J, Gordijn R, *et al.*: Diagnostic value of T-cell receptor beta gene rearrangement analysis on peripheral blood lymphocytes of patients with erythroderma. *J Invest Dermatol* 1991, 97:782–786.

12. Seymour JL, Keswick BH, Hanifin JM, *et al.*: Clinical effects of diaper types on the skin of normal infants and infants with atopic dermatitis. *J Am Acad Dermatol* 1987, 17:988–997.

13.•• Phillips TJ, Dover JS: Leg ulcers. *J Am Acad Dermatol* 1991, 24:965–987.

SELECT BIBLIOGRAPHY

Cooper KD: Atopic dermatitis: recent trends in pathogenesis and therapy. *J Invest Dermatol* 1994, 102:128–137.

Hopkins T, Clark RAF: The other eczemas. In *Dermatology*, edn 3. Edited by Moschella SL, Hurley HJ. Philadelphia: WB Saunders; 1992: 465–504.

Katsambas A, Antonion CH, Frangouli E, *et al.*: A double-blind trial of treatment of seborrheic dermatitis with 2% ketoconazole cream with 1% hydrocortisone cream. *Br J Dermatol* 1989, 121(3):353–357.

Kay J, Gawkrodger DJ, Mortimer MJ, Jaron AG: The prevalence of childhood atopic eczema in a general population. *J Am Acad Dermatol* 1994, 30:35–39.

Acne Vulgaris and Related Diseases 10

Guy F. Webster

Key Points
- Acne is a two-stage disease, with comedonal and inflammatory stages.
- Cleanliness, dirt, and diet have no role in acne pathogenesis or management.
- Comedonal and papular inflammatory acne may be treated topically.
- Isotretinoin should be reserved for therapy-resistant, disfiguring (usually nodular) acne.
- Long-term oral antibiotic therapy is safe and effective for most inflammatory acne patients.

ACNE VULGARIS

Acne vulgaris is an extraordinarily common disease, with nearly every individual affected at some time in their life. The process is centered around the pilosebaceous units of the face, upper back, and chest and is a true multifactorial condition (Table 10-1). The primary lesion is termed a *comedo* and results from the impaction and distention of the follicle with improperly desquamated follicular epithelium. Instead of being shed as small particles, the epithelium produces large sheets, not unlike scales, which are shed into the follicle and result in an impaction. Another factor in the development of acne is the onset of sebum secretion that follows the puberal surge of androgen levels, which not only further distends the follicle but also provides nutrition for *Propionibacterium acnes*, an anaerobic diphtheroid that lives within the follicle. Although of very little infectious potential, *P. acnes* is very inflammatory and in certain individuals provokes a vigorous inflammatory and immune response. The patients with the most severe acne may reasonably be said to be hypersensitive to *P. acnes* in a classical immunologic sense (Fig. 10-1) [1,2•,3•].

Some patients are predisposed to severe acne because of an underlying hormonal abnormality (Fig. 10-2). It was once thought incorrectly that everyone with severe acne was hyperandrogenic: this is clearly not true, and in fact hyperandrogenism is common only in a small subset of patients with acne, namely adult women with therapeutically resistant acne.

Treatment

Acne vulgaris is a very treatable disease. Using currently available drugs and techniques, the patient whose disease cannot be well controlled is rare.

Because of the many misconceptions about acne, no discussion of its treatment would be complete without a section on patient instructions (Table 10-2). Whatever treatment is chosen, there are several instructions that generally apply. Above all, patients should be instructed not to pop their pimples. Manipulation of acne lesions can force inflammatory comedonal contents into the tissue and prolong inflammation, producing a scar where none would have formed. A second very important issue is that acne is not caused by dirt or bad hygiene.

TABLE 10-1 ETIOLOGIC FACTORS IN ACNE
Major
Comedo formation
Sebum secretion-*Propionibacterium acnes* populations
Hypersensitivity to *P. acnes*
Minor
Hyperandrogenism

Excessive or vigorous face washing can have the same effect as squeezing pimples and generally results in more severe skin disease.

The role of cosmetics in causing acne is a matter of some debate. In the past it was certain that many cosmetics, especially oily ones, could cause comedones to form. In recent years acnegenic components have been eliminated from most cosmetics, and makeup can be judiciously applied. Finally, diet has no known influence on the acne process.

Comedonal Acne

The comedo is the primary acne lesion [1,3•]. It may be present as a visible blackhead or whitehead, or exist as a microcomedo at the center of an inflammatory lesion. Reduction in follicular plugging is a major goal of acne therapy and a key to long-lasting remission. In the past,

agents that induced desquamation (peeling agents) were used to accomplish this goal. For the past decade or so most dermatologists have favored using topical vitamin A (tretinoin), usually in a cream form. The medication is very safe and does not produce detectable changes in circulating vitamin A levels. The single adverse effect that may be expected is mild irritation of the skin to which it is applied. The skin will be somewhat reddish and perhaps have the appearance of being windburned, and patients often complain of an associated dryness. When this occurs, topical moisturizing lotions may be applied. These lotions should be noncomedogenic (*ie*, not induce acne).

Inflammatory Acne

Most patients have a significant number of inflammatory papules in addition to comedones. Although topical tretinoin will eventually reduce the number of inflammatory lesions, this does not happen quickly. Patients with inflammatory acne should receive either topical or systemic antibiotic treatment. The more mild and superficial the inflammatory lesion, the more suitable the patient is for topical therapy (Table 10-3). Benzoyl peroxide in 2.5% to 10% concentrations is of great value; however, a percentage of the population is severely irritated by this medication. Combination products of benzoyl peroxide and erythromycin seem to be better tolerated and quite effective. Other topical products include clindamycin phosphate and erythromycin preparations. Although lotions and gels

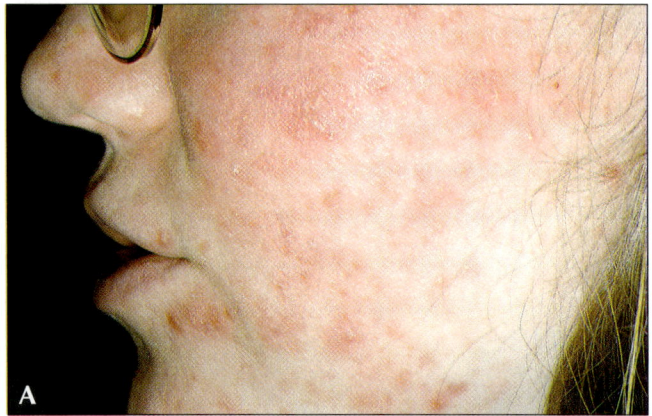

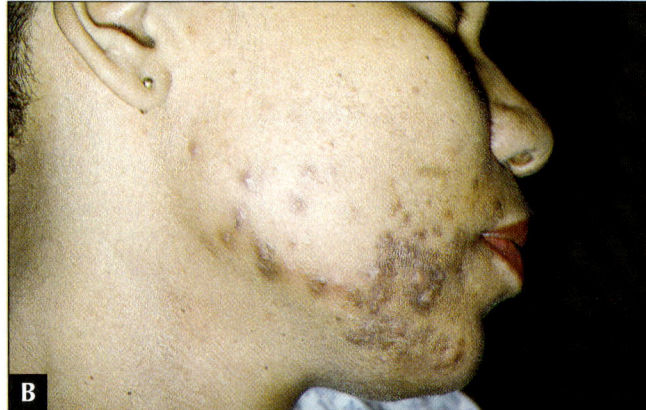

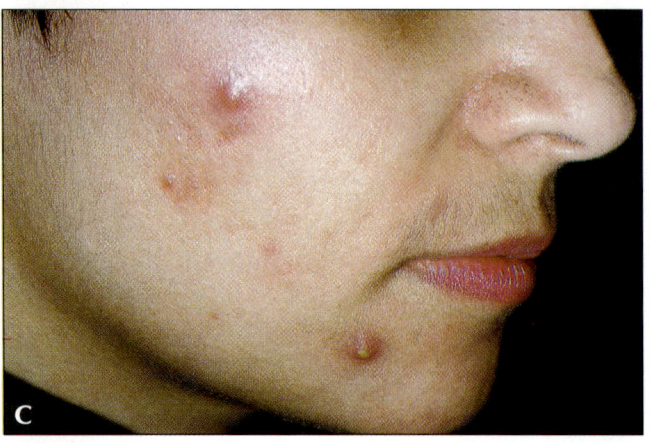

FIGURE 10-1 **A**, Severe papulopustular acne in a young woman. A few closed comedones are present. Scaling resulted from overvigorous washing. **B**, Papulonodular acne. Note the severe hyperpigmentation that may result in dark-skinned patients. **C**, Patients may have very few lesions and still be badly disfigured.

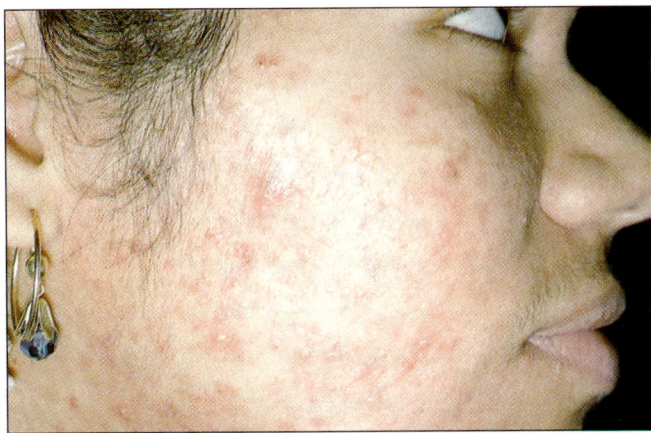

FIGURE 10-2 Papulopustular acne in a woman with polycystic ovaries. Note facial hirsuitism.

TABLE 10-2 PATIENT INSTRUCTIONS
Clean *gently* (dirt has no role in the acne process)
No popping, picking, or emptying of lesions
Diet has no role in acne
Minimize but do not eliminate cosmetics

are available, I generally prefer topical antibiotics in aqueous or alcoholic solutions.

Systemic treatment for acne should be considered when a large body-surface area is involved (for example, the face and the back or when acne in any area is more severe than superficial papules or pustules). Patients may be treated safely and successfully for many years using typical oral regimens. Systemic antibiotics appear to work through two mechanisms: suppression of *P. acnes* populations, and direct inhibition of components of the inflammatory response (Table 10-4). The tetracyclines and erythromycin are most commonly used and are generally well tolerated. Typical dosages are found in Table 10-5. Penicillins and cephalosporins are of little benefit in treating acne. In general, erythromycin and tetracycline are adequate for mild-to-moderate acne, but more severe disease requires doxycycline or minocycline for improvement. Although many doctors recommend minocycline for the most severe forms of acne, I find doxycycline to be as effective and significantly less expensive. The incidence of photosensitivity while taking the drug is a consideration with the use of doxycycline. For this reason, patients should be counseled to avoid sun exposure and to use sunscreens liberally.

Application of topical tretinoin is a useful adjunct to oral antibiotic therapy. Its use should be considered in most patients with acne who are taking systemic or topical antibiotics.

Patients whose disease is predominantly composed of deep nodules that result in scars or patients who have significant acne that is refractory to oral antibiotic therapy should be considered for isotretinoin treatment. Isotretinoin (13-*cis*-retinoic acid) is a metabolite of vitamin A that has profound effects on the skin. In the majority of patients isotretinoin will produce a permanent cure of their acne after a 6-month treatment period. This cure is accomplished through a suppression of sebum secretion, a change in the formation of comedones by the follicular epithelium, and a modulation of the follicular inflammatory response. Isotretinoin is an extraordinarily important and useful drug that has greatly changed the course of severe acne. At this time there is little reason for a patient to be significantly disfigured because of acne.

Unfortunately, the great benefits of isotretinoin are balanced by a significant side-effect profile. The side effects of all oral retinoids are identical to the effects of chronic

TABLE 10-4 ANTI-INFLAMMATORY ACTIVITY OF ANTIBIOTICS IN ACNE
Decreased *Propionibacterium acnes* stimulus
Decreased *P. acnes* chemotactic factor production
Inhibition of neutrophil motility
Inhibition of chronic acne inflammation

TABLE 10-5 ORAL ANTIBIOTICS IN ACNE
Commonly used treatments
Tetracycline (250 to 500 mg bid to qid)
Erythromycin (250 mg bid to qid)
Doxycycline (50 to 100 mg qd to bid)
Minocycline (50 to 100 mg qd to bid)
Occasionally used treatments
Trimethoprim-sulfamethoxazole (single or double strength qd to bid)
Ciprofloxacin (500 mg bid or tid)
bid—Twice a day; qd—every day; qid—four times a day; tid—three times a day.

TABLE 10-3 TOPICAL ACNE THERAPY
Benzoyl peroxide—cream, 2.5% to 10.0% one to two times daily
Erythromycin or clindamycin, 2% solution one to two times daily
Benzoyl peroxide–erythromycin gel (Benzamycin; Dermik, Collegeville, PA) one to two times daily
Retin-A (Ortho, Raritan, NJ), 0.025% to 0.1% gel or cream one to two times daily

vitamin A intoxication. Dryness of the skin and mucous membranes is expected, with the lips, nasal mucosa, and conjunctiva most severely affected. Some patients note a thinning of scalp hair, which tends to be reversible. Few patients complain of muscle and joint pain, and a syndrome of diffuse idiopathic skeletal hyperostosis has been reported in a few patients on long-term retinoid treatment. This latter condition is usually asymptomatic. Decreased night vision is rarely noticed, but can be measured in a significant number of patients. An elevation in triglyceride levels is seen in about one third of patients, and increases of two to three times normal levels are not rare. These elevations usually resolve with modification in diet or dosage, and on the whole seem to be well tolerated. In very rare instances an elevation in liver transaminases has been noted, as has the release of creatinine kinase from skeletal muscle, a process which may be exercise-related.

The most serious concern regarding oral retinoid treatment is the potential for birth defects [4,5]. Women of childbearing age must take extreme care to avoid conception while taking the drug, because the birth of a normal child is extremely unlikely. There is no adverse effect on subsequent pregnancies. The manufacturer of Accutane (Roche, Nutley, NJ) has gone to great lengths to see that proper counseling is given before the treatment is instituted in women. It is recommended that these guidelines be scrupulously followed. Isotretinoin has no adverse effects on male fertility.

Typical isotretinoin dosages are between 0.5 and 1.0 mg/kg/d. Lower dosages may have some benefit, but are associated with an increased frequency of relapse following discontinuation of treatment. Lower dosages do produce fewer side effects, but also necessitate a longer period of treatment than 5 or 6 months.

Other treatments for acne are occasionally used. Some women have significant elevations of circulating androgens that worsen their acne. Normalization of androgen levels, using low-progestin oral contraceptives or low daily dosages of oral corticosteroids, may aid the control of acne. Likewise, spironolactone is occasionally used because of its ability to block the binding of testosterone to sebaceous gland receptors. Neither of these maneuvers is usually enough to completely control severe acne alone or in combination with oral antibiotics. Oral corticosteroids in anti-inflammatory dosages (eg, 30 or 40 mg/d) are sometimes used for severe exacerbations of inflammatory acne: situations where this is appropriate are very rare.

ROSACEA

Rosacea is a chronic skin problem that is usually limited to the central portions of the face. It occurs most commonly in fair-skinned adults, often those who have had significant acne as children. Severity is very variable, with manifestations that range from red cheeks and telangiectasia to crops of pustules and inflammatory nodules (Fig. 10-3). Follicular

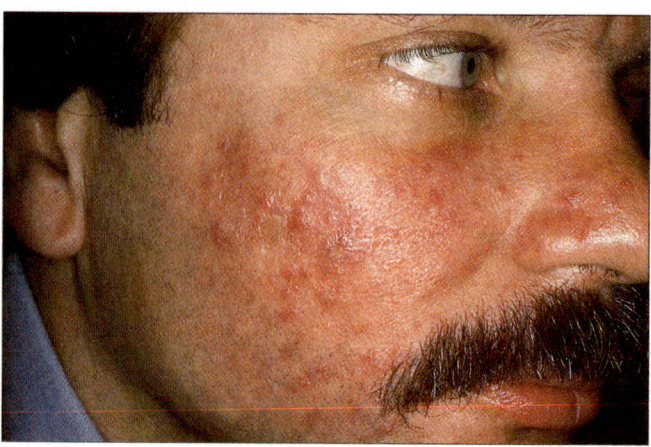

FIGURE 10-3 Papular rosacea.

impaction (comedones) are not a part of rosacea. Left untreated, the most severe cases may trigger a sebaceous hyperplasia, particularly on the nose, a reaction which is termed *rhinophyma* (Fig. 10-4).

It is sometimes difficult to distinguish rosacea from the malar eruption of lupus erythematosus (LE). No single criterion is suitably sensitive or specific. Both diseases occur in similar age groups, and both may have prominent telangiectasia. If papules or pustules are present, the diagnosis is usually rosacea. Small, white, atrophic scars favor LE. Erythema that waxes and wanes over several hours is more likely to be seen in rosacea. A confluent induration favors LE. To complicate matters, some LE patients may also develop rosacea. Evaluation by a dermatologist is often required.

The cause of rosacea is not known. It is certain that individuals with abnormal vascular reactivity on their cheeks, that is, people who flush and blush readily, tend to get rosacea. Compounds that promote facial redness, such as alcohol and spicy food, can exacerbate the rosacea process. There is also clearly a role for the follicular bacterium *P. acnes* in the pustular and nodular forms of the disease. It has long been suspected that the *Demodex* mite that is a normal inhabitant of the sebaceous glands has some role in rosacea. Although that is a widely held belief, supporting evidence is scanty, and treatment with antiparasitic drugs is of no proven benefit.

Many patients with rosacea also have evidence of chronic blepharitis, dry eyes, or recurrent styes. This is certainly part of the rosacea process and may be seen in up to 50% of patients. Treatment of the rosacea with systemic medication usually produces a great improvement in symptoms.

Rosacea is treated by two general approaches. Low-potency corticosteroids may be used alone or in combination with 3% precipitated sulfur. This treatment seems to work best in patients whose rosacea is predominantly vascular. A major problem with topical corticosteroid therapy for rosacea is the tendency of facial skin to accommo-

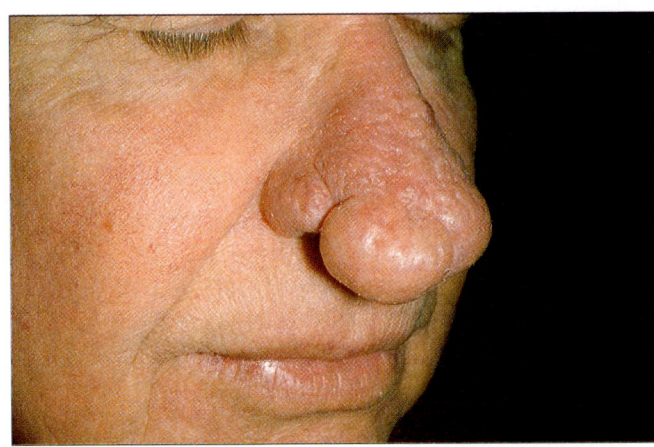

FIGURE 10-4 Rhinophyma, a sebaceous hyperplasia triggered by the rosacea process.

date to the corticosteroid, requiring an increase in drug potency for the same clinical effect. This phenomenon has a great potential to lead to the use of inappropriately strong steroids on the face, which invariably results in a worsening of the rosacea and a severe, potentially permanent, facial atrophy. Topical antibiotics are of some use in treating rosacea and are very safe, but in the hands of most dermatologists are not completely effective in more than moderately severe disease.

Systemic therapy for rosacea is often the most satisfactory, especially in disease with a significant papulopustular component. Tetracyclines are generally superior to erythromycin, although both are effective. I prefer to use doxycycline, 100 mg, one to three times daily, in most situations. Patients who report significant conjunctival symptoms often benefit greatly from systemic treatment.

REFERENCES AND RECOMMENDED READING

Recently published papers of particular interest have been highlighted as:

- • Of interest
- •• Of outstanding interest

1. Kligman AM: An overview of acne. *J Invest Dermatol* 1974, 62:268–287.

2.• Webster GF: Inflammatory acne. *Int J Dermatol* 1990, 29:313–317.

3.• Pochi PE, and Members of Consensus Panel: Report of the consensus conference on acne classification. *J Am Acad Dermatol* 1991, 24:1–6.

4. Rothman KF, Pochi PE: Use of oral and topical agents for acne in pregnancy. *J Am Acad Dermatol* 1988, 19:431–442.

5. Dai WS, Hsu M-A, Itri LM: Safety of pregnancy after discontinuation of isotretinoin. *Arch Dermatol* 1989, 125:362–365.

11 *Pruritus*

Seth G. Kates
Jeffrey D. Bernhard

Key Points

- Pruritus, which is the most common dermatologic complaint, has an extensive differential diagnosis.
- Pruritus can be present with diagnostic or nondiagnostic skin eruptions, or without skin eruptions.
- A positive diagnosis is frequently based on careful patient history, physical examination, and, if necessary, laboratory evaluation.
- Primary dermatologic conditions associated with pruritus include inflammatory conditions, infestations or infections, and neoplastic conditions.
- Systemic disorders associated with pruritus include drug reactions, hepatobiliary, endocrinolgic, and hematologic disorders.
- Management of pruritus is best achieved by alleviating the underlying cause, but if this is not possible, many other treatments are available.

Pruritus, or itching, is defined as the sensation that provokes the urge to scratch. It is the most common dermatologic symptom. Itching can be described as deep or superficial, can provoke a desire to rub or scratch the skin, and can be associated with specific eruptions, nonspecific rashes (*eg*, excoriations), or no eruption whatsoever. It can arise from a primary dermatologic etiology; a complication of pharmacologic therapy; an underlying psychogenic pathology; or a systemic cause, including infection, metabolic disorders, malignancy, hematologic disease, and senescence. Pruritus is a symptom of underlying systemic disease in an estimated 10% to 50% of patients [1]. When a patient complains of pruritus, there is a rational way to assemble the myriad of etiologies into finite groups, to evaluate the patient in a cost-effective and thoughtful manner, and to then correct the underlying cause or treat the pruritus [2••].

The history and physical examination are crucial in the evaluation of a patient with pruritus. The history must include duration, quality (*eg*, burning, tingling, crawling), intensity (*eg*, nocturnal wakening), location, aggravating factors (*eg*, after exposure to water, while at work, in the sun), time of day, careful drug history, and general review of symptoms. A primary eruption, if present, can frequently be diagnostic to the trained eye. A secondary eruption consisting of excoriations, changes caused by rubbing, or cutaneous infection can indicate an obscured primary eruption or an underlying systemic etiology [3] (Fig. 11-1).

PRURITUS WITH CUTANEOUS ERUPTION

Pruritus is a very common feature of dermatologic conditions; therefore, the differential diagnosis of itching with a rash is complex (Table 11-1). It becomes easier if the quality of the cutaneous eruption can be characterized and if the

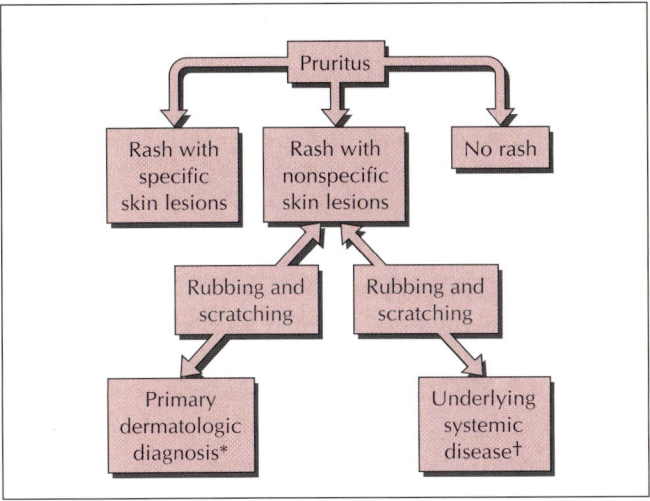

FIGURE 11-1 Clinical algorithm for evaluation of pruritus. *See Table 11-2; †see Table 11-3. (For a more extensive algorithm, see Champion [3].)

TABLE 11-1 MOST COMMON PRIMARY SKIN ERUPTIONS THAT ITCH	
Inflammatory conditions	**Infestations or infections**
Atopic eczema	Scabies
Contact allergic and irritant dermatitis	Pediculosis
Urticaria	Arthropod bites
Dermatitis herpetiformis	Parasitic infestations
Bullous pemphigoid	Varicella
Lichen planus	Cutaneous fungal infections
Photosensitivity reactions	Impetigo
Psoriasis	**Neoplastic**
Drug hypersensitivity reactions	Mycosis fungoides
	Urticaria pigmentosa (mastocytosis)

Adapted from Bernhard [1]; with permission.

distribution can be appreciated. An urticarial eruption, if transient, can signify urticaria from many causes or, if the lesions are of a longer duration, can signify an urticarial vasculitis or an early form of bullous pemphigoid. Vesicular, bullous, or pustular lesions can be diagnostic of different conditions. The presence of excoriations in a flexural pattern in a patient with a history of seasonal allergies or asthma (although not primary lesions) strongly suggests the diagnosis of atopic eczema (Fig. 11-2). Multiple excoriations and erythematous papules on the lower extremities or arms in a patient with a pet at home, even during the winter, frequently result from flea bites, although patients generally protest the diagnosis (Fig. 11-3).

Drugs can cause either a primary cutaneous eruption or itching without any other cutaneous effects. The pruritus from drugs can be localized, as in a fixed drug eruption, or diffuse. The itching can result from hypersensi-

tivity to the drug itself or from complications from medications such as estrogen-induced cholestasis. Table 11-2 is a partial list of common medications that can cause pruritus, although any drug can cause pruritus through idiosyncratic mechanisms, no matter how long the drug has been used.

PRURITUS WITHOUT RASH

Pruritus secondary to underlying systemic pathology is frequently generalized, although some conditions are associated with a localized presentation. Table 11-3 provides a partial list of systemic disorders associated with pruritus.

Diabetes Mellitus

Diabetes mellitus was once thought to be a cause of diffuse pruritus, but more recently it has been recognized as a

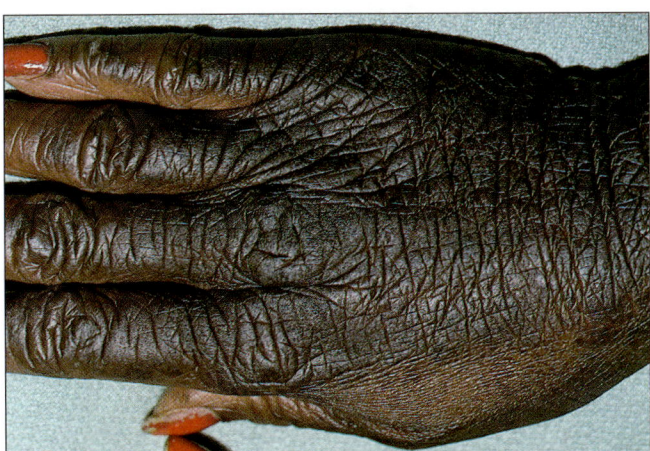

FIGURE 11-2 Lichenification of the skin resulting from chronic scratching in a patient with atopic dermatitis.

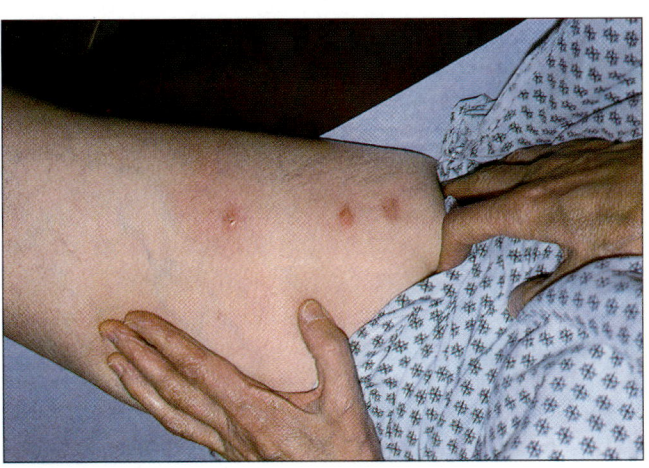

FIGURE 11-3 Typical "breakfast, lunch, dinner" configuration of insect bites.

| TABLE 11-2 DRUGS ASSOCIATED WITH PRURITUS |

Opiates and opiate derivatives
Phenothiazines
Tolbutamide
Erythromycin estolate
Anabolic steroids
Estrogens
Progestins
Testosterone
Aspirin
Quinidine
Vitamin B complex
Psoralens with ultraviolet A radiation
Antimalarials

Adapted from Bernhard [4•]; with permission.

TABLE 11-3 SYSTEMIC DISORDERS ASSOCIATED WITH PRURITUS

Hepatobiliary disorders	Visceral carcinoma
Primary biliary cirrhosis	Central nervous system
Biliary obstruction	tumors
Cholestasis during pregnancy	Mycosis fungoides
	Multiple myeloma
Endocrine disorders	
Hyperthyroidism	**Parasitic infestations**
Hypothyroidism	Hookworm
Diabetes mellitus	Onchocerciasis
Carcinoid syndrome	Ascariasis
Adrenal insufficiency	Trichinosis
Hematologic disorders	**Infections**
Polycythemia vera	HIV*
Iron deficiency	Hepatitis B virus
Paraproteinemia	
Waldenström's macroglobu-	**Psychogenic states**
linemia	Psychogenic pruritus
	Delusions of parasitosis
Renal disorders	Neurotic excoriations
Chronic renal failure	
Chronic hemodialysis	**Senescense**
Malignant disorders	**Aquagenic pruritus**
Lymphoma	
Leukemia	

*Data from Shapiro and coworkers [5], and Liautaud and coworkers [6].
Adapted from Bernhard [4•]; with permission.

frequent cause of localized pruritus, especially of the anogenital area [7]. Diffuse pruritus in diabetes is usually associated with chronic renal failure.

Chronic Renal Failure and Chronic Hemodialysis

Pruritus is usually a late finding in patients with renal failure and rarely heralds its onset. It is frequently most marked in patients during or immediately after dialysis and can affect up to 75% of patients [8]. Pruritus can be both generalized and persistent, as well as localized and intermittent. The precise molecule or molecules responsible for itching in chronic renal failure are not known. Pruritus is not a feature of acute renal failure. Other factors in chronic renal failure that may contribute to pruritis include secondary hyperparathyroidism [9], xerosis, and hypermagnesemia [10] (Fig. 11-4).

Cholestasis

Pruritus is a hallmark of obstructive liver disease. The pathophysiology of the itching is unclear, and although elevated bile salts have been implicated, doubt that bile salts are responsible is increasing [11]. Itching is unusual in infective hepatitis or hemolytic anemias, although it is common in drug-induced cholestasis. It is commonly the presenting complaint in primary biliary cirrhosis [12].

Polycythemia Vera and Aquagenic Pruritus

Case series have disclosed greater than 50% incidence of pruritus in patients with polycythemia vera [13,14]. It typically occurs after bathing, and is frequently described as severe and prickling, lasting for 15 to 60 minutes. The skin examination is normal, and the history and quality of the pruritus is very similar to those of aquagenic pruritus. Aquagenic pruritus of the elderly most commonly occurs in women and is described as a prickling pruritus lasting approximately 15 minutes after bathing. Xerosis is some-

times present. No underlying systemic abnormality exists. Because water-induced pruritus can precede the onset of polycythemia vera by several years, long-term follow-up is suggested [15]. The pruritus of polycythemia vera frequently improves with treatment.

Malignancies

Patients with Hodgkin's disease can have associated pruritus as the presenting complaint. Frequently, the pruritis can have bizarre patterns that are localized or diffuse and occasionally migratory. Severe pruritus may portend a poor prognosis [16]. Pruritus can also be severe in cutaneous T-cell lymphoma, in which it is frequently associated with a rash. Itching occurs in internal occult malignancies, especially multiple myeloma, adenocarcinoma, and squamous cell carcinoma. However, the actual incidence is probably rare.

Senescence

Pruritus in the elderly is extremely common and increases in incidence with age. Although it is important to rule out an underlying systemic etiology, a large number of patients are left with advancing age as the only etiology. Xerotic or winter itch, or dry skin with fine cracking, is common in the elderly.

TABLE 11-4 LABORATORY EVALUATION OF A PRURITIC PATIENT*
Routine screening tests
Complete blood count with differential
Liver function
Thyroid function panel
Renal panel and urine
Blood glucose
Chest radiograph
Other tests, as indicated by above, or by history and physical examination
Stool for occult blood
Stool for ova and parasites
Papanicalaou smear
Serum protein electrophoresis
Erythrocyte sedimentation rate
Serum iron and ferritin
Blind skin biopsy with or without immunoflorescence
Additional radiologic or serologic investigations
*As indicated by history and physical examination. *Adapted from* Bernhard [1]; with permission.

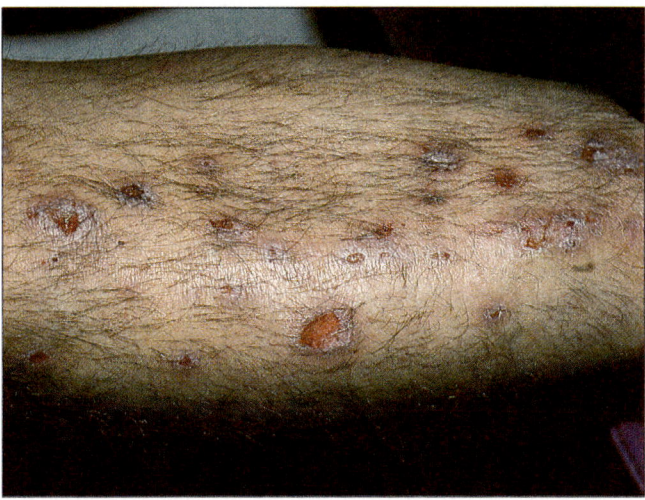

FIGURE 11-4 Excoriations in a patient with chronic renal failure on dialysis.

Age-related degenerative changes in cutaneous nerve endings may cause "phantom" pruritus in elderly patients in whom no other explanation exists for itching [17].

EVALUATION

The evaluation of a patient presenting with pruritus should proceed in a logical manner. The history, review of systems, and physical examination should provide a differential diagnosis. An initial laboratory evaluation should include a complete blood count with differential, liver function tests with a chemistry battery, thyroid function studies, and a chest radiograph (Table 11-4). Further studies can be performed but should be tailored to the patient's history. Performing a very large panel of laboratory studies with a small pretest index of suspicion is generally not helpful and can be misleading. Therefore, if the test results are negative initially, the patient can be treated symptomatically and re-evaluated at regular intervals (Table 11-4). If a primary cutaneous eruption is present, a dermatology consultation is indicated. Beware of allowing patients to fall out of contact when they are sent for evaluation because the collaborative efforts of the dermatologist and primary care physician may be required to make a diagnosis over time.

TREATMENT

Ideally, the best way to treat pruritus is to identify the underlying etiology and to correct it. Commonly, no underlying etiology is found during the initial evaluation, and treatment must be instituted for symptomatic relief [18].

Emollients are the easiest, least expensive, and most reliably successful treatments. They can be curative in patients with xerosis, atopic dermatitis, aquagenic pruritus of the elderly, and many other disorders. They can be compounded with 0.25% menthol, 0.125% phenol, or both, which may increase their efficacy. Cool soaks or a cool shower before bed can also be very effective.

Low-potency topical corticosteroids can be used, although their use should be restricted over the long term, especially when there is no definite diagnosis. Similarly, high-potency corticosteroids should be avoided unless a clear inflammatory condition is being treated. Systemic corticosteroids have no role in the treatment of pruritus of undetermined origin.

Aside from their soporific effect, H_1-blocking antihistamines are not particularly effective unless a histamine disorder, such as urticaria, is present. Again, caution should be used in the dispensing of these agents if the etiology of the pruritus is unclear. Drugs that work both peripherally and centrally, although more effective, can be very sedating. The newer nonsedating agents are not usually effective for the treatment of generalized pruritus, which is to be expected. H_2-blockers alone or in combination with H_1-blockers add little, if at all, to the treatment of pruritus.

Cholestyramine, activated charcoal, psoralens plus ultraviolet A or ultraviolet B light, and aspirin can be effective in the treatment of specific types of pruritus. It is important to remember that, in all cases of pruritus in which a cause has not been identified or in cases in which an etiology has been determined but appropriate treatment has failed, periodic re-evaluation is required.

References and Recommended Reading

Recently published papers of particular interest have been highlighted as:
- Of interest
- •• Of outstanding interest

1.   Bernhard JD: Itching as a manifestation of noncutaneous disease. *Hosp Pract* 1987, 22:81–95.

2.•• Bernhard JD: *Mechanism and Management of Pruritus.* New York: McGraw Hill; 1994.

3.   Champion RH: Generalized pruritus. *Br Med J* 1984, 289:751–753.

4.•   Bernhard JD: Pruritus: Pathophysiology and clinical aspects. In *Dermatology*, edn 4. Edited by Moschella SL, Hurley HJ. Philadelphia: WB Saunders; 1992:2042–2047.

5.   Shapiro RS, Samorodin C, Hood AF: Pruritus as a presenting sign of acquired immunodeficiency syndrome. *J Am Acad Dermatol* 1987, 16:1115–1117.

6.   Liautaud B, Pape JW, DeHovitz JA, *et al.*: Pruritic skin lesions. A common initial presentation of acquired immunodeficiency syndrome. *Arch Dermatol* 1989, 125:629–632.

7.   Neilly JB, Martin A, Simpson N, MacCuish AC: Pruritus in diabetes mellitus: investigation of prevalence and correlation with diabetes control. *Diabetes Care* 1986, 9:273.

8.   Gilchrest BA, Stern R, Steinman TI, *et al.*: Clinical features of pruritus among patients undergoing maintenance hemodialysis. *Arch Dermatol* 1982, 118:154–156.

9.   Massry SG, Popovtzer MM, Coburn JW, *et al.*: Intractable pruritus as a manifestation of secondary hyperparathyroidism in uremia. Disappearance of itching after subtotal parathyroidectomy. *N Engl J Med* 1968, 279:697–700.

10.   Graf J, Kovarik J, Stumjmvoll HK, *et al.*: Disappearance of uremic pruritus after lowering dialysate magnesium concentration. *Br Med J* 1979, ii:1478–1479.

11.   Jones EA, Bergasa NV: Hypothesis. The pruritus of cholestasis: From bile acids to opiate agonists. *Hepatology* 1990, 11:884–887.

12.   Ghent CN, Carruthers SG: Treatment of pruritus in primary biliary cirrhosis with rifampin. Results of a double-blind, crossover, randomized trial. *Gastroenterology* 1988, 94:488–493.

13.   Berlin NI: Diagnosis and classification of the polycythemias. *Semin Hematol* 1975, 12:339–351.

14.   Fjellner B, Hagermark O: Pruritus in polycythemia vera: Treatment with aspirin and possibility of platelet involvement. *Acta Derm Venereol (Stockh)* 1979, 59:505–512.

15.   Kligman AM, Greaves MW, Steinman H: Water-induced itching without cutaneous signs. Aquagenic pruritus. *Arch Dermatol* 1986, 122:183–186.

16.   Feiner AS, Mahmood J, Wanner SF: Prognostic importance of pruritus in Hodgkin's disease. *JAMA* 1978, 240:2738–2740.

17.   Bernhard JD: Phantom itch, pseudophantom itch, and senile pruritus. *Int J Dermatol* 1992:856–857.

18.   Bernhard JD: Pruritus: advances in treatment. *Adv Dermatol* 1991, 6:57–71.

Leg Ulcers 12

Jeffrey B. Pardes
Vincent Falanga

Key Points

- Venous ulcers occur frequently in areas affected by lipodermatosclerosis, which is manifest in its acute phase by redness, scaling, induration, and intense pain on the medial aspect of the leg.

- Biopsies of the edge of venous ulcers heal to the original margin.

- The androgenic steroid stanozolol is an effective treatment for acute lipodermatosclerosis and for ulcers caused by cryofibrinogenemia.

- Compressive bandages should not be used without first ensuring that there is adequate arterial flow in the lower extremities.

- Patients with cholesterol embolization generally have palpable pulses in the lower extremities.

- Topical agents should be avoided in patients with venous disease because of their frequent potential for sensitization.

- Although bacterial organisms are cultured from chronic ulcers regularly, systemic antibiotics should only be prescribed if cellulitis is present.

- Occlusive dressings help leg ulcers by decreasing pain, stimulating granulation tissue, and causing painless débridement.

Ulceration of the lower extremity is an increasingly common clinical problem as our population ages, and it is responsible for significant morbidity. Noninflammatory vascular disease is responsible for the vast majority of leg ulcers, with venous disease accounting for nearly 75% of cases [1]. Arterial and neuropathic disease are responsible for most other cases of leg ulcers. Table 12-1 lists many causes of leg ulcers that should be considered in a differential diagnosis.

DIAGNOSIS

Because most leg ulcers are the result of structural abnormalities in large vessels, knowledge of the vascular system is important. Physicians should look for the presence of venous, arterial, or neuropathic disease in any patient who presents with a leg ulcer. A comprehensive evaluation is required. In a given patient, ulcers may be caused by a combination of factors. The gross appearance of the lower extremities should be noted: leg deformities or scars may provide clues about past pathologic processes or surgical intervention that may have led to structural damage in the vascular or nervous system, thereby contributing to ulcer development. Typical venous, arterial, or neuropathic ulcers are often easy to diagnose. Table 12-2 illustrates features of the history and physical examination that help distinguish between the three most common causes of leg ulcers. It should be noted that the presence, quality, or intensity of pain within an ulcer is not sufficiently specific for a diagnosis,

TABLE 12-1 CLASSIFICATION OF LEG ULCERS

Vascular (noninflammatory)
Venous disease
Arterial disease
   Atherosclerosis
   Buerger's disease
Cholesterol emboli
Antiphospholipid antibody syndrome
Hemoglobinopathies

Vascular (inflammatory)
Vasculitis
   Chronic hypersensitivity angiitis
   Polyarteritis nodosa
   Necrobiosis lipoidica diabeticorum
   Wegener's granulomatosis
   Connective tissue disease
      Systemic lupus erythematosus
      Rheumatoid arthritis
      Scleroderma
Cryofibrinogenemia, cryoglobulinemia

Neuropathic
Diabetes mellitus
Hansen's disease
Syringomyelia

Neoplastic
Squamous cell carcinoma
Basal cell carcinoma
Cutaneous lymphoma
Kaposi's sarcoma
Metastases

Infectious
Bacterial
Mycotic
Mycobacterial
Syphilitic gumma

Physical
Factitial
Postirradiation

Pyoderma gangrenosum

although arterial ulcers are generally more painful than venous ulcers, and neuropathic ulcers are often painless.

COMMON CAUSES OF LEG ULCERS

Venous Ulcers

Venous disease and ulceration are more frequent in older women than in men, even when the greater longevity of women is taken into account [1]. A characteristic finding in patients with venous disease is the presence of dermatitis in the affected extremity (Fig. 12-1). In addition to the typical clinical features of venous disease, which include hyperpigmentation surrounding the ulcer (Table 12-2; Figs. 12-2 and 12-3), the physician often obtains a history of intense pain, redness, and scaling preceding the development of the ulcer. These clinical features suggest the diagnosis of lipodermatosclerosis. The acute phase of lipodermatosclerosis does not occur in every patient who develops a venous ulcer, and is often misdiagnosed as morphea or a cellulitis unresponsive to antibiotic treatment [2••]. Chronic lipodermatosclerosis often results in depression and induration on the medial aspect of the leg (Fig. 12-4). It may cause the lower leg to assume a shape similar to an inverted bottle. A palpa-

TABLE 12-2 DISTINGUISHING FEATURES OF SELECTED LEG ULCERS

Feature	Venous	Arterial	Neuropathic
History	Previous deep venous thrombosis or vein stripping	Risk of atherosclerosis	Diabetes or neurologic disease
Symptoms	Dull leg pain, heaviness, relief with leg elevation	Claudication; pain with leg elevation	None or paresthesias
Ulcer location	Medial and lateral malleoli	Toes or areas of pressure	Malleolar or plantar surfaces
Ulcer appearance	Shallow, irregular exudative	Deep, regular, dry, necrotic, exposed tendons	Deep, often surrounded by callus
Associated findings	Edema, venous dermatitis (scaling, redness, hyperpigmentation), venous dilatation, lipodermatosclerosis	Xerosis, fissures, alopecia, dependent rubor, decreased pulses	Evidence of deformity, muscle atrophy, sensory deficit

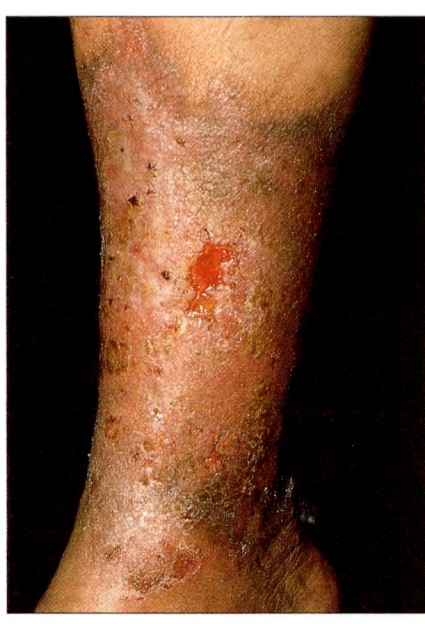

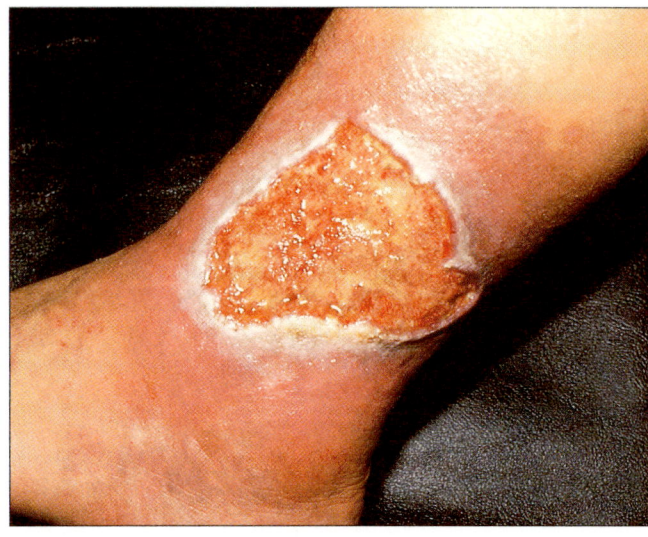

FIGURE 12-2 Venous ulcer with surrounding dermatitis.

ble abrupt transition is detectable between the indurated and the normal skin, reminiscent of a cliff drop. We stress clinical recognition of lipodermatosclerosis because biopsy incisions in the indurated skin may not heal and may become venous ulcers. However, if a biopsy does become necessary, direct immunofluorescence studies of the ulcer's edge will show the presence of pericapillary fibrin [1]. Interestingly, after biopsy specimens are obtained from the edge of venous ulcers, remaining tissue heals up to the original margin [3].

Arterial Ulcers

Patients with known risk factors for atherosclerosis and the cutaneous findings displayed in Table 12-2 often have arterial ulcers (Fig. 12-5). With advanced arterial disease, elevation of the leg for less than 1 minute leads to limb pallor; return of the elevated leg to a dependent position results in diffuse erythema. It is important to realize that palpable distal pulses do not absolutely exclude the presence of arterial disease. Doppler ultrasonography is a quick, effective method of measuring systolic blood pressure in the leg and of excluding arterial insufficiency. The ratio of the ankle systolic blood pressure to the brachial systolic blood pressure (ankle–brachial index) is a widely used parameter [4]. The presence of an index greater than 0.8 is a reliable indicator that significant arterial disease is not present in a given patient. Figure 12-6 demonstrates the method of

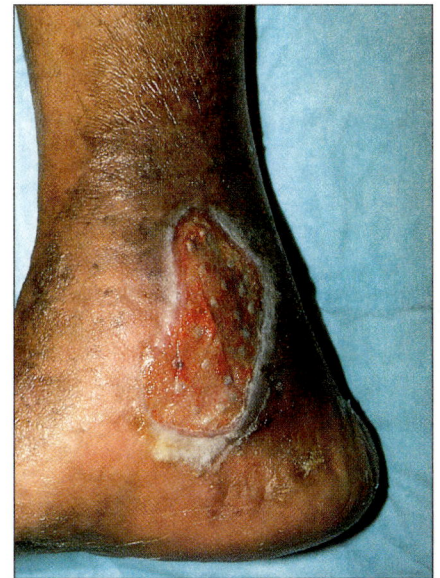

FIGURE 12-3 Venous ulcer overlying the medial malleolus. Ulcers in this location are difficult to heal.

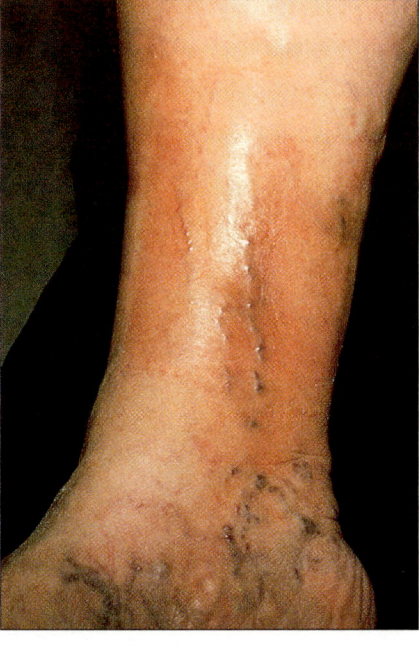

FIGURE 12-4 Lipodermatosclerosis.

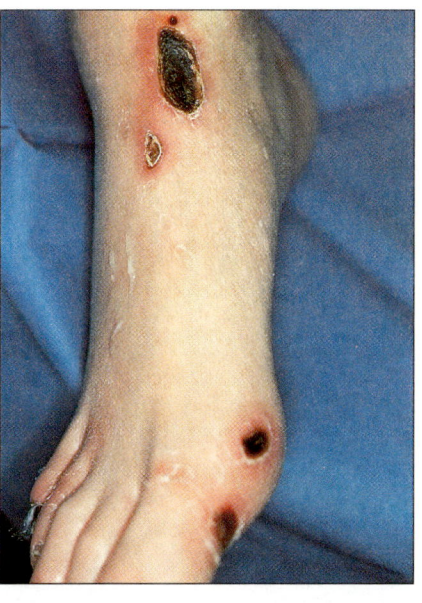

FIGURE 12-5 Arterial ulcers covered by necrotic eschar. Notice the presence of alopecia.

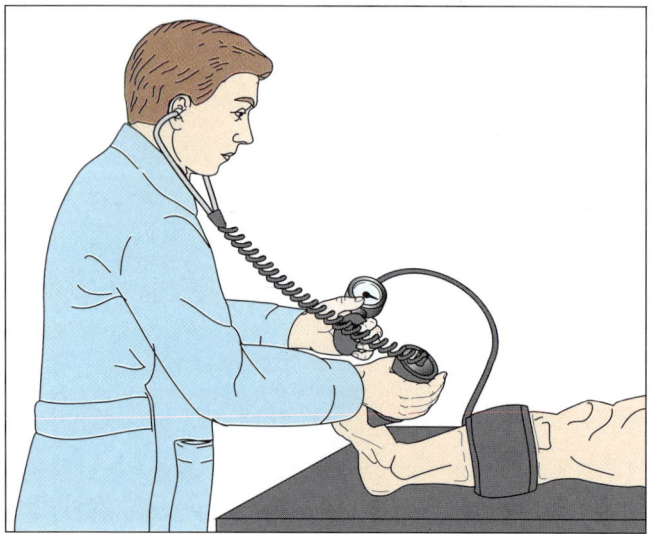

FIGURE 12-6 Method of obtaining ankle systolic blood pressure.

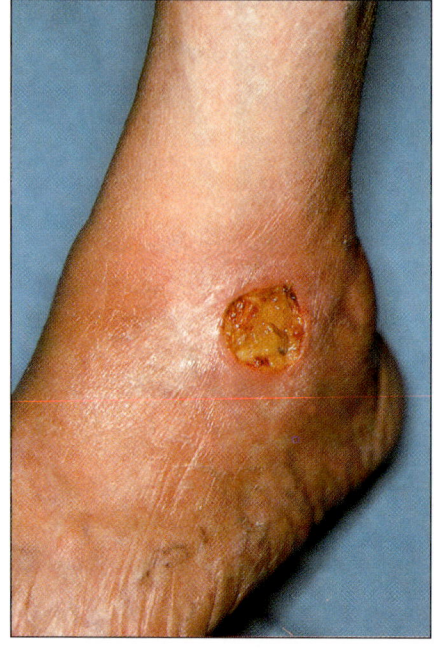

FIGURE 12-7 Combined arterial and venous disease led to ulcer formation.

obtaining the ankle systolic blood pressure. Patients with suspected arterial disease should be evaluated further for corrective vascular surgery. Up to 20% of patients have combined venous and arterial disease (Fig. 12-7).

Neuropathic Ulcers

Patients with neuropathies (*eg*, from diabetes mellitus) often have considerable leg deformity. This deformity is the result of constant trauma from loss of or alteration in sensory function and failure to maintain normal neurologic impulses to the musculature of the lower extremity [5]. The development of new pressure points unaccustomed to pressure can lead to the findings shown in Table 12-2. Ulcers developing as a result of pressure are often surrounded by a

callus and are typically larger than suggested by the overlying skin defect: subcutaneous tissue may be necrotic with little clinical evidence. In patients with diabetes, vascular deficits may combine with the neuropathy to produce complex ulcers (Figs. 12-8 and 12-9).

LESS COMMON CAUSES OF LEG ULCERS

Patients often present with ulcers whose appearance and location are atypical for vascular and neuropathic etiologies, leading to consideration of less common causes of ulceration. Table 12-3 suggests a diagnostic framework in which to view leg ulcers that are not caused by large arterial disease, venous insufficiency, or neuropathy.

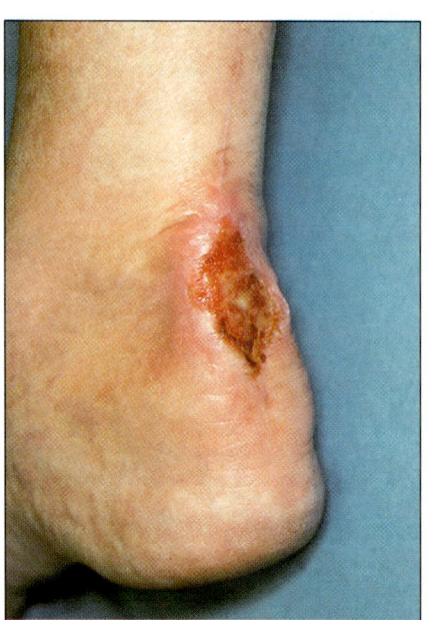

FIGURE 12-8 Neuropathic ulcer overlying the Achilles tendon region after previous surgery in that location.

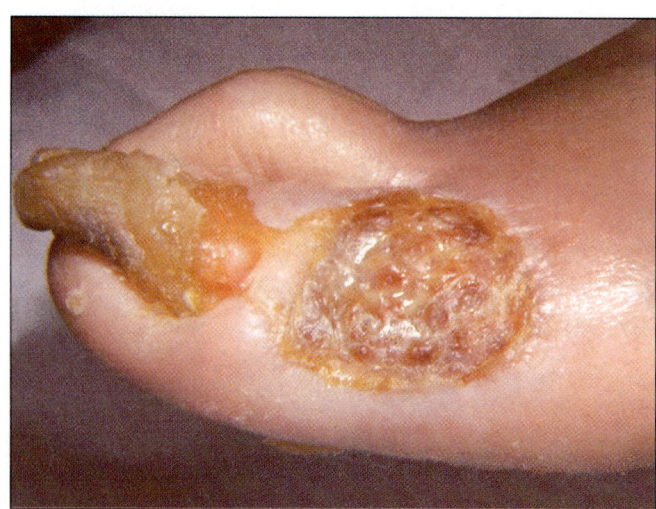

FIGURE 12-9 Distal ulcer in a patient with diabetes and severe arterial disease.

TABLE 12-3 DIFFERENTIAL FEATURES OF SELECTED CAUSES OF LEG ULCERS

Finding	Cryoproteins	Cholesterol emboli	Antiphospholipid antibody syndrome	Vasculitis	Pyoderma gangrenosum
Pulses	+	+	+	+	+
Purpura	+	+	+	+	-
Livedo reticularis	+	+	+	+	-
Punched-out ulcer	-	-	-	-	-
Eschar over ulcer	+	+	+	+	+
Undermined edges	-	-	-	-	+
Violaceous edges	+	-	-	-	+
Cribriform healing	-	-	-	-	+
Raynaud's phenomenon	+	-	+/-	+/-	-
Intractable pain	+	-	+	-	-
Associated diseases	Carcinoma, infections, connective tissue disease, embolic processes	Atherosclerosis	Systemic lupus erythematosus and other connective tissue diseases, recurrent abortions	Connective tissue disease, neoplasia	Inflammatory bowel disease, rheumatoid arthritis, IgA gammopathy

+—common; - —uncommon; +/-—sometimes.

Physicians should look for several cutaneous symptoms that may provide clues to the etiology of the ulceration. Purpura, which represents extravasation of blood into the skin, suggests the possibility of inflammatory vascular disease (*ie*, vasculitis). Livedo reticularis, a fixed reddish-blue mottling of the skin in a netlike pattern, is often prominent on the lower extremities. Livedo reticularis is commonly seen in association with underlying vascular occlusion, connective tissue disease, or vasculitis. The following sections discuss selected causes of leg ulcers that are less common, but often prove to be diagnostic dilemmas for the physician.

Cryoproteinemia

Cryofibrinogenemia may occur either as a primary disease or in association with underlying connective tissue disease, neoplasm, acute infection, or thromboembolic disorders [6,7]. Characteristically, ulcers caused by cryofibrinogenemia are exquisitely painful. During our examination of patients with this condition, we have repeatedly observed that they constantly rub the surrounding skin in an effort to get pain relief. The skin surrounding the ulcers is often a violaceous color and may show purpura and livedo reticularis (Figs. 12-10 and 12-11). Histologically, intravascular fibrin thrombi are typically seen in the dermis. The use of

FIGURE 12-10 Multiple, crusted necrotic ulcers with surrounding erythema in a patient with cryofibrinogenemia.

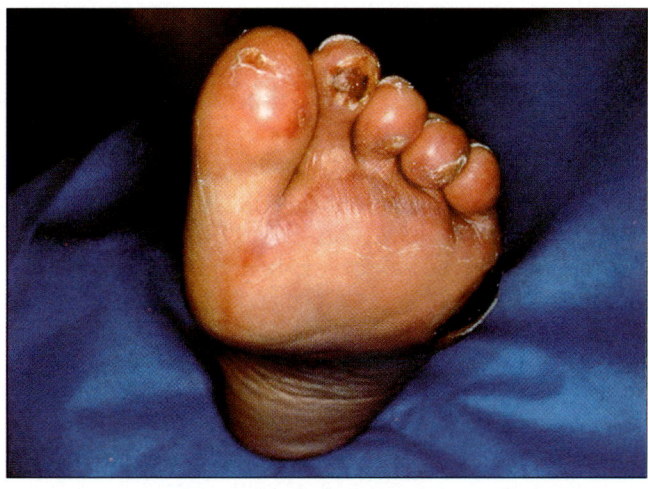

FIGURE 12-11 Distal purpura and necrotic toe ulcers in a patient with cryofibrinogenemia secondary to lymphoblastic leukemia.

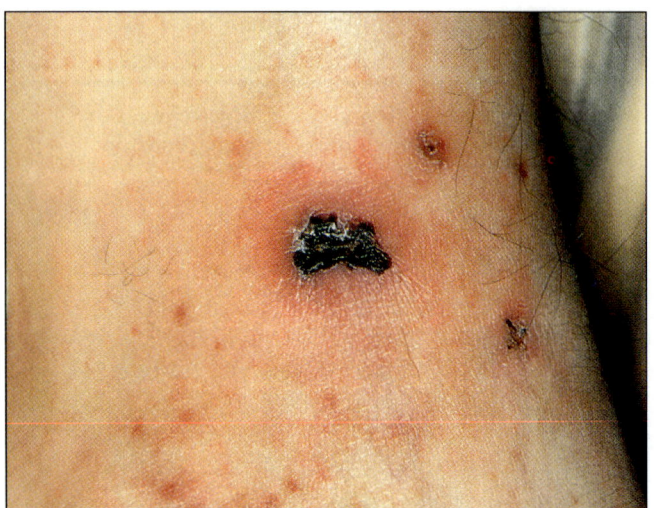

Figure 12-12 Necrotic ulcer and purpura secondary to cholesterol emboli.

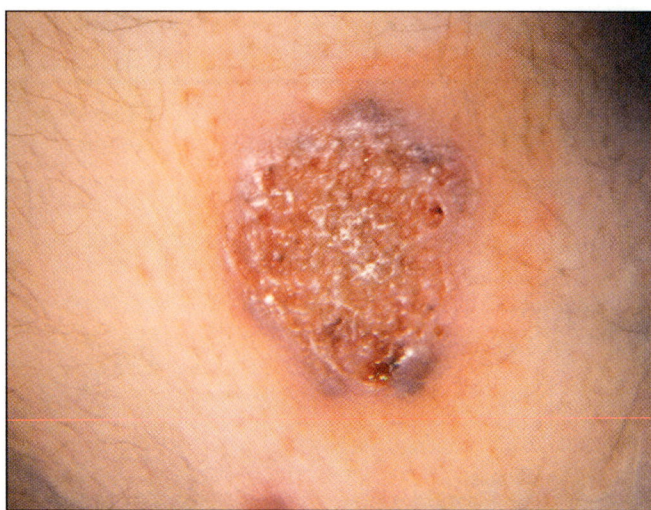

Figure 12-13 Pyoderma gangrenosum. Note the violaceous borders and evidence of cribriform healing.

stanozolol, an anabolic steroid with fibrinolytic properties, leads to dramatic pain relief and ulcer healing in these patients [6,7].

Cholesterol Emboli

Ulcers due to cholesterol emboli typically occur when atheromatous material is dislodged from the abdominal aorta. Cholesterol embolization often occurs after anticoagulant therapy, vascular surgery, or arteriography. Patients may be quite ill, with nonspecific findings including fever, central nervous system changes, sudden arterial hypertension, and myalgia [8]. Leg ulcers due to cholesterol emboli may be associated with extensive livedo reticularis, purpura, and characteristic purple toes (Fig. 12-12). Cholesterol clefts within arterioles are the expected histopathologic finding, but serial subsectioning of biopsy material may be necessary for detection. Interestingly, despite extensive atherosclerotic disease, distal pulses are readily palpable in patients with cholesterol emboli.

Antiphospholipid Antibody Syndrome

Patients with antiphospholipid antibody syndrome develop vascular thromboses, recurrent fetal loss, and thrombocytopenia. The syndrome is not restricted to patients with systemic lupus erythematosus. Positive or reactive testing for Venereal Disease Research Laboratory (test), anticardiolipin antibody, and lupus anticoagulant help confirm the diagnosis of this syndrome [9]. Leg ulcers, livedo reticularis, and purpura are not uncommon in these patients.

Pyoderma Gangrenosum

Rapidly enlarging ulcers with violaceous, undermined edges and cribriform healing (ie, with sievelike perforations of the re-epithelializing wound bed) are typical of pyoderma gangrenosum (Figs. 12-13 and 12-14). Many patients develop ulcers at sites of trauma (pathergy), and lesions often begin as pustules. Although often idiopathic, pyoderma gangrenosum may be associated with ulcerative colitis, rheumatoid arthritis, IgA gammopathies, and multiple myeloma [10]. Mycotic and atypical mycobacterial infection must be excluded. Histology does not aid the diagnosis.

Factitial Ulcers

Manipulation of the skin by the patient can result in the development of leg ulcers that are often atypical in appearance. Such ulcers have odd geometric or linear shapes (Fig. 12-15).

Necrobiosis Lipoidica Diabeticorum

Necrobiosis lipoidica diabeticorum refers to characteristic circumscribed, atrophic, yellow-brown patches that rarely

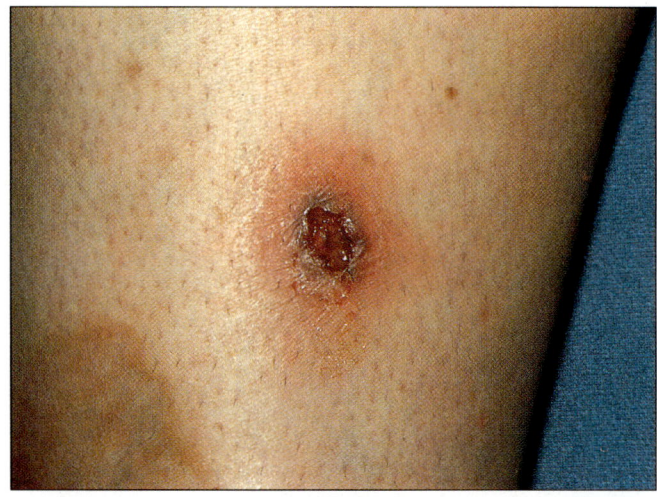

Figure 12-14 Healing pyoderma gangrenosum in a patient with Behçet's syndrome. Previously healed hypopigmented plaque is also present.

ulcerate (Fig. 12-16). Patients with necrobiosis lipoidica diabeticorum either have diabetes, will develop diabetes, or have a strong family history of diabetes.

Neoplasia

A chronic ulcer that is refractory to treatment may be caused by a cutaneous neoplasm. The most common neoplasms arising from a venous ulcer are basal cell carcinoma and rarely, squamous cell carcinoma [11]. The physician should be particularly suspicious of ulcers with exuberant granulation tissue, which is a presentation common in basal cell carcinoma.

TREATMENT

Certain fundamental principles are followed in the treatment of any leg ulcer. Correction of or improvement in underlying illnesses that impair wound healing should be undertaken. Common systemic diseases in which this approach is feasible are diabetes mellitus, anemia, nutritional deficiency, systemic hypertension, and congestive heart failure. Systemic agents that may impair wound healing include corticosteroids and other immunosuppressive drugs, nonsteroidal anti-inflammatory medications, and antineoplastic drugs. Topical agents, including antiseptics and various home remedies (eg, soap), may have a deleterious effect on wound healing. The damage caused by antiseptics is often overlooked [3,12].

Chronic wounds often become infected and have copious malodorous drainage. Although bacterial organisms are cultured from chronic ulcers regularly, we do not prescribe antibiotics unless signs of cellulitis are present. Topical antibiotics have little effect in patients with venous ulcers who also have a high frequency of allergic contact dermatitis. Moreover, the use of topical antibiotics leads to the development of resistant organisms [3].

The goals of ulcer treatment include cleansing of the wound bed, stimulation of granulation tissue formation, and re-epithelialization.

Cleansing

Irrigation of ulcers with normal saline or water, followed by gentle patting, is recommended. The use of antiseptic solutions (eg, hydrogen peroxide or povidone-iodine) is not recommended because of their toxicity to the cells within the wound bed. Hydrogen peroxide is also quite ineffective in the presence of serum.

Granulation Tissue Formation
Occlusive dressings
Occlusive dressings include hydrocolloids, hydrogels, and films. Occlusive dressings promote painless débridement and granular tissue formation, and they also reduce pain associated with the ulcer [3]. They should not be used in the presence of cellulitis, but any fear of causing infection with the use of these agents is unwarranted. Patients must be warned that within a few days of the application of an occlusive dressing, a foul-smelling and considerable exudate may occur. This is not a sign of infection and is expected, particularly with hydrocolloid dressings, which melt into the wound and form a brown or green exudate (Fig. 12-17). Occlusive dressings should be removed and changed only when they start to peel away from the wound, a process that may take days to occur. With the continued use of these dressings, the initial, exudative phase of occlusive therapy is generally followed by

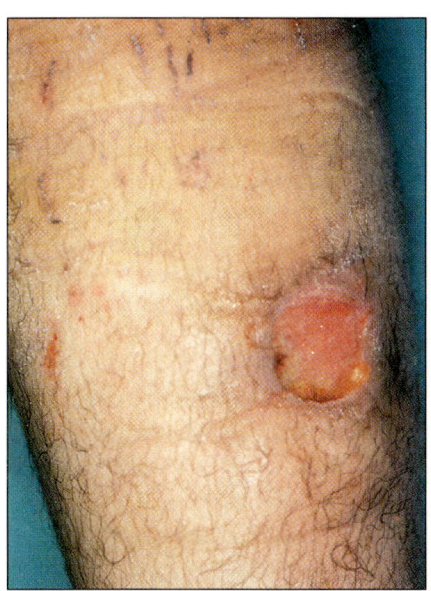

FIGURE 12-15 Factitial ulcer. Proximal, crusted linear excoriations were produced with a stick in an attempt to manipulate the ulcer that was under an Unna boot.

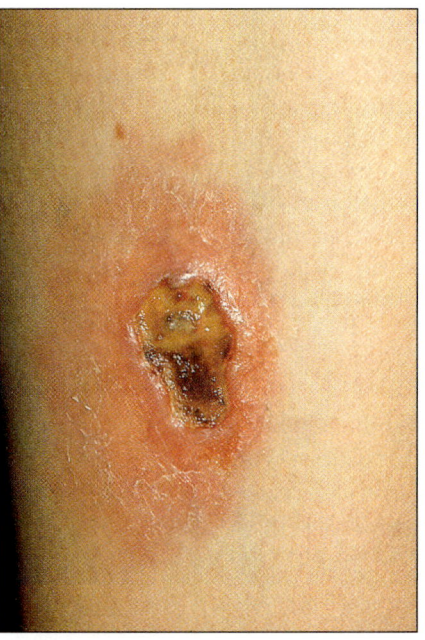

FIGURE 12-16 Necrobiosis lipoidica diabeticorum with ulceration.

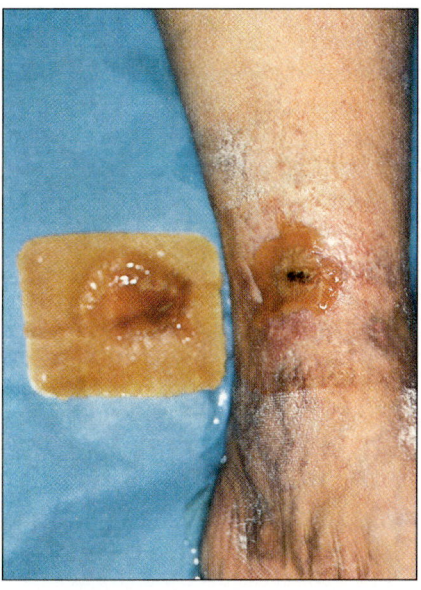

FIGURE 12-17 Removal of a hydrocolloid dressing demonstrates the expected brown exudate several days after dressing application.

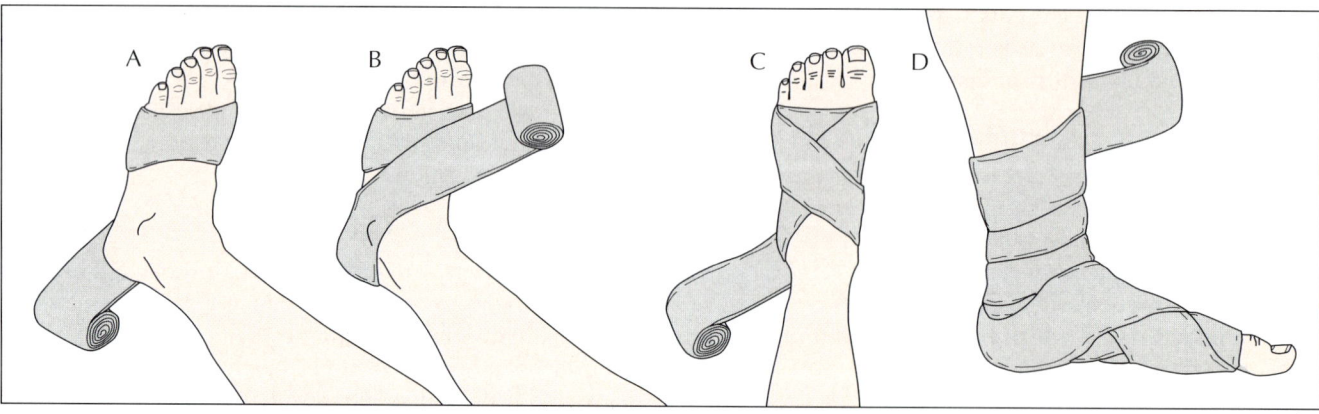

FIGURE 12-18 Unna boot application.

less exudate production. Hasty removal of an occlusive dressing may disrupt fragile, nascent epithelium.

Vitamin A derivatives

Vitamin A or retinoic acid is particularly useful in immunosuppressed patients with ulcers. In this setting, ulcers typically have poor granulation tissue. The once-daily application of retinoic acid lotion to the wound bed often promotes good granulation tissue. The skin surrounding the ulcer should be protected from the irritant action of retinoic acid with petrolatum. If irritation does develop, alternate-day therapy may be better tolerated.

SPECIFIC TREATMENTS

Venous Ulcers

The main goal of therapy is improved venous return and treatment of edema. Specifically, bed rest and leg elevation are recommended, but this may be not practical advice for all patients. Compressive occlusive therapy with an Unna boot or tight, self-adherent bandages is highly efficacious in controlling edema and promoting ulcer healing [12]. Compressive bandages, such as the Unna boot, should be changed weekly. Figure 12-18 demonstrates the method of Unna boot application. It is important to exclude arterial disease before compression therapy is used.

Arterial Ulcers

Referral to a physician skilled in determining the feasibility of vascular reconstruction is recommended for patients with arterial ulcers. If patients are not eligible for bypass procedures, conservative management includes cessation of smoking, weight loss, reduction of systemic blood pressure, and treatment of hyperlipidemia.

Neuropathic Ulcers

Diseases underlying the neuropathy that causes these ulcers should be treated. Patients should examine or should have a trained person examine their legs and feet periodically to prevent the development of new ulcers. Educating the patient about the avoidance of external pressure on the ulcer is essential to ulcer healing. Often, neuropathic ulcers contain deep necrotic tissue, akin to the configuration of an iceberg under the surface of a body of water. Thus, deep débridement and a high index of suspicion for osteomyelitis are often necessary [5,13]. Treatment with pressure-relief hydrocolloid dressings has proved to be useful.

Therapies for Less Common Leg Ulcers

Treatments useful for selected rarer causes of leg ulcers are found in Table 12-4.

TABLE 12-4 UNCOMMON CAUSES OF LEG ULCERS AND SPECIFIC RECOMMENDED THERAPIES	
Disease process causing ulcer	**Treatment**
Cholesterol embolization	No effective treatment
Antiphospholipid antibody syndrome*	Intralesional or systemic corticosteroids
Pyoderma gangrenosum*	Corticosteroids (intralesional or systemic [orally or intravenous pulse])
	Sulfones, clofazimine, cyclosporine
Cryofibrinogenemia*	Stanozolol
	Directed at underlying disease
Vasculitis associated	Steroids
Neoplasia	Excision and referral
Infection	Microbial chemotherapy
Factitial*	Physical occlusion with bandages (Unna boot)

*In the absence of arterial insufficiency, compression therapy may be helpful. The concomitant presence of venous disease should be treated with compression.

Systemic Agents

Stanozolol is an anabolic steroid that has shown promise in the treatment of patients with ulcers caused by cryofibrinogenemia [7]. Similarly, patients with acute lipodermatosclerosis often respond dramatically to stanozolol (at a dosage of 2 to 4 mg twice a day). This agent should not be used in patients with arterial hypertension, congestive heart failure, renal failure, prostatic hypertrophy or cancer, lipid disorders, and liver function test abnormalities.

Ulcers That Fail to Heal

On occasion, despite proper treatment and the development of good granulation tissue, ulcers do not re-epithelialize. Split-thickness skin grafting (eg, with pinch grafts or keratome sheets) can be used in refractory cases as a rapid method of wound closure (Fig. 12-19). When an ulcer does not heal, the diagnosis must be reconsidered. The possibility that the ulcer has a factitial or neoplastic component should be considered. Inquiry about the use of topical or systemic agents that can adversely affect wound healing is very important in such cases. Hospitalization may be necessary to gain control over topical treatment.

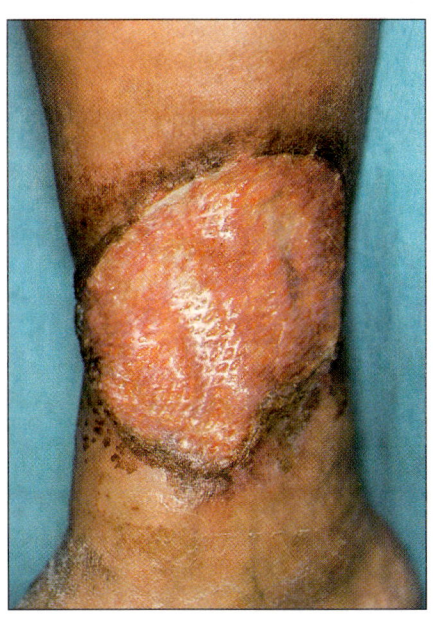

FIGURE 12-19
Split-thickness skin graft applied to a venous ulcer.

REFERENCES AND RECOMMENDED READING

Recently published papers of particular interest have been highlighted as:

• Of interest

•• Of outstanding interest

1. Katz MH, Falanga V, Eaglstein WH: Leg ulcers: a wound-healing model. In *Recent Advances in Dermatology*. Edited by Champion RH, Pye RJ. Edinburgh: Churchill Livingstone; 1992: 199–218.

2.•• Kirsner RS, Pardes JB, Eaglstein WH, Falanga V: The clinical spectrum of lipodermatosclerosis. *J Am Acad Dermatol* 1993, 28:623–627.

3. Falanga V, Eaglstein WH: A therapeutic approach to venous ulcers. *J Am Acad Dermatol* 1986, 14:777–784.

4. Yao ST, Hobbs JT, Irvine WT: Ankle systolic pressure measurements in arterial disease affecting the lower extremities. *Br J Surg* 1969, 56:676–679.

5. Boulton AJM: The diabetic foot. *Med Clin North Am* 1988, 72:1513–1530.

6. Falanga V, Kirsner RS, Eaglstein WH, *et al.*: Stanozolol in treatment of leg ulcers due to cryofibrinogenemia. *Lancet* 1991, 338:347–348.

7. Kirsner RS, Eaglstein WH, Katz MH, *et al.*: Stanozolol causes rapid pain relief and healing of ulcers caused by cryofibrinogenemia. *J Am Acad Dermatol* 1993, 28:71–75.

8. Falanga V, Fine MJ, Kapoor WN: The cutaneous manifestations of cholesterol crystal embolization. *Arch Dermatol* 1986, 122:1194–1198.

9. Stephens CJM: The antiphospholipid syndrome: clinical correlations, cutaneous features, mechanisms of thrombosis and treatment of patients with the lupus anticoagulant and anticardiolipin antibodies. *Br J Dermatol* 1991, 125:199–206.

10. Matis WL, Ellis CN, Griffiths CEM, Lazarus GS: Treatment of pyoderma gangrenosum with cyclosporine. *Arch Dermatol* 1992, 128:1060–1064.

11. Harris B, Eaglstein WH, Falanga V: Basal cell carcinoma arising in venous ulcers and mimicking granulation tissue. *J Dermatol Surg Oncol* 1993, 19:150–152.

12. Mayberry JC, Moneta GL, Taylor LM, Porter JM: Fifteen-year results of ambulatory compression therapy for chronic venous ulcers. *Surgery* 1991, 109:575–581.

13. LoGerfo FW, Coffman JD: Current concepts: vascular and microvascular disease of the foot in diabetes. *N Engl J Med* 1984, 311:1615–1619.

SELECT BIBLIOGRAPHY

Cheatle TR, Sarin S, Coleridge Smith PD, Scurr JH: The pathogenesis of skin damage in venous disease: a review. *Eur J Vasc Surg* 1991, 5:115–123.

Falanga V: Occlusive wound dressings: why, when, which? *Arch Dermatol* 1988, 124:872–877.

Falanga V, Moosa HH, Nemeth AJ, *et al.*: Dermal pericapillary fibrin in venous disease and venous ulceration. *Arch Dermatol* 1987, 123:620–623.

Phillips TJ, Dover JS: Leg ulcers. *J Am Acad Dermatol* 1991, 25:965–987.

13 *Photosensitivity*

Yardy Tse
Henry W. Lim

Key Points

- Evaluation of photosensitive patients should include history, physical examination, and photobiologic studies.
- Polymorphous light eruption is the most common idiopathic photodermatosis.
- Solar urticaria is characterized by development of urticaria after exposure to sunlight.
- Photoallergy and phototoxicity require the concomitant presence of photosensitizers and radiation.
- Chronic actinic dermatitis consists of a spectrum of chronic photosensitivity disorders, known previously under other terminologies.

Solar radiation can be classified according to wavelength (Table 13-1). Ultraviolet (UV)C is absorbed in the atmosphere and does not reach the surface of the earth. Common side effects of sun exposure, ranging from sunburn to skin cancers, are the result of acute and chronic exposure to UVB (Fig. 13-1). UVA may potentiate the photocarcinogenic effect of UVB and is responsible for the development of most types of photoallergy and phototoxicity. UV light may also induce the development of idiopathic dermatoses (*eg*, polymorphous light eruption [PMLE], solar urticaria, and chronic actinic dermatitis [CAD]), and exacerbate other disorders, such as lupus erythematosus, pellagra, pemphigus, and Hartnup disease (for porphyrias, *see* Werth and McKinley Grant, Cutaneous Manifestations of Endocrine and Metabolic Disorders).

APPROACH TO THE PATIENT WITH PHOTOSENSITIVITY

A detailed history must be obtained when evaluating patients with photosensitivity. Particular attention should be paid to 1) age at onset of the eruption; 2) length of exposure, and whether reaction is immediate or delayed (Table 13-2); 3) persistence of reactions (recurrent or chronic); 4) seasonal variation; and 5) the effect of window glass (which blocks out most UVB). Questioning with regard to exposure to photosensitizers, either systemic or topical (the latter including sunscreens, cosmetics, plants or occupational agents), is essential. Current systemic medication, as well as medication to which the patient was exposed at the time of the initial episode of photosensitivity, should be reviewed. A history of exposure to oral contraceptives or ingestion of ethanol is important in patients who may have porphyria. Of particular interest in the review of systems is multiple organ involvement in connective tissue disease (*ie*, arthralgia, oral ulcers, hair loss, and neurologic symptoms associated with the hepatic porphyrias).

TABLE 13-1 CLASSIFICATION OF ELECTROMAGNETIC RADIATION FROM SUNLIGHT	
Wavelength range, *nm*	**Type**
290–320	UVB
320–400	UVA
400–800	Visible
800–17,000	Infrared

nm—nanometer; UV—ultraviolet.

Physical Examination

Physical examination should include evaluation of the morphology and distribution of the eruption. The classic "sun-exposed distribution" includes the face, "V" of the neck with submental and upper-lip sparing, dorsal hand and forearm involvement with sharp cutoff at areas covered by clothing, and sparing of skin folds on the neck (Fig. 13-2). In severe eruptions, covered areas may also be involved, albeit to a lesser extent.

Laboratory Studies

Skin biopsy for histologic examination and direct immunofluorescence is an integral part of the diagnostic work-up. The diagnosis of connective tissue disease, especially lupus erythematosus, must also include examination of serum for autoimmune antibodies (ANA, Anti-Ro, and Anti-La tests). The porphyrias can be properly evaluated only by examination of the complete porphyrin profile (erythrocytes, plasma, urine, and feces).

Photobiological Studies

Photobiological studies are needed to confirm that photosensitivity is present and to define the spectrum of the sensitivity. Photo tests to determine the minimal erythema dose (MED) to UVA, UVB, and visible light, and photopatch tests to evaluate photocontact sensitivity, should be performed by an experienced dermatologist.

POLYMORPHOUS LIGHT ERUPTION

Polymorphous light eruption is the most common idiopathic photodermatosis, occurring in 10% of the population

TABLE 13-2 TIMING OF ERUPTION
Immediate
Solar urticaria
Erythropoietic protoporphyria*
Delayed
Polymorphous light eruption
Photoallergic contact dermatitis
Photosensitivity to systemic agents
Lupus erythematosus
Chronic/seasonal
Chronic actinic dermatitis
Porphyria cutanea tarda*

*See **Werth and Grant, Cutaneous Manifestations of Endocrine and Metabolic Disorders.**

(Table 13-3). Young adults are usually affected within hours to days following sun exposure. The eruption assumes a varied morphology of pruritic papules, papulovesicles, nodules, or plaques on sun-exposed skin (Fig. 13-3). However, in each patient a single morphology usually predominates and remains constant.

The eruption typically presents in the spring and gradually improves in the summer. Tolerance is attributed anecdotally to thickening of the stratum corneum and increased pigmentation or tanning ("hardening"). Attacks of PMLE may recur after each exposure to sunlight, and the disease usually follows a chronic, progressive course.

Histopathologically, PMLE is characterized by a dense perivascular lymphocytic infiltrate in the upper and mid dermis. Epidermal spongiosis may also be present.

Because there are no specific chemical or serologic tests for PMLE, the diagnosis is often made by exclusion. Serologic and immunofluorescent tests for lupus erythematosus, photo tests to UVA, UVB, and visible light, and photopatch tests are usually negative. Provocative photo tests, where test sites are exposed to UVA and UVB for 3 to 4 consecutive days, are known to result in the induction of classic lesions.

Treatment of PMLE consists of photoprotection and topical corticosteriods. To prevent further episodes, patients

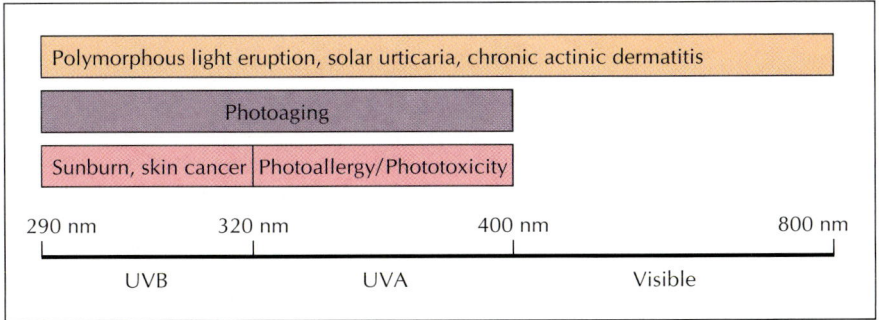

FIGURE 13-1 Predominant action spectra of the acute and chronic effects of sunlight and photodermatoses. nm—nanometer.

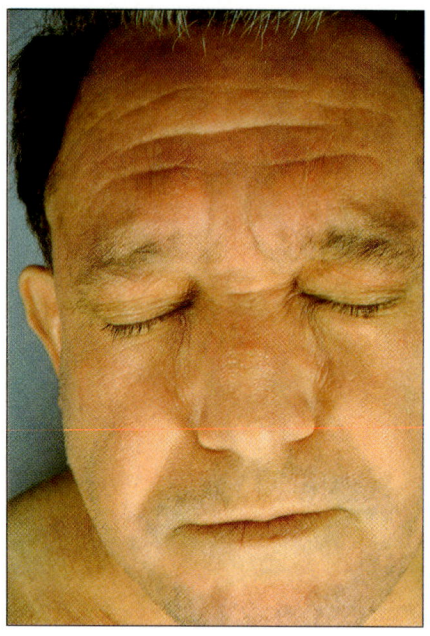

FIGURE 13-2 A patient with photodistributed eruption, with sparing of the nasolabial folds and eyelids.

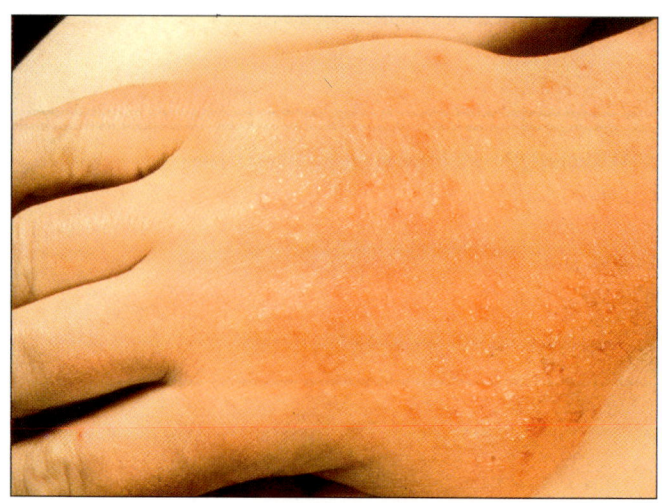

FIGURE 13-3 A patient with polymorphous light eruption. There are multiple erythematous papules on the dorsum of the hand after sun exposure.

can be treated with sunscreens with a sun protection factor of 15 or higher. β-carotene, 60 to 120 mg/day for 4 to 6 weeks before anticipated exposure, has been reported as an effective prophylactic treatment of PMLE [1,2]. Antimalarials (chloroquine and hydroxychloroquine) are effective in some patients but, because of their potential toxicity, they should be reserved for patients whose disease cannot be controlled by other means [3•]. Induction of "hardening" by phototherapy (UVB) can be very effective. Treatment with 8-methoxypsoralen plus UVA (PUVA) is the most effective therapy and has prevented recurrence of lesion development in more than 75% of patients treated [1,4,5].

SOLAR URTICARIA

Solar urticaria is a relatively rare form of photosensitivity characterized by the development of urticaria following exposure to sunlight (Table 13-3). The peak age of onset is young adulthood, and slightly more women are affected than men. Clinically, the exposed skin reddens, scattered wheals appear and coalesce, and an erythematous and edematous flare develops around the wheals (Fig. 13-4). Pruritus is often intense. The reaction almost always occurs within minutes of exposure to sunlight, and subsides completely after one to several hours.

The pathogenesis of solar urticaria appears to involve hypersensitivity to a specific photoallergen generated in the skin or plasma following irradiation [6]. Serum histamine and mast cell–derived chemotactic factors have been detected in blood obtained from the irradiated skin of patients, indicating the important role of mast cells in the pathogenesis [7].

Diagnosis of solar urticaria can be confirmed by photo testing. Urticaria can develop within minutes after irradiation with the appropriate wavelength (UVB, UVA, or visible). The remainder of the diagnostic workup is negative, including photo tests, which are read at 24 hours. Solar urticaria may also be seen in patients with systemic lupus erythematosus.

Treatment includes photoprotection with clothing and sunscreens along with antihistamines to suppress symptoms. Oral β-carotene is ineffective [8], while the induction

		Photo tests			
Condition	**Action spectrum**	**MED-A**	**MED-B**	**Visible**	**Photopatch tests**
Polymorphous light eruption	UVA, UVB, visible	NL	NL	NL	Negative
Solar urticaria	UVA, UVB, visible	NL*	NL*	NL*	Negative
Photoallergy	UVA	Decreased†	NL	NL	Positive
Phototoxicity	UVA	Decreased†	NL	NL	Not done

*Lesions may be induced within minutes of irradiation; †decreased only in patients exposed to systemic photosensitizers.
MED—minimal erythema dose; NL—normal; UV—ultraviolet.

TABLE 13-3 COMMON PHOTODERMATOSES

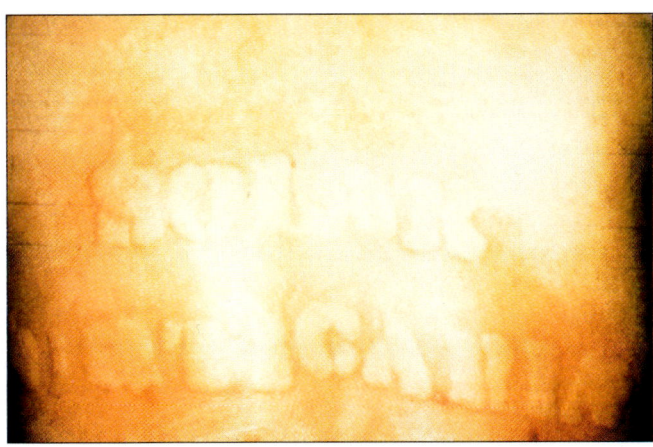

FIGURE 13-4 Urticaria on the back appearing within minutes of sun exposure in a patient with solar urticaria. (*From* Hawk and Norris [24]; with permission.)

of tolerance by UVB or PUVA has been moderately successful [9].

CHEMICAL PHOTOSENSITIVITY

Photoallergy and phototoxicity (Table 13-3) both require the concomitant presence of a photosensitizer and the appropriate radiation for the development of skin lesions.

Photoallergy

Photoallergy is by definition an immune-mediated response [10•]. The photoallergen in the skin absorbs photons and is converted to a stable or unstable photo product, which then binds to a carrier protein to form an antigen. After the initial sensitization, a delayed hypersensitivity response ensues, which causes the cutaneous lesions on subsequent exposures (Fig. 13-5).

Photoallergic reactions can occur following exposure to either a systemic or topical photosensitizer, and can be induced by a relatively minute quantity of photoallergen. The reaction usually occurs in a sensitized individual 24 to 48 hours after the combined exposure to both the photoallergen and UV light.

Clinically, photoallergic reactions are eczematous in morphology, resembling the types of allergic contact dermatitis caused by poisoning. Histopathologically, epidermal spongiosis and a pronounced dermal infiltrate made up predominantly of lymphocytes and histiocytes is present.

The list of agents causing photoallergic dermatitis is exhaustive. Table 13-4 lists commonly encountered agents inducing photoallergy.

Photopatch testing of patients with photoallergic dermatitis is always positive and confirms the diagnosis. Patients with photoallergy to systemic agents have a lowered MED to UVA; however, those with photoallergy to topical agents have a normal MED to UVA if photo testing is performed on sites unexposed to the agents.

Treatment of photoallergic dermatitis rests on recognition of the photosensitizer and its elimination from the patient's environment. Sun exposure should be avoided; topical corticosteriods can offer symptomatic relief.

Phototoxicity

In contrast to photoallergy, phototoxicity is not an immune-mediated response. Rather, the mechanism of phototoxic reactions is a direct toxic one, with the pathways involved varying in an agent-specific manner. For example, furo-coumarins react with UV light to induce monoadducts and

FIGURE 13-5 Mechanism of photoallergic reactions.

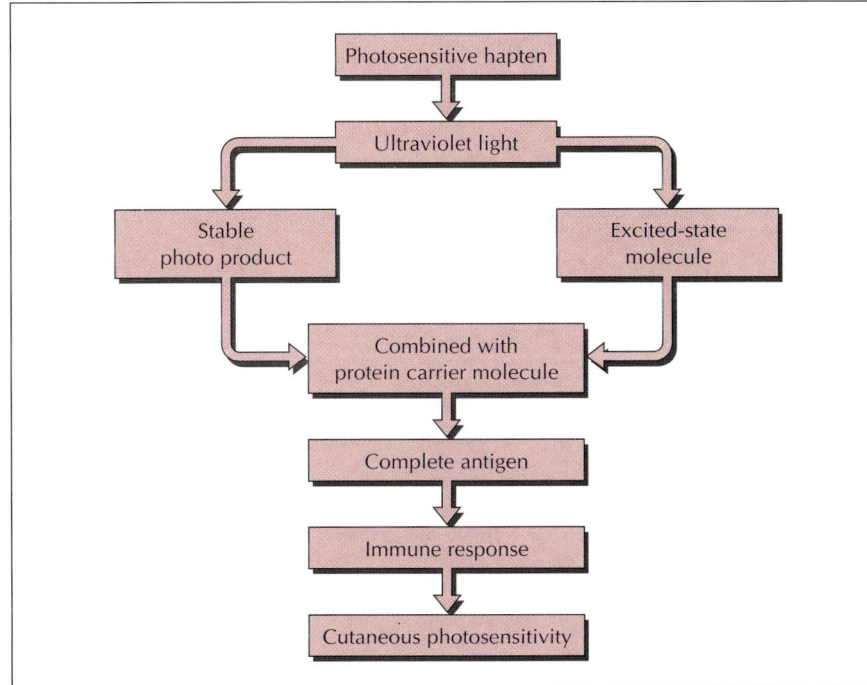

TABLE 13-4 COMMON AGENTS INDUCING PHOTOALLERGIC DERMATITIS	
Antibacterials	**Sunscreens**
Sulfanilamide	PABA, PABA ester
Chlorhexidine	Benzophenones
Hexachlorophene	Cinnamates
Fragrances	**Therapeutic agents**
Musk ambrette	Diphenhydramine
6-methylcoumarin	Thiazides
Sandalwood oil	Sulfonylureas
	Chlorpromazine
	Promethazine

PABA—para-aminobenzoic acid.

TABLE 13-5 COMMON AGENTS INDUCING PHOTOTOXICITY	
Coal tar derivatives	**Furocoumarins**
Anthracene	8-methoxypsoralen
Phenanthrene	4,5,8-trimethylpsoralen
Crude coal tar	
	Plants
Drugs	Lime, lemon
Phenothiazines	Celery
Sulfonamides	Parsley
Doxycycline	Parsnip
Minocycline	Fig
Tetracycline (rarely)	

cross-linking of DNA, while other photosensitizers such as tars and porphyrins induce cellular membrane damage through the production of excited oxygen species [11]. Table 13-5 lists the common agents inducing phototoxicity.

Phototoxic reactions can occur in all individuals if they have been exposed to a sufficient amount of photosensitizing chemical and radiation. However, to elicit a phototoxic reaction, a considerably greater amount of photosensitizer is necessary than in photoallergic reactions. In contrast to photoallergic reactions, no prior sensitization is required; patients may develop phototoxicity after the first exposure to the photosensitizers (Table 13-6).

The onset of phototoxic reactions can be within minutes to hours of exposure to the photosensitizer. Clinically, an exaggerated sunburn response is present, with erythema, edema, and possibly bullae on involved skin (Fig. 13-6). Histopathologically, epidermal spongiosis with necrotic keratinocytes is present.

As in photoallergic dermatitis, the action spectrum of phototoxic reactions is in the UVA range. However, photopatch testing should not be performed, since the agents inducing phototoxicity are photoirritants and will produce positive results in all individuals. Thus, the diagnosis of phototoxicity must be made on the basis of history and morphology.

Treatment of phototoxicity is similar to that of photoallergic dermatitis: avoidance of the photosensitizer, photoprotection, and topical corticosteroids for symptomatic relief.

CHRONIC ACTINIC DERMATITIS

Chronic actinic dermatitis consists of a spectrum of chronic photosensitivity disorders described previously under other terminologies, including persistent light reactivity, photosensitive eczema, and actinic reticuloid [12•] (Table 13-7). Clinical presentation ranges from erythematous patches and plaques to lichenified papules and plaques on sun-exposed areas (Fig. 13-7). Transition within the spectrum of CAD, although not invariable, does occur in some patients.

TABLE 13-6 COMPARISON OF PHOTOALLERGY AND PHOTOTOXICITY		
	Photoallergy	**Phototoxicity**
Occurrence on first exposure	No	Yes
Onset after UV exposure	24–48 h	Min to h
Clinical morphology	Eczematous	Sunburn
Histology	Spongiotic dermatitis	Necrotic kertinocytes
Action spectrum	UVA	UVA
Photo tests	↓ MED to UVA*	↓ MED to UVA*
Photopatch tests	Positive	Not done
Diagnosis	Photopatch testing	History and clinical picture

*Caused by systemic agents. Those caused by topical agents have normal MED to UVA.
↓—decreased; MED—minimal erythema dose; UV—ultraviolet.

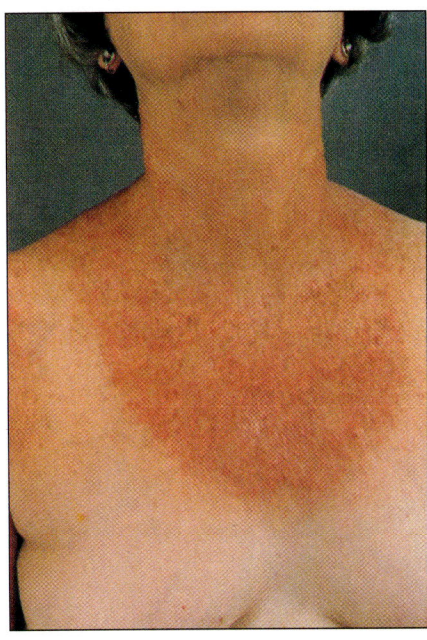

FIGURE 13-6 Phototoxicity presenting as erythema on the upper chest, with sharp cutoff at areas covered by clothing.

protein which binds the photoallergen is altered by UV radiation, resulting in the formation of a neoantigen (an altered carrier protein) which initiates a delayed hypersensitivity response. Sensitivity to contact allergens such as *Compositae oleoresins*, fragrances and lichens, an impaired ability to repair tissue damage induced by oxygen-free radicals, and possible persistence of photoallergens in the skin, have all been postulated to play a role in the pathogenesis of CAD.

Management of patients with CAD consists of restriction of UV light exposure, with the use of broad-spectrum sunscreens and topical corticosteroids for symptomatic relief. If these are ineffective, PUVA, hydroxychloroquine, azathioprine, or cyclosporin A are efficacious in some patients [15–17].

Persistent light reactivity usually begins as a photocontact dermatitis, but patients remain exquisitely sensitive to sunlight for many years. Photopatch tests in these patients are usually positive, although negative results have been observed. In contrast to photoallergy to topical agents, photo testing reveals lowered MEDs to UVB, UVA, or visible light. A skin biopsy specimen of persistent light reactivity demonstrates a spongiotic dermatitis with a lymphohistiocytic infiltrate.

Patients with photosensitive eczema present with an eczematous eruption, lowered MED to UVB, and negative photopatch tests. Histopathologic findings are similar to those seen with persistent light reactivity.

Like patients with persistent light reactivity, patients with actinic reticuloid also have lowered MEDs to UVB, UVA, or visible light. Photopatch tests may be either positive or negative. Diagnosis of actinic reticuloid is confirmed by histologic evidence of atypical mononuclear cells in the epidermis and dermis, changes which are indistinguishable from those seen in cutaneous T-cell lymphoma.

The pathophysiology of CAD is only partially understood [13,14]. It has been postulated that the carrier

PHOTOAGGRAVATED DERMATOSES

Photoaggravated dermatoses are a group of heterogeneous diseases which share the common feature of being induced or exacerbated by exposure to sunlight. Photoaggravation occurs in only a minority of affected patients; for the most part, the action spectra have not been clearly defined. Selected examples of these dermatoses are described below.

Lupus Erythematosus

Photosensitivity is one of the 11 major criteria in the diagnosis of systemic lupus erythematosus (SLE). One third to one half of all patients with SLE are photosensitive. New cutaneous lesions with the morphologic, histologic, and immunofluorescence characteristics of LE may develop after exposure to solar or artificial UV light. The action spectrum for induction of cutaneous lesions in LE includes both UVA and UVB wavelengths [18•].

The pathogenic role of UV radiation is uncertain, but evidence exists to suggest that it can act as a stimulus to immune complex formation. UV light has been shown to increase the immunogenicity of DNA, induce expression of nuclear and cytoplasmic antigens on keratinocyte cell membranes, induce expression and release of proinflammatory factors from keratinocytes, and enhance the activity of a clastogenic factor found in lymphocytes of LE patients [19–22].

TABLE 13-7 SPECTRUM OF CHRONIC ACTINIC DERMATITIS			
Clinical entity	**MED**	**Photopatch test**	**Histology**
Persistent light reactivity	↓ UVB, UVA, visible	+	Spongiotic dermatitis, lymphohistiocytic infiltrate
Photosensitive eczema	↓ UVB	–	Spongiotic dermatitis, lymphohistiocytic infiltrate
Actinic reticuloid	↓ UVB, UVA, visible	±	Atypical mononuclear cells in dermis and epidermis

+—positive; -—negative; ↓—decreased; ±—positive in some patients. MED—minimal erythema dose; UV—ultraviolet.

TABLE 13-8 PHOTOAGGRAVATED DERMATOSES

Acne vulgaris	Herpes simplex
Atopic dermatitis	Lupus erythematosus
Bloom's syndrome	Pellagra
Darier's disease	Pemphigus foliaceus
Disseminated superficial actinic porokeratosis	Pemphigus erythematosus
Benign familial pemphigus (Hailey-Hailey disease)	Transient acantholytic dermatosis
	Hartnup disease

Pellagra

Pellagra results from a deficiency of niacin or its precursor, the essential amino acid tryptophan. It is characterized by the triad of dermatitis (erythema, desquamation, hyperpigmentation), gastroenteritis, and encephalopathy. Prominent skin changes are precipitated by sun exposure, with a tendency to appear in the spring and summer and to improve in the winter.

Niacin, in the form of nicotinamide, is necessary for the synthesis of nicotinamide adenine dinucleotide (NAD) and NAD phosphate. A deficiency of niacin causes decreased availability of these cofactors, which appear to be essential for oxidation and reduction reactions to repair epidermal damage after UV exposure.

Hartnup Disease

Hartnup disease, inherited as an autosomally recessive trait, is a disorder of tryptophan absorption from the gastrointestinal tract and renal tubule. Clinically, it is characterized by pellagralike photosensitivity dermatitis, cerebellar ataxia, and mental retardation. The pellagralike dermatitis appears to be the result of a defect in niacin production due to the decreased tryptophan absorption.

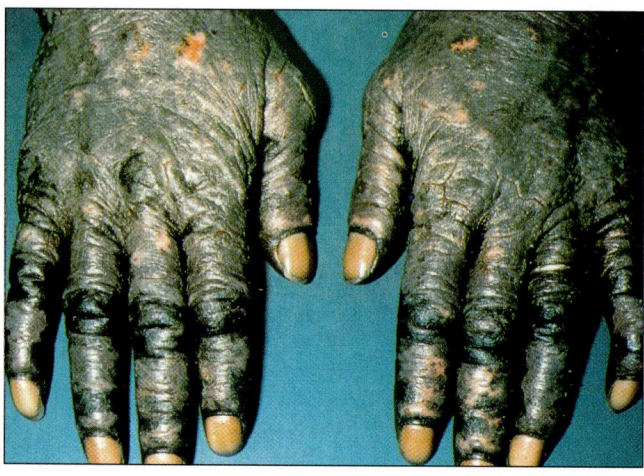

FIGURE 13-7 Lichenification and excoriation on the dorsum of the hands of a patient with chronic actinic dermatitis.

Pemphigus Foliaceus and Pemphigus Erythematosus

Pemphigus foliaceus and erythematosus are chronic, autoimmune, blistering dermatoses characterized by deposition of intercellar IgG throughout the epidermis. Sun exposure has been shown to induce cutaneous lesions [23].

REFERENCES AND RECOMMENDED READING

Recently published papers of particular interest have been highlighted as:
• Of interest
•• Of outstanding interest

1. Parrish JA, Levine MJ, Morison WL, *et al.*: Comparison of PUVA and beta-carotene in the treatment of polymorphous light eruption. *Br J Dermatol* 1979, 100:187–191.

2. Hölzle E, Plewig G, von Kries R, Lehmann P: Polymorphous light eruption. *J Invest Dermatol* 1987, 88:32s–38s.

3.• Hönigsmann H: Polymorphous light eruption. In *Clinical Photomedicine*. Edited by Lim HW, Soter NA. New York: Marcel Dekker; 1993:167–180.

4. Molin L, Volden G: Treatment of polymorphous light eruption with PUVA and prednisolone. *Photodermatol* 1987, 4:107–108.

5. Murphy GM, Logan RA, Lorell CR *et al.*: Prophylactic PUVA and UVB therapy in polymorphic light eruption—a controlled trial. *Br J Dermatol* 1987, 116:531—538.

6. Leenutaphong V, Hölzle E, Plewig G: Pathogenesis and classification of solar urticaria: a new concept. *J Am Acad Dermatol* 1989, 21:237–240.

7. Neittaanmaki H, Jaaskelainen T, Harvima RJ, Fraki JE: Solar urticaria: demonstration of histamine release and effective treatment with doxepin. *Photodermatol* 1989, 6:52–55.

8. Kobza Black A: Oral beta-carotene therapy in actinic reticuloid and solar urticaria. Failure to demonstrate a photoprotective effect against long-wave UV and visible radiation. *Br J Dermatol* 1973, 88:157–166.

9. Addo HA, Sharma SC: UVB phototherapy and photochemotherapy (PUVA) in the treatment of polymorphic light eruption and solar urticaria. *Br J Dermatol* 1987, 116:539–547.

10.• DeLeo VA: Photoallergy. In *Clinical Photomedicine*. Edited by Lim HW, Soter NA. New York: Marcel Dekker, 1993:227–239.

11. Gange RW, Lim HW: Photobiology and pathophysiology of cutaneous responses to electromagnetic radiation. In *Pathophysiology and Dermatologic Diseases*, edn 2. Edited by Soter NA, Baden HP. New York: McGraw Hill, 1990:395–423.

12.• Lim HW, Morison W, Kamide R, *et al.*: Chronic actinic dermatitis: an analysis of 51 patients evaluated in the United States and Japan. *Arch Dermatol* 1994, 130:1284–1289.

13. Norris PG, Hawk JLM: Chronic actinic dermatitis: a unifying concept. Arch Dermatol 1990, 126:376–378.

14. Addo HA, Sharma SC, Ferguson J, *et al.*: A study of compositae plant extract reactions in photosensitivity dermatitis. *Photodermatol* 1985, 2:68–79.

15. Yokel B, Morison WL: PUVA therapy of chronic photosensitive eczema. *Arch Dermatol* 1990, 126:1283–1285.

16. Haynes HA, Bernhard JD, Gange RW: Actinic reticuloid: response to combination treatment with azathioprine, hydroxychloroquine, and prednisone. *J Am Acad Dermatol* 1984, 10:947–952.

17. Norris PG, Camp RDR, Hawk JLM: Actinic reticuloid: response to cyclosporine. *J Am Acad Dermatol* 1989, 21:301–309.

18.• Lehmann P, Hölze E, Kind P, *et al.*: Experimental reproduction of skin lesions in lupus erythematosus by UVA and UVB radiation. *J Am Acad Dermatol* 1990, 22:181–187.

19. Lee LA, Norris DA: Mechanisms of cutaneous tissue damage in lupus erythematosus. *Immunol Series* 1989, 46:359–386.

20. Furukawa F, Kashihara-Sawami M, Lyons MB, Norris DA: Binding of antibodies to the extractable nuclear antigens SS-A/Ro and SS-B/La is induced on the surface of human keratinocytes by ultraviolet light (UVL): implications for the pathogenesis of photosensitive cutaneous lupus. *J Invest Dermatol* 1990, 94:77–85.

21. Golan TD, Elkon KB, Gharavi AE, Krueger JG: Enhanced membrane binding of autoantibodies to cultured keratinocytes of systemic lupus erythematosus patients after ultraviolet B/ultraviolet A irradiation. *J Clin Invest* 1992, 90:1067–1076.

22. Steinberg AD, Gourley MF, Klinman DM, et al.: NIH conference. Systemic lupus erythematosus. *Ann Intern Med* 1991, 115:548–559.

23. Deschamps P, Pedailles S, Michel M, Leroy D: Photoinduction of lesions in a patient with pemphigus erythematosus. *Photodermatol* 1984, 1:38–41.

24. Hawk JLM, Norris PG: Abnormal responses to ultraviolet radiation: idiopathic. In *Dermatology in General Medicine*, edn 4. Edited by Fitzpatrick TB, Eisen AZ, Wolff K, *et al.* New York: McGraw Hill; 1993:1661—1677.

14 Collagen-Vascular Diseases

Jeffrey P. Callen

Key Points
- Cutaneous disease is a common feature of lupus erythematosus, dermatomyositis, and sclerodermoid syndromes.
- The skin changes can be the initial feature of these disorders and the most prominent feature.
- Recognition of subsets of cutaneous lupus erythematosus can aid in the prognostic prediction.
- Dermatomyositis, while predominantly a disease of the skin and muscle, can be associated with multisystem changes.
- Appropriate testing to evaluate for malignancy should occur in the patient with dermatomyositis.
- Any treatment of these disorders should be tailored to the specific findings in each disorder.

The term *collagen-vascular diseases* is widely used to encompass systemic disorders with prominent musculoskeletal abnormalities. These disorders have been linked to immunologic aberrations. There is frequent cutaneous involvement, and in fact, many of the diseases were described and named based on the dermatologic findings. In this chapter, we discuss the three more common types of these disorders in which skin disease is an important feature: lupus erythematosus, dermatomyositis, and sclerodermoid syndromes.

LUPUS ERYTHEMATOSUS

Lupus erythematosus is a multisystem disorder that spans from a relatively benign, self-limited cutaneous eruption to a severe, often fatal, systemic disease. The American College of Rheumatology has developed a set of criteria to be used for the classification of systemic lupus erythematosus (SLE) (Table 14-1) [1]. When a patient meets four or more of the criteria either concurrently or serially during any period of observation, the patient is classified as having SLE.

In the 1940s and 1950s, dermatologists first recognized that most of their patients with chronic, scarring, discoid lupus erythematosus (DLE) lesions had few, if any, systemic findings, whereas those with photosensitivity, malar erythema, or both frequently had systemic disease. They also recognized a middle group in whom the skin lesions were more transient, resolved without scarring, and in whom there was frequent, non–life-threatening systemic disease. The classification of cutaneous subsets was stressed by Gilliam and Sontheimer [2], who proposed that patients be classified into two groups by the type of skin disease present: those that are histopathologically lupus erythematosus specific or those that are not histopathologically specific (Table 14–2).

TABLE 14-1 CRITERIA FOR THE DIAGNOSIS OF SYSTEMIC LUPUS ERYTHEMATOSUS*

Malar rash

Discoid lupus erythematosus lesions

Photosensitivity, by history or observation

Oral ulcers, usually painless, observed by physician

Nonerosive arthritis involving two or more joints

Serositis and pleuritis or pericarditis

Renal disorder: proteinuria (> 500 mg/d) or cellular casts

Central nervous system disorder: seizures or psychosis (absence of known cause)

Hematologic disorder: hemolytic anemia, leukopenia (< 4000/mm^3) or thrombocytopenia (< 10,000/mm^3)

Immunologic disorder: positive lupus erythematosus preparation, abnormal titer of antinative DNA and anti-Sm, false-positive result on VDRL test

Antinuclear antibody

*If four or more criteria are present serially or simultaneously during any observation, the patient is said to have systemic lupus erythematosus.

VDRL—Venereal Disease Research Laboratory.

From Tan and coworkers [1]; with permission.

LE-specific histopathology

Chronic cutaneous LE

  Discoid LE (widespread vs localized)

  Hypertrophic or verrucous LE

  Palmar or plantar LE

  Oral discoid LE

  LE panniculitis

SCLE

  Polymorphous light eruption-like lesions

  Annular lesions

    Oriental SCLE (annular erythema of primary Sjögren's syndrome)

  Papulosquamous lesions (photosensitive psoriasis?)

  Neonatal LE

  C2-deficient LE-like syndrome

  Drug-induced SCLE

Acute cutaneous LE

  Malar erythema

  Photosensitivity dermatitis

  Generalized erythema

LE-nonspecific histopathology

Vasculopathy

  Urticaria

  Vasculitis

  Livedo reticularis or leg ulcerations

Mucosal lesions

Nonscarring alopecia

Bullous LE or epidermolysis bullosa acquisita

Associated mucocutaneous problems

  Mucinous infiltrations

  Porphyrias

  Lichen planus

  Psoriasis

  Sjögren's syndrome

  Squamous cell carcinomas

LE—lupus erythematosus; SCLE—subacute cutaneous LE.

Chronic cutaneous lupus erythematosus can be manifested in several clinical variations. The commonest subset is that with DLE lesions [3]. These patients may be classified as having localized DLE, when lesions are only on the head and neck, or widespread DLE, when lesions are on other body surfaces as well as on the head and neck. Other, less common forms of chronic cutaneous lupus erythematosus include hypertrophic or verrucous (wartlike) lesions, lesions on the palms or soles, oral discoid lupus erythematosus, and lupus panniculitis (lupus profundus).

The discoid lupus erythematosus lesion is characterized by erythema; telangiectasia; adherent scale, varying from fine to thick; follicular plugging; dyspigmentation; and atrophy and scarring (Fig. 14-1). The lesions are usually sharply demarcated and can be round, thus giving rise to the term *discoid* (or disklike). The presence of scarring or atrophy is the characteristic that separates these lesions from those of subacute cutaneous lupus erythematosus (SCLE). The differential diagnosis most often includes papulosquamous diseases, such as psoriasis, lichen planus, secondary syphilis, superficial fungal infection, polymorphous light eruption, and sarcoidosis. Histopathologic examination is usually very helpful in confirming a diagnosis, and only rarely is immunofluorescence microscopy necessary.

Hypertrophic or verrucous DLE is a unique subset in which an unusual lesion occurs [4]. The thick, adherent scale is replaced by massive hyperkeratosis, and the lesions look like warts or squamous cell carcinomas (Fig. 14-2). These lesions usually occur in the setting of other, more typical DLE lesions. These patients tend to have

chronic disease, to have few systemic symptoms or laboratory findings, and to be extremely difficult to treat with conventional therapy.

The DLE-SLE subset defines a small group of patients (approximately 5% to 10%) who by the nature of their selection have systemic disease in association with scarring cutaneous disease. Patients who progress from pure cutaneous disease into this group are characterized by widespread DLE, the presence of clinically appreciable periungual telangiectasias, persistent elevated sedimentation rates, leukopenia, and positive antinuclear antibody (ANA). These patients with DLE-SLE rarely have renal disease,

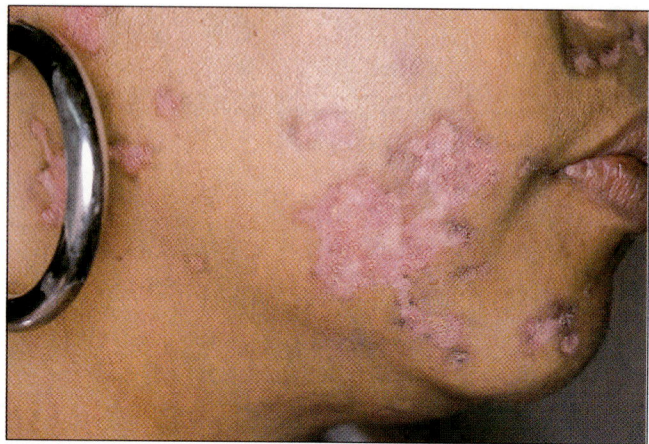

FIGURE 14-1 Discoid lupus erythematosus. This young black woman demonstrates multiple features of discoid lupus erythematosus, including follicular plugging, scarring, atrophy, and dyspigmentation.

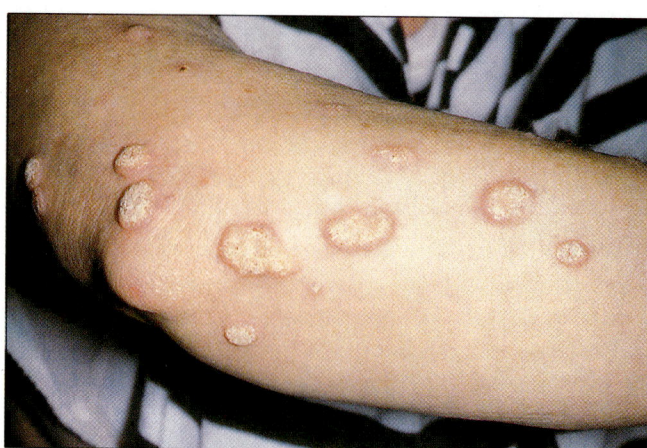

FIGURE 14-2 Hypertrophic (verrucous) lupus erythematosus. These wart-like lesions were present in a patient with typical discoid lupus erythematosus elsewhere. They simulate warts, keratoacanthoma, or squamous cell carcinoma.

and even when they do, it is most often transient and mild. DLE-SLE is a distinct lupus erythematosus subset because of its relatively benign, albeit chronic, course.

Subacute cutaneous lupus erythematosus is a skin lesion that has all the features of DLE without the scarring or atrophy [5•]. Patients whose major cutaneous manifestation is SCLE lesions have been classified as having a subset called SCLE. However, a patient in the SCLE subset can also have scarring lesions of DLE or can have lesions generally associated with SLE, such as a malar rash or vasculitic lesions. Many of the SCLE patients (approximately 50%) fulfill four or more of the American College of Rheumatology criteria for SLE; thus, some authorities have not recognized these patients as forming a distinct subset.

Subacute cutaneous lupus erythematosus skin lesions are of at least two types: annular or papulosquamous. Annular SCLE lesions are characterized by erythematous rings with central clearing (Fig. 14-3). Often a slight scale is present. Lesions of annular SCLE must be differentiated from other figurate erythemas. Papulosquamous SCLE lesions are characterized by plaques and papules with scale (Figs. 14-4 and 14-5). The differential diagnosis of papulosquamous SCLE lesions includes psoriasis and lichen planus. In both annular and papulosquamous SCLE, the lesions often begin as erythematous papules or plaques in a photosensitive distribution (Fig. 14-6). SCLE may be associated with Sjögren's syndrome, idiopathic thrombocytopenic purpura, cutaneous vasculitis, or deficiency of the second component of complement (C2d). SCLE has also been reported to be induced by hydrochlorothiazide.

Malar erythema is the classic butterfly rash from which the name *lupus erythematosus* (wolflike redness) was coined

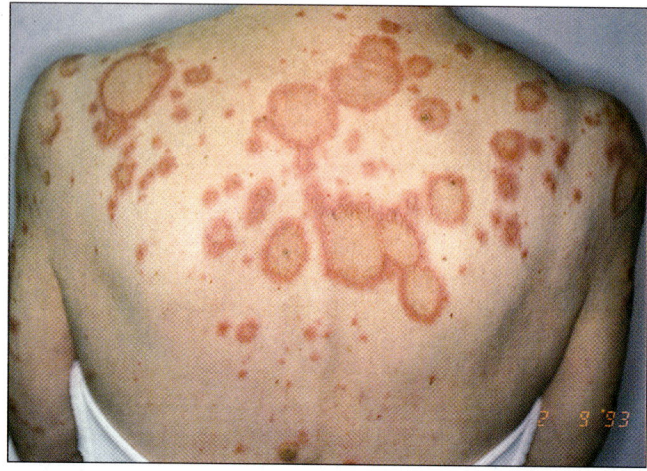

FIGURE 14-3 This erythematosus, annular lesion lacks scarring or atrophy yet represents a histologically specific pattern of lupus erythematosus.

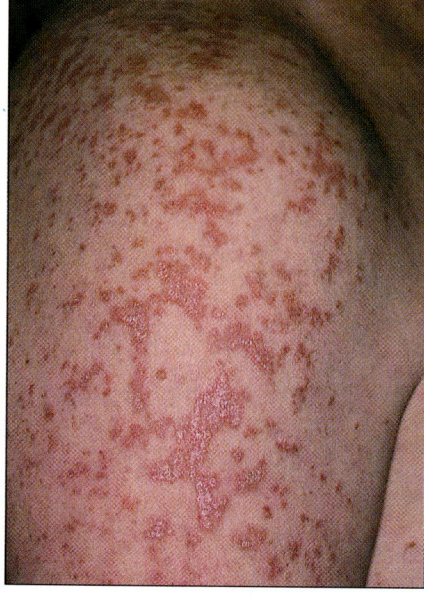

FIGURE 14-4 Subacute cutaneous lupus erythematosus, papulosquamous variant. This patient developed an exquisitely photosensitive eruption with minimal sun exposure.

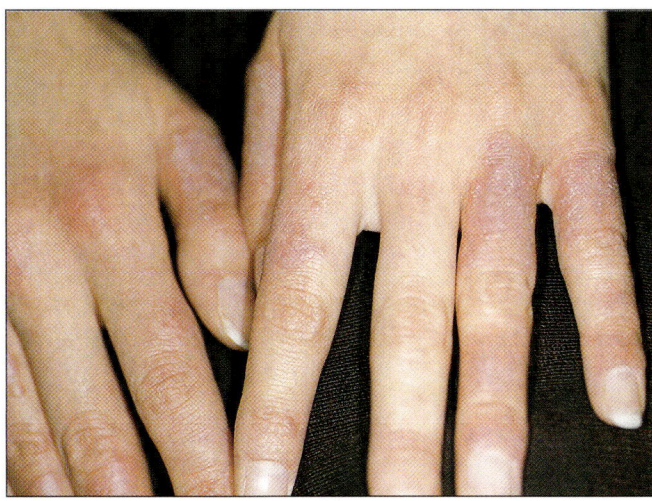

FIGURE 14-5 Lichen planus–like lesions of subacute cutaneous lupus erythematosus.

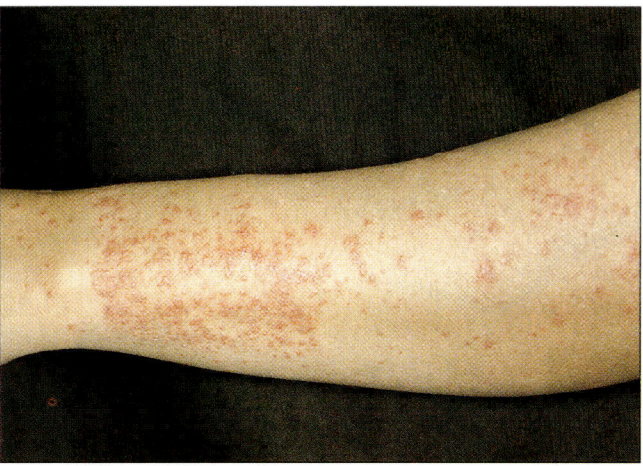

FIGURE 14-6 Erythematous papular lesion of polymorphous light eruption representing a clinical picture similar to that seen in subacute cutaneous lupus erythematosus.

(Fig. 14-7). The rash is induced by sun exposure, usually by ultraviolet B light ranging from 290 to 320 nm. Patients with an active malar butterfly rash usually have active systemic disease, but no specific organ system is involved.

Livedo reticularis, pyoderma gangrenosum–like leg ulcerations, or both may occur in patients with antiphospholipid antibodies (anticardiolipin and lupus anticoagulant) [6•]. Many such patients have lupus erythematosus, but some have primary antiphospholipid antibody syndrome. These patients have arterial occlusions, which can result in transient ischemic attacks, cerebrovascular accidents, and recurrent fetal loss; venous occlusion, which can result in thrombophlebitis, renal or hepatic vein occlusion, or pulmonary embolism; thrombocytopenia; and cardiac valvular vegetations and dysfunction.

Laboratory Abnormalities in Patients With Cutaneous Lupus Erythematosus

The ANA is a system that represents many antibodies to multiple substrates [7••]. The frequency of a positive ANA correlates with the substrate used. The reported pattern of the ANA may also correlate with specific antibodies; however, except when interpreted by experts, the ANA pattern is not highly specific. Table 14-3 represents the frequency of these antibodies in the subsets discussed. Antinative (double-stranded) DNA correlates with active SLE and, in particular, active renal disease. Anti-Ro (SS-A) was initially described in patients with ANA-negative lupus erythematosus and Sjögren's syndrome. However, it is also present in mothers who have babies with neonatal lupus erythmatosus, individuals with cutaneous vasculitis associated with SCLE, those with C_2 deficient lupus erythematosus syndromes, and patients with hydrochlorothiazide -induced SCLE. Therapy should not be based solely on these laboratory abnormalities.

Cutaneous immunofluorescence was applied as a diagnostic and prognostic tool that led to a better understanding of lupus erythematosus. Lesional immunofluorescence may be helpful when the clinical and histopathologic diagnosis is in question. However, one must realize that normal facial skin can demonstrate 10% to 20% false-positive reactions [8•]. The use of noninvolved, "nonexposed" skin in the lupus band test is believed to correlate with active renal disease. Refined antibody testing has reduced the need for immunofluorescence testing.

Therapy for Cutaneous Lupus Erythematosus

Before therapy is begun, the clinician must evaluate the patient thoroughly to determine the extent of disease and to be able to reassure the patient of the benign nature of the process. Table 14-4 lists the testing that should be ordered, and Table 14-5 the therapeutic options available.

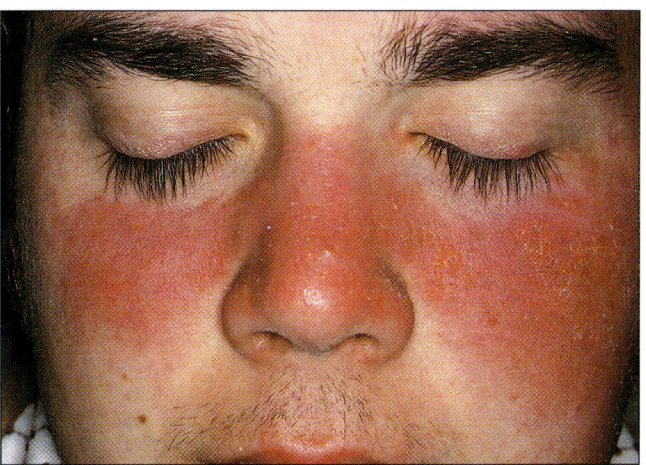

FIGURE 14-7 Systemic lupus erythematosus. This young man has a very typical butterfly eruption of systemic lupus erythematosus.

TABLE 14-3 FREQUENCY OF AUTOANTIBODIES IN VARIOUS CLINICAL SUBSETS OF LUPUS ERYTHEMATOSUS*

Test	DLE	HLE	DLE/SLE	SCLE	NLE	ACLE
ANA	5–10	5	75	50–75	60–90	95
Anti-ssDNA	35	25	75	20–50	?	90
Anti-nDNA	< 5	< 5	10	10	10–50	70
Anti-RNP (U₁RNP)	< 5	25	?	10	?	40
Anti-Sm	< 5	5	5	10	?	25
Anti-Ro (SS-A)	5	5–10	5	40–95	90	30
Anti-La (SS-B)	5	5	5	15	15–20	10

*All numbers given are percentages.

ACLE—acute cutaneous lupus erythematosus; ANA—antinuclear antibody; DLE—discoid lupus erythematosus; HLE—hypertrophic lupus erythematosus; nDNA—native DNA; NLE—neonatal lupus erythematosus; RNP—ribonucleoprotein; SCLE—subacute cutaneous lupus erythematosus; SLE—systemic lupus erythematosus; ssDNA—single-stranded DNA.

Photosensitivity is a major factor in all types of cutaneous lupus erythematosus. Almost all SCLE patients are photosensitive, and approximately 60% to 75% of SLE patients demonstrate photosensitivity. This reaction is induced by ultraviolet B light, but in some individuals, ultraviolet A light (320 to 360 nm) can be involved as well [9••]. Therefore, one of the most important therapeutic manipulations is the use of sunscreens and sun avoidance. Sunscreens with a sun protective factor of at least 15 are to be used every day. Topical corticosteroids should be prescribed in conjunction with other agents. The specific agent used is chosen based on the clinical lesion and area of the body affected. The prescribing physician must remember that these agents can produce atrophy, which is also a sign of the disease. Lesions that do not respond to topical agents can be injected intralesionally with a corticosteroid, such as triamcinolone acetonide (3 to 4 mg/mL).

Antimalarial agents form a mainstay of systemic therapy of cutaneous lupus erythematosus. The mechanism of action of these agents is unknown, but it may relate to photoprotection, immunomodulation, or both. The agents available include hydroxychloroquine hydrochloride and

TABLE 14-4 EVALUATION OF THE PATIENT WITH CUTANEOUS LUPUS ERYTHEMATOSUS

Standard testing

Careful history and physical examination
Skin biopsy for routine histology
Complete blood count with differential and platelet count
Serum multiphasic analysis
Antinuclear antibody
Serological tests
Antinative DNA
Anti-RNP (U₁RNP)
Anti-Ro (SS-A)
Erythrocyte sedimentation rate
Urinalysis
Total hemolytic complement (if abnormal, C3, C2, C4 levels)
Creatinine clearance

Optional tests

Serum protein electrophoresis
Circulating immune complexes
Immunofluorescence skin biopsy
Antiphospholipid antibodies

RNP—ribonucleoprotein.

TABLE 14-5 THERAPEUTIC AGENTS USED TO TREAT CUTANEOUS LUPUS ERYTHEMATOSUS

Standard therapy

Sunscreens
Topical corticosteroids
Intralesional corticosteroids (avoid atrophy)
Antimalarials
    Hydroxychloroquine: potential ocular toxicity
    Chloroquine: potential ocular toxicity

Alternatives

Dapsone (best for bullous lupus erythematosus, vasculitis)
Auranofin (oral gold)
Accutane (13-*cis*-retinoic acid)
Clofazimine
Low-dose cytotoxic agents, *eg*, azathioprine or methotrexate
Systemic corticosteroids (poorly effective for chronic lesions)
Interferon (recombinant interferon α)

chloroquine phosphate. Chloroquine and hydroxychloroquine may be associated with retinopathy. Hydroxychloroquine is given orally in a dosage of 200 to 400 mg/d.

DERMATOMYOSITIS

Dermatomyositis is a condition that combines an inflammatory myopathy with a characteristic cutaneous disease. This disorder is related to polymyositis, which has similar features to the muscle disease caused by dermatomyositis but lacks the characteristic cutaneous findings. These disorders are of unknown etiology, but immune-mediated muscle damage is believed to be an important pathogenetic mechanism. Dermatomyositis appears to be characterized by an increased frequency of internal malignancy, whereas the association with malignancy in patients with polymyositis is less well resolved. Both dermatomyositis and polymyositis may occur in children, and both disorders are associated with morbidity and occasional mortality; therefore, a prompt and aggressive approach to therapy is indicated.

Bohan and Peter [10] suggested the use of five criteria to define the entities of polymyositis and dermatomyositis and also suggested a classification system. The criteria include:

Proximal symmetric muscle weakness that progresses over
a period of weeks to months
Elevated serum levels of muscle-derived enzymes
Abnormal electromyographic results
Abnormal muscle biopsy results
The presence of cutaneous disease compatible with
dermatomyositis

The following system of classification has been useful in differentiating groups of patients:

Dermatomyositis
Polymyositis
Myositis with malignancy
Childhood myositis
Overlap syndromes with other collagen vascular disease
and myositis
Inclusion body myositis
Dermatomyositis-sine-myositis (amyopathic dermato-
myositis)

Clinical Manifestations

The characteristic and possibly pathognomonic cutaneous features of dermatomyositis are the heliotrope rash and Gottron's papules. Several other cutaneous features that occur in patients who have dermatomyositis are characteristic of the disease despite not being pathognomonic and include malar erythema, poikiloderma in a photosensitive distribution, violaceous erythema on the extensor surfaces, and periungual and cuticular changes.

The heliotrope rash consists of a dark lilac discoloration or a violaceous to dusky erythematous rash with or without edema in a symmetric distribution involving periorbital skin

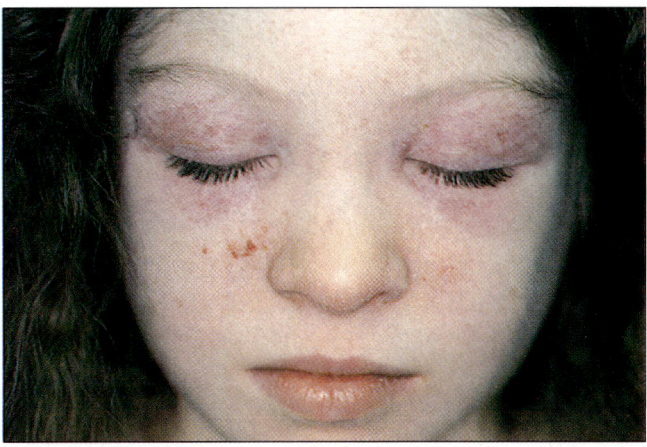

FIGURE 14-8 Dermatomyositis. This young girl developed inflammatory myopathy in conjunction with a very typical heliotrope eruption around the eyelids and typical lesions elsewhere on her body.

(Fig. 14–8). Gottron's papules are found over bony prominences, particularly over the metacarpal-phalangeal joints, the proximal interphalangeal joints, or the distal interphalangeal joints (Fig. 14–9). They may also be found over bony prominences, such as the elbows, knees, and feet. Nail fold changes consist of periungual telangiectasias and a characteristic cuticular change with hypertrophy of the cuticle and small, hemorrhagic infarcts within this hypertrophic area (Fig. 14–10). Poikiloderma can occur within Gottron's papules or on exposed skin, such as the extensor surfaces of the arm or "V" of the neck (Fig. 14–11).

Dermatomyositis-sine-myositis is diagnosed when typical cutaneous disease is present without clinical weakness and with normal serum muscle enzyme levels. A small subset of patients never develop myositis, despite having prominent cutaneous changes [11•]. A larger group exists in whom the myositis resolves with therapy,

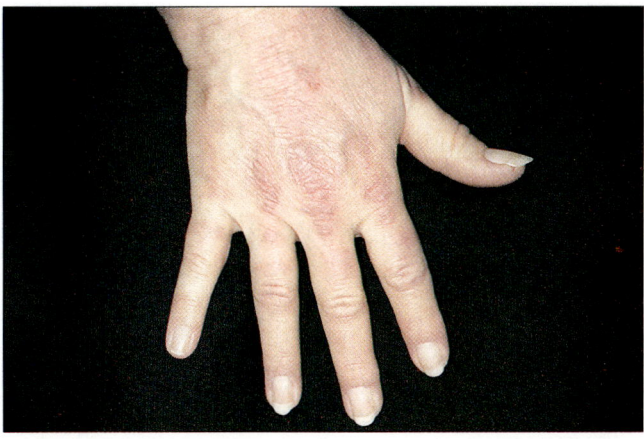

FIGURE 14-9 Gottron's papules. Typical erythematous to violaceous lesions over the bony prominences on the extensor surfaces of the hands.

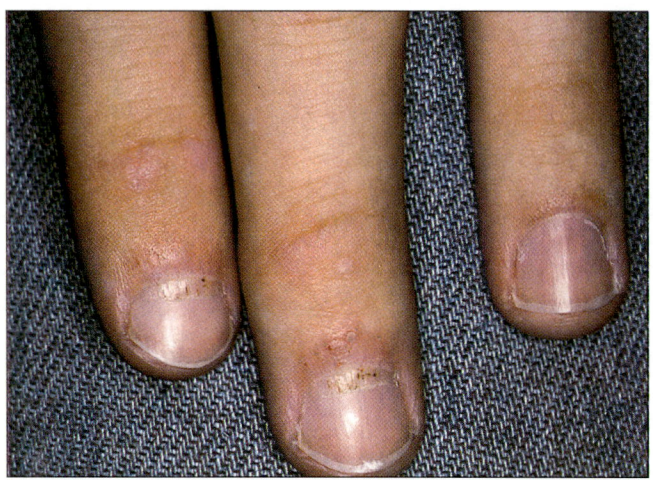

FIGURE 14-10 Cuticular hypertrophy, splinter hemorrhages, and periungual telangiectasias are present in this patient with dermatomyositis.

and the skin disease becomes the most important feature of the disease.

Clinical and laboratory abnormalities suggestive of muscle disease are characteristic features of dermatomyositis and polymyositis. Even in patients who initially have only skin disease, myositis often eventually follows. The myopathy affects mainly proximal muscle groups of the shoulder and pelvic girdle muscles, and the disease is usually symmetric. Initial complaints include weakness, fatigue, an inability to climb stairs, an inability to raise the arms for actions like hair grooming or shaving, an inability to rise from a squatting or sitting position, or a combination of these features. The progression of disease is variable but usually occurs over a period of weeks to months. An inability to swallow and symptoms of aspiration may reflect the involvement of striated muscle of the pharynx or upper esophagus. Dysphagia often signifies a rapidly

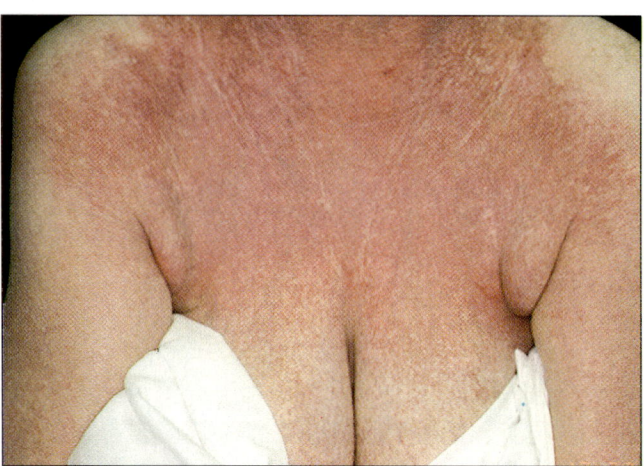

FIGURE 14-11 Poikilodermatous eruption in the photosensitive distribution is present in this woman with dermatomyositis.

progressive course and may be associated with a poor prognosis.

The laboratory abnormalities are enzyme elevations, disturbances of electrical action, histopathologic changes, or all of these. Muscle enzyme levels are frequently elevated in patients with inflammatory myopathy. The enzymes that are commonly elevated are creatine kinase, aldolase, lactic dehydrogenase, and serum transaminases. Creatine kinase determination seems to be the most practical and available test for measuring activity of muscle disease. Occasionally, patients may have normal muscle enzyme levels, and in these individuals, the measurement of creatine excretion in the urine may be reflective of active muscle disease.

Electromyography characteristically shows sharp or positive waves, insertional irritability, fibrillation, and short polyphasic motor units. Innervation remains intact; thus, neuropathic changes do not occur. Muscle biopsy specimens show typical features, including II fiber atrophy, necrosis, regeneration, centralization of the nuclei, and a lymphocytic infiltrate in a perifascicular or perivascular region. Other assessments that may be used are various imaging techniques, in particular, magnetic resonance imaging. In children, levels of von Willebrand factor VIII–related antigen or neopterin may predict a more severe dermatomyositis variant with vasculopathy. However, the use of these tests, particularly the von Willebrand factor VIII–related antigens, adds little to the information obtained with enzyme testing and clinical examination [12•].

Dermatomyositis and polymyositis are multisystem disorders, as is reflected by the high frequency of other clinical features in patients with these diseases. Arthralgias and arthritis may be present in up to 25% of patients with inflammatory myopathy. Esophageal disease, as manifested by dysphagia, is estimated to be present in 15% to 50% of patients with inflammatory myopathy. The dysphagia can be of two types: proximal dysphagia or distal dysphagia. Pulmonary disease occurs in dermatomyositis, and polymyositis, in approximately 15% to 30% of patients. Cardiac disease may also occur in patients with polymyositis, as manifested by myocarditis or pericarditis. Calcinosis of the skin or muscle is unusual in adults but may occur in up to 40% of children with dermatomyositis.

Myositis and Malignancy

The issue of the relationship of dermatomyositis and polymyositis to malignancy remains controversial. The frequency of malignancy in dermatomyositis has varied from 6% to 60% in various studies. This variation is probably related to differing methodology. In 1992, Siguregeirsson and coworkers [13••], in a well-controlled study, clearly documented the increased frequency of malignancy in patients with dermatomyositis over that in the general population. Although polymyositis patients had a slight increase in cancer frequency, it was not highly significant and could be explained by the more aggressive cancer search in these patients. Malignancies may occur before the onset of myositis, concurrently with myositis, or after the onset of dermatomyositis. In addition, the myositis may follow the course of the malignancy (a paraneoplastic course) or its own course independent of the treatment of the malignancy. Siguregeirsson and coworkers also suggested that ovarian cancer might be overrepresented in their group. Other investigators have also reported this finding [14•]. Studies demonstrating benefits of cancer surgery on myositis as well as those showing no relationship of the myositis and malignancy have been reported.

Evaluation

The diagnosis of myositis is one of exclusion (Table 14-6). A complete history should be taken, with particular attention to drugs or toxins that may be involved [15•]. It should include a history of previous malignancies, previous travel, changes in diet, and any symptoms of associated phenomena, such as dysphagia, dyspnea, or arthritis. A thorough review of systems is necessary, which will aid in the evaluation of patients with dermatomyositis for malignancies.

Course and Therapy

Several general measures are helpful in treating patients with dermatomyositis and polymyositis. Bed rest is often valuable in the individual with progressive weakness; however, this measure must be combined with a range-of-motion exercise program to prevent contractures. Nutrition is important because of a negative nitrogen balance that exists in inflammatory myopathy. This feature of treatment is particularly important in children. Patients who have evidence of dysphagia should have the head of their bed elevated and should avoid eating meals before retiring.

The mainstay of therapy for dermatomyositis is the use of systemic corticosteroids. Traditionally, prednisone is given in a dosage of 0.5 to 1 mg/kg/d as the initial therapy [16•]. Approximately 25% to 30% of patients with dermatomyositis or polymyositis do not respond to systemic corticosteroids or develop significant steroid-related side effects. In these patients, immunosuppressive agents (methotrexate, azathioprine, cyclophosphamide, chlorambucil, or cyclosporine) may be an effective means of inducing or maintaining a remission [17•]. The most recent therapeutic maneuver for immunosuppressive-resistant dermatomyositis is the use of intravenous immunoglobulin. Dalakas and coworkers [18••] demonstrated that the myopathy as well as the cutaneous disease improved with this therapy.

Therapy for cutaneous disease in patients with dermatomyositis is often difficult because even though the myositis may respond to treatment with corticosteroids, immunosuppressives, or both, the cutaneous lesions often persist. Although cutaneous disease may be of minor importance in patients with serious fulminant myositis, in many patients cutaneous disease becomes an important aspect of their disorder. Most patients with cutaneous lesions are photosensitive [19]; thus, as in patients with lupus erythematosus, the daily use of a sunscreen with a sun protective factor of at least 15 is recommended. Some may require a broader-spectrum sunscreen. Hydroxychloroquine in dosages of 200 to 400 mg/d is effective in approximately 80% of patients treated as a means of partially controlling their cutaneous disease and allowing a decrease in the corticosteroid dosage [20]. In some patients, the use of low-dose methotrexate has been effective.

TABLE 14-6 EVALUATION OF THE PATIENT WITH MYOSITIS
Careful history
Previous malignancy
Associated symptoms
History of toxins, infections, travel, drug intake, bovine collagen implants, or breast augmentation surgery
Complete physical examination
Dermatologic evaluation
Pelvic and breast examinations in women
Rectal examination in men
Evaluation of muscle disease
Creatine kinase or phosphokinase, aldolase, urinary creatine EMG (if results of laboratory tests are normal)
Muscle biopsy (if EMG and laboratory results are abnormal)
MRI/MRS
Skin disease evaluation
Biopsy
Routine laboratory studies
Complete blood count, serum multiphasic analysis, urinalysis
Chest radiograph
Thyroid function
Stool hematest
Electrocardiogram
Papanicolaou smear, mammography in women
Pulmonary function tests
Esophageal studies
Manometry
Cineradiography
Optional
Holter monitor
Echocardiogram
Autoantibody studies, *eg*, Jo-1, PM, Ku, Mi-2
Viral serologies
Further testing
Based on abnormalities discovered in above tests
EMG—electromyography. MRI—magnetic resonance imaging; MRS—magnetic resonance spectroscopy.

The prognosis of dermatomyositis and polymyositis varies greatly, depending on the series of patients studied. Factors that affect the prognosis include the patient's age, the type and severity of myositis, the presence of dysphagia, the presence of an associated malignancy, duration of disease prior to treatment, and the response to corticosteroid therapy. The fact that therapy alters prognosis seems to be well established by retrospective reports on the benefits of corticosteroids and immunosuppressives.

SCLERODERMA

Scleroderma is a term used to describe a specific clinical disease spectrum represented by cutaneous involvement, multisystem involvement, or both. In addition, several disorders are associated with sclerodermoid changes (Table 14-7). Scleroderma is a disorder of unknown cause and pathogenesis that can be subdivided into two major categories: localized scleroderma and systemic sclerosis.

Localized Scleroderma

Localized scleroderma refers to primary involvement of the skin, with minimal if any systemic features. Only rarely have patients with localized scleroderma developed systemic sclerosis or SLE. Three major types of localized scleroderma exist: morphea, generalized morphea, and linear scleroderma. Morphea is manifested by indurated dermal or subcutaneous plaques (Fig. 14-12). The disease is commonest in young women. Morphea sometimes overlaps or coexists with another cutaneous condition known as *lichen sclerosus et atrophicus*. In contrast, a small number of patients develop numerous and larger lesions, which coalesce (Fig. 14-13). These individuals are said to have *generalized morphea*. Patients with morphea usually have a benign course, characterized by softening of their lesions with time.

TABLE 14-7 SCLERODERMA AND SCLERODERMOID CONDITIONS

Localized scleroderma

Morphea (dermal, subcutaneous and pransclerotic variants)
Linear scleroderma
Generalized morphea

Systemic sclerosis (scleroderma)

Limited (acrosclerosis, CREST variant)
Diffuse
Overlap with another collagen vascular disease (lupus erythematosus or dermatomyositis)
Mixed connective tissue disease

Idiopathic syndromes possibly related to scleroderma

Eosinophilic fasciitis
Eosinophilia myalgia syndrome

Mucinoses

Scleredema
Scleromyxedema (lichen myxedematosus or papular mucinosis)

Chemical or drug-induced sclerosis

Polyvinylchloride
Silicone (breast implants, injectable) or collagen injections
Bleomycin
Spanish rapeseed oil

Metabolic

Porphyria cutanea tarda
Carcinoid syndrome

Immunologic

Chronic graft-vs-host disease

Vibratory injury

CREST—calcinosis, Raynaud's phenomenon, esophageal dysmotility, sclerodactyly, and telangiectasia.

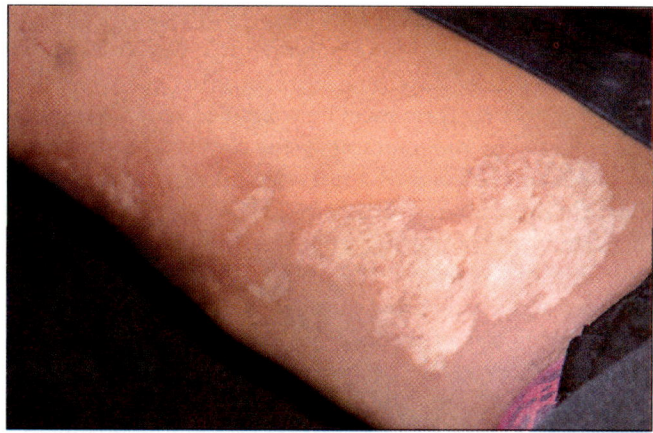

FIGURE 14-12 Morphea. Note discrete sclerotic plaques.

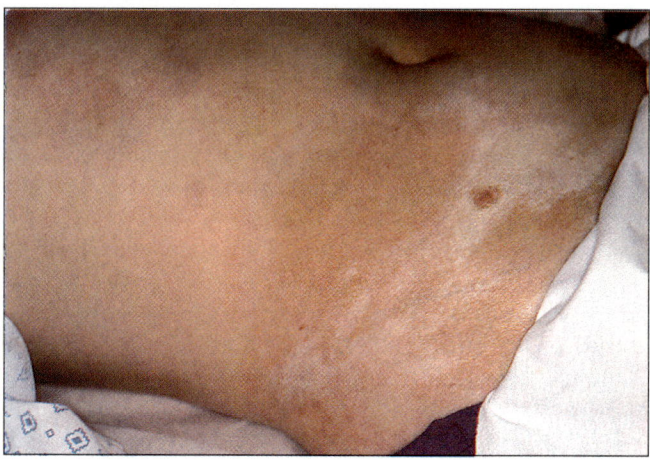

FIGURE 14-13 Generalized morphea. Note coalescent plaques of induration on the trunk.

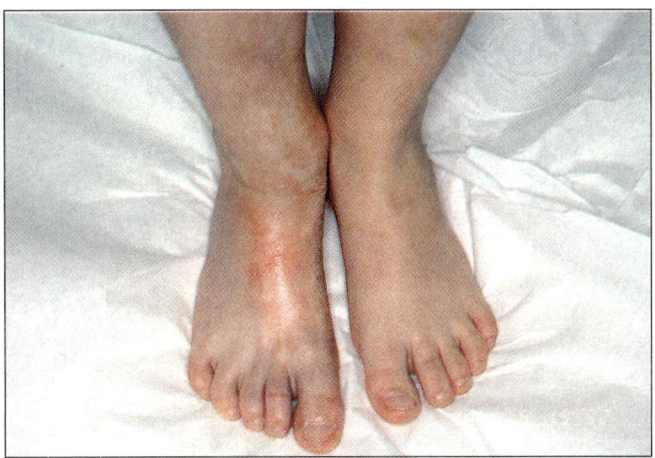

FIGURE 14-14 Linear scleroderma. When this abnormality occurs across a joint, contracture is possible.

Linear scleroderma is most often a single sclerotic linear lesion. This variant is also more common in young women. The disease frequently occurs on the extremities (Fig. 14-14) or the forehead. When on the forehead, the term *en coup de sabre* has been applied (Fig. 14-15). When the disease crosses a joint, limitation of motion is possible, as well as decreased growth [21•]. In addition, facial disfigurement can occur. Linear scleroderma also appears to soften over time, but treatment with physical therapy to reduce the likelihood of permanent contracture is indicated.

Raynaud's Phenomenon and Raynaud's Disease

Classic Raynaud's phenomenon is a triphasic color reaction, usually involving the digits, that is induced by cold or emotional distress. Initial pallor is followed by cyanosis and then a reactive hyperemia. In addition to the color changes, either numbness or pain may occur. Rewarming relieves not only the color changes but also the symptoms. As the disorder progresses, repeated ischemic episodes can result in small pitted areas on the distal digits (Fig. 14-16), ulcerations, or gangrene.

The process is termed *Raynaud's disease* when there is no identifiable cause. However, there are frequent reports of patients with long-standing Raynaud's disease who later develop SLE or systemic sclerosis. The diagnoses that need to be considered in a patient with Raynaud's phenomenon are listed in Table 14-8.

Management of Raynaud's phenomenon is directed at prevention, removal of exacerbating factors, and vasodilatation. Patients may wear gloves and avoid situations that are known to precipitate an episode, such as cold exposure. The use of tobacco (smoking or chewing) should be stopped, and drugs that cause vasoconstriction should be avoided. Drugs that allow for vasodilation are often helpful in reducing the severity or number of episodes that the patient may have. Agents such as topical nitroglycerin, calcium channel blockers (*eg*, nifedipine, diltiazem), and prostacyclin analogues (*eg*, iloprost) have been useful in many patients.

Systemic Sclerosis

Systemic sclerosis (progressive systemic sclerosis) is characterized by cutaneous and internal organ fibrosis. Almost all patients have Raynaud's phenomenon, which is a common presenting manifestation. Systemic sclerosis is much more common in women than in men. The pathogenesis of systemic sclerosis is not known, but theories involve a dysregulation of collagen synthesis, endothelial cell injury, and abnormal immunity.

Patients with systemic sclerosis may be subclassified as having diffuse disease or limited disease. In the limited form, the primary involvement is on acral skin (hands, forearms, legs, and face), whereas in the diffuse form, extensive sclerosis of the proximal portions of the extremities as well as the truncal skin is present. The prognosis generally is poorer in patients with diffuse disease. Sclero-

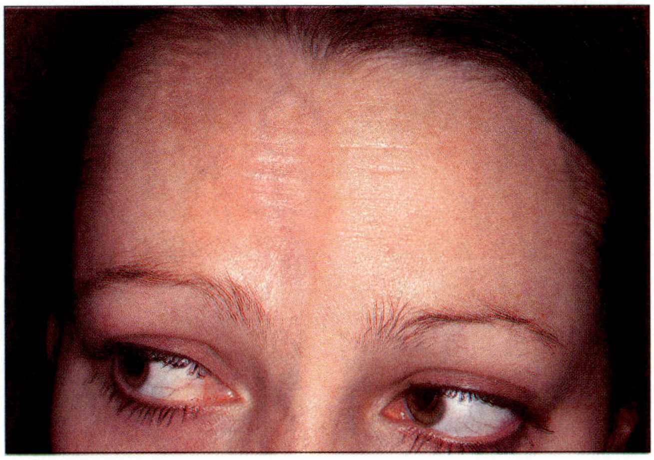

FIGURE 14-15 En coup de sabre. Linear scleroderma involving the facial skin.

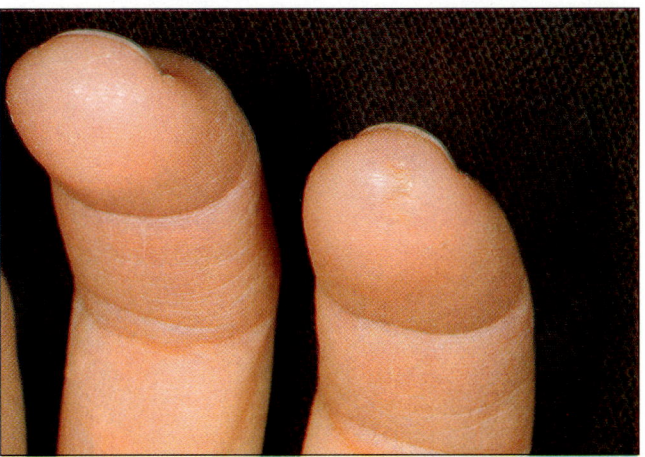

FIGURE 14-16 Pitting of the fingertips is the result of ischemia from severe Raynaud's phenomenon.

TABLE 14-8 CONDITIONS ASSOCIATED WITH RAYNAUD'S PHENOMENON

Collagen-vascular diseases—scleroderma, lupus erythematosus, rheumatoid arthritis, dermatomyositis, vasculitis (polyarteritis nodosa), mixed connective tissue disease

Hematologic disorders—cryoglobulinemia (particularly type I), cryofibrinogenemia, cold agglutinin, macroglobulinemia, hyperglobulinemic purpura, polycythemia, thrombocythemia

Arterial disease—thromboangitis obliterans, atherosclerosis, embolic disease

Drugs—ergots, β-blockers, bleomycin, caffeine, nicotine

Neurovascular compression—thoracic outlet syndrome, carpal tunnel syndrome

Vibratory injury

Malignancy

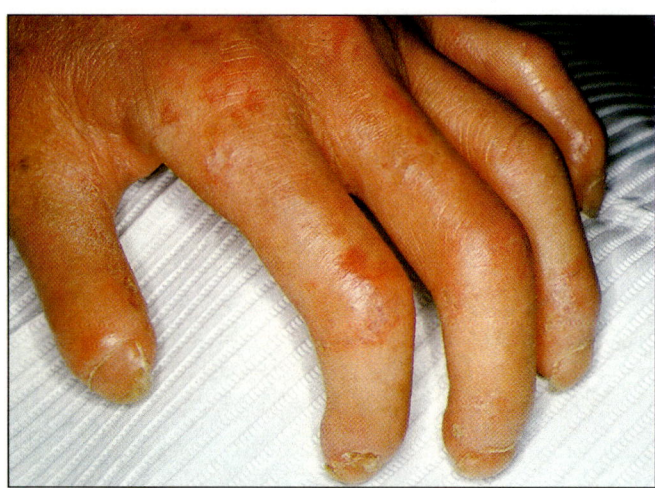

FIGURE 14-17 Sclerodactyly is one of the characteristic findings in systemic sclerosis.

dactyly is a hallmark of the disease in both forms (Fig. 14-17). In addition, abnormal pigmentation is a common finding (Fig. 14-18), as are telangiectasia and nail fold capillary abnormalities (Fig. 14-19). The term *CREST* has been developed to denote a subset of patients with systemic sclerosis and refers to calcinosis, Raynaud's phenomenon, esophageal dysmotility, sclerodactyly, and telangiectasia. These patients tend to possess anticentromere antibodies and often have a slowly progressive course of disease [22]. Pulmonary hypertension is also common in this group of patients.

Systemic disease is a common feature of systemic sclerosis. Pulmonary function is frequently decreased, and esophageal dysmotility and gastrointestinal dysmotility are common. Renal dysfunction is fortunately uncommon, but when present, it can be life-threatening. Patients with diffuse disease frequently possess anti–topoisomerase I antibodies.

No cure exists for scleroderma; therefore, treatment is directed at symptomatic relief [23]. Therapy for Raynaud's phenomenon is discussed in an earlier section. Prevention of aspiration pneumonitis in patients with esophageal disease is indicated.

Eosinophilic Fasciitis and Eosinophilia Myalgia Syndrome

Eosinophilic fasciitis is characterized by the sudden onset of progressive induration of the skin. Patients often report that the disease followed an unusual amount of exertion. The patients do not have Raynaud's phenomenon, sclerodactyly, or autoantibodies but frequently have hyperglobulinemia and eosinophilia. Histologically, they have a fasciitis. Patients may respond to prednisone or methotrexate therapy, or both.

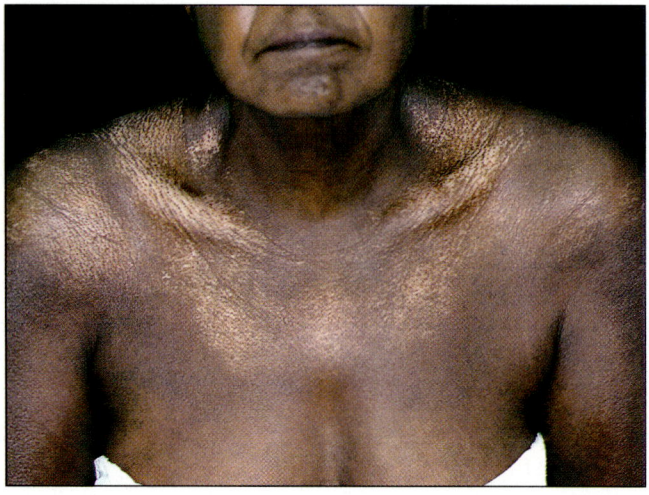

FIGURE 14-18 Abnormal pigmentation with retention of pigment in the perifollicular areas is common in systemic sclerosis.

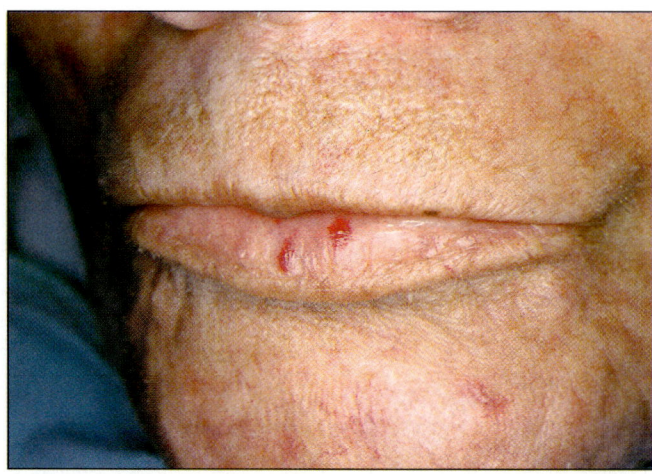

FIGURE 14-19 Mat-like telangiectasia in a patent with the CREST (calcinosis, Raynaud's phenomenon, esophageal dysmotility, sclerodactyly, and telangiectasia) variant of scleroderma.

A syndrome characterized by eosinophilia, myalgia, cutaneous sclerosis, neuropathy, and pulmonary dysfunction developed in patients taking contaminated L-tryptophan. Some of the features closely mimic eosinophilic fasciitis, but the patients often fail to respond to therapy and may have progressive debilitation, or death may even occur [24•].

Mixed Connective Tissue Disease

Mixed connective tissue disease is an overlap syndrome that is frequently characterized by cutaneous sclerosis with features of another collagen-vascular disease, such as lupus erythematosus or inflammatory myopathy. Patients with this disease commonly possess high levels of anti–U_1 ribonucleoprotein antibodies. Despite this antibody marker, follow-up of the patient presumed to have mixed connective tissue disease usually allows classification within one of the more traditional categories.

REFERENCES AND RECOMMENDED READING

Recently published papers of particular interest have been highlighted as:
• Of interest
•• Of outstanding interest

1. Tan EM, Cohen AS, Fries JF, *et al.*: The 1982 revised criteria for the classification of systemic lupus erythematosus. *Arthritis Rheum* 1982, 25:1271–1277.

2. Gilliam JN, Sontheimer RD: Distinctive cutaneous subsets in the spectrum of lupus erythematosus. *J Am Acad Dermatol* 1981, 4:471–475.

3. Callen JP: Chronic cutaneous LE. *Arch Dermatol* 1982, 118:412–416.

4. Spann CR, Callen JP, Klein JB, *et al.*: Clinical, serologic and immunogenetic studies in patients with chronic cutaneous (discoid) lupus erythematosus who have verrucous and/or hypertrophic skin lesions. *J Rheumatol* 1988, 15:256–261.

5.• David-Bajar KM: Subacute cutaneous lupus erythematosus. *J Invest Dermatol* 1993, 100:2S–8S.

6.• Petri M: Antiphospholipid antibodies: lupus anticoagulant and anticardiolipin antibody. *Curr Probl Dermatol* 1992, 4:171–201.

7.•• Sontheimer RD, McCauliffe DP, Zappi E, *et al.*: Antinuclear antibodies: clinical correlations and biologic significance. *Adv Dermatol* 1991, 7:3–53.

8.• Fabré VC, Lear S, Reichlin M, *et al.*: Twenty percent of biopsy specimens from sun-exposed skin of normal young adults demonstrate positive immunofluorescence. *Arch Dermatol* 1991, 127:1006–1011.

9.•• Lehmann P, Hölzle E, Kind P, *et al.*: Experimental reproduction of skin lesions in lupus erythematosus by UVA and UVB radiation. *J Am Acad Dermatol* 1990, 22:181–187.

10. Bohan A, Peter JB: Polymyositis and dermatomyositis. *N Engl J Med* 1975, 292:344–347.

11.• Stonecipher MR, Jorizzo JL, White WL, *et al.*: Cutaneous changes of dermatomyositis in patients with normal muscle enzymes: dermatomyositis sine myositis? *J Am Acad Dermatol* 1993, 28:951–956.

12.• Guzmán J, Petty RE, Malleson PN: Monitoring disease activity in juvenile dermatomyositis: the role of von Willebrand factor and muscle enzymes. *J Rheumatol* 1994, 21:739–743.

13.•• Sigurgeirsson B, Lindelöf B, Edhag O, *et al.*: Risk of cancer in patients with dermatomyositis or polymyositis. *N Engl J Med* 1992, 326:363–367.

14.• Cherin P, Piette JC, Herson S, *et al.*: Dermatomyositis and ovarian cancer: a report of 7 cases and literature review. *J Rheumatol* 1993, 20:1897–1899.

15.• Cukier J, Beauchamp RA, Spindler JS, *et al.*: Association between bovine collagen implants and a dermatomyositis or polymyositis-like syndrome. *Ann Intern Med* 1993, 118:920–928.

16.• Fafalak RG, Peterson MGE, Kagen LJ: Strength in polymyositis and dermatomyositis: best outcome in patients treated early. *J Rheumatol* 1994, 21:643–648.

17.• Sinoway P, Callen JP: Chlorambucil: an effective corticosteroid sparing agent for patents with recalcitrant dermatomyositis. *Arthritis Rheum* 1993, 36:319–324.

18.•• Dalakas MC, Illa I, Dambrosia JM, *et al.*: A controlled trial of high-dose intravenous immune globulin infusions as a treatment for dermatomyositis. *N Engl J Med* 1993, 329:1993–2000.

19. Callen JP: Photodermatitis in a 6-year-old child. *Arthritis Rheum* 1993, 36:1483–1485.

20. Woo TY, Callen JP, Voorhees JV, *et al.*: Cutaneous lesions of dermatomyositis are improved by hydroxychloroquine. *J Am Acad Dermatol* 1984, 10:592–600.

21.• Uziel Y, Krafchik BR, Siverman ED, *et al.*: Localized scleroderma in childhood: a report of 30 cases. *Sem Arthr Rheum* 1994, 23:328–340.

22. Steen VD, Ziegler GL, Rodnan GP, *et al.*: Clinical and laboratory associations of anticentromere antibody in patients with progressive systemic sclerosis. *Arthritis Rheum* 1984, 27:125–131.

23. Siebold JR, Furst DE, Clements PJ: Why everything (or nothing) seems to work in the treatment of scleroderma. *J Rheumatol* 1992, 19:673–676.

24.• Swygert LA, Back EE, Auerbach SE, *et al.*: Eosinophilia-myalgia syndrome: mortality data from the US national surveillance system. *J Rheumatol* 1993, 20:1711–1717.

SELECT BIBLIOGRAPHY

Bohan A, Peter JB, Bowman RL, *et al.*: A computer-assisted analysis of 153 patients with polymyositis and dermatomyositis. *Medicine* 1977, 56:255–286.

Callen JP: Lupus erythematosus. In *Clinical Dermatology*, rev 19. Edited by Demis DJ. Philadelphia: JB Lippincott; 1992: 5–1,1–28.

Callen JP, Tuffanelli DL, Provost TT: Collagen-vascular disease: an update. *J Am Acad Dermatol* 1993, 28:477–484.

Campbell PM, Leroy EC: Raynaud phenomenon. *Semin Arthritis Rheum* 1986, 16:92–103.

Falanga V: Localized scleroderma. *Med Clin North Am* 1989, 73:1143–1156.

Lee LA, David KM: Cutaneous lupus erythematosus. *Curr Probl Dermatol* 1989, 1:161–200.

Targoff IN: Dermatomyositis and polymyositis. *Curr Probl Dermatol* 1991, 3:131–180.

15 Urticaria and Other Reactive Dermatoses

Carol L. Kulp-Shorten

Key Points

- Urticaria, erythema multiforme, and erythema nodosum represent hypersensitivity phenomena.
- Laboratory testing should be directed by pertinent history and physical examination findings.
- With all hypersensitivity states, the ideal treatment is identification and elimination of the antigenic stimulus.
- An etiology cannot be determined in more that 75% of cases of chronic urticaria (urticaria greater than 6 weeks' duration).
- Herpes simplex virus infections are responsible for the majority of erythema multiforme cases in the United States.
- Oral contraceptives are a leading cause of erythema nodosum.

URTICARIA

General Considerations

Urticaria and angioedema are transient reactive erythemas to substances systemically distributed. Raised evanescent erythematous wheals secondary to superficial dermal edema are known as urticaria (Fig. 15-1), whereas angioedema develops when the deep dermal, subcutaneous, or submucosal layers are involved (Fig. 15-2). Individual lesions arise suddenly, rarely persist for longer than 12 to 24 hours, and are intensely pruritic.

Urticarial reactions are common: they are experienced by 20% to 25% of the population at least once during a lifetime [1]. Patients may experience urticaria alone (40%), angioedema alone (10%), or combined urticaria and angioedema (50%) [2••]. The final endpoint in the pathogenesis of urticaria centers on the local increased permeability of capillaries and postcapillary venules secondary to mediators such as histamine, kinins, prostaglandins, complement, and leukotrienes. Extravasation of protein-rich fluid produces the characteristic wheals.

Classification

There are many ways to classify urticaria. One schema involves the duration of an attack. Acute urticaria is often IgE mediated, evolves over days to weeks, and then completely resolves. Episodes persisting longer than 6 weeks are termed chronic urticaria. Approximately 50% of patients with urticaria alone will be free of lesions within 1 year, whereas 20% have involvement for more than 20 years. Of patients who have both urticaria and angioedema, 75% continue to have episodes for more than 5 years and 20% continue to have them for more than 20 years [3••].

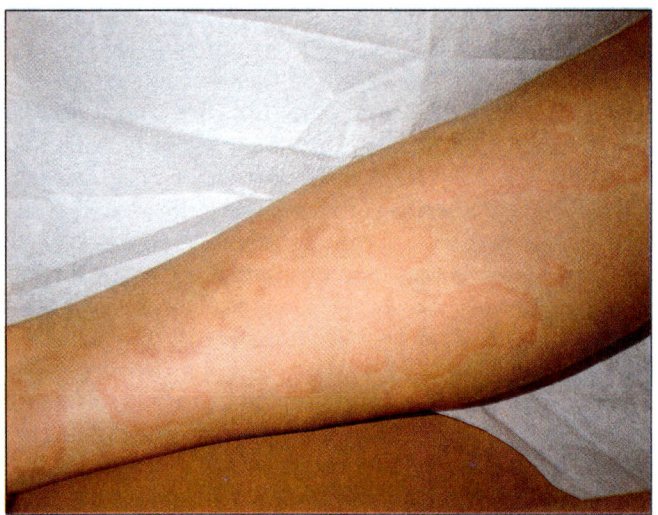

FIGURE 15-1 Erythematous wheals typical of urticaria.

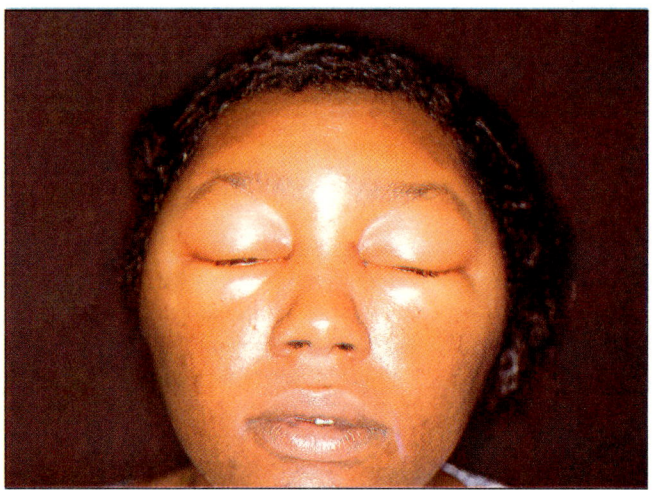

FIGURE 15-2 Periorbital angioedema with deep dermal and subcutaneous edema.

Urticaria can also be classified with respect to etiology, that is, as immunologic, nonimmunologic, or idiopathic urticaria (Table 15-1). IgE-dependent (type I hypersensitivity) mechanisms are often involved in urticarial reactions

---

TABLE 15-1 CLASSIFICATION OF URTICARIA

Immunologic

IgE dependent (type I hypersensitivity)
  Specific antigen sensitivities
  Physical urticarias
Complement mediated (type III hypersensitivity)
  Hereditary angioedema
  Acquired C1 esterase inhibitor deficiency (lymphomas,
    myelomas, systemic lupus erythematosus)
  Serum sickness
  Urticarial vasculitis

Nonimmunologic

Direct mast cell degranulators
  Opiates
  Polymyxin
  Tubocurarine
  Radiocontrast dye
Indirect mast cell degranulators via arachidonic acid
  pathway alteration
  Aspirin
  Nonsteroidal anti-inflammatory drugs
  Tartrazine (yellow food dye)
  Benzoate (food preservative)

Idiopathic

ie, etiology cannot be determined

---

to food, drugs, therapeutic agents, infections, inhalants, and venoms. IgE is also believed to play a role in many of the physical urticarias (Table 15-2). Deficiency of the inhibitor of the activated first component of the complement system (C1 esterase inhibitor) may be hereditary (autosomal dominant) or may be acquired with systemic disease. Direct degranulators cause the release of histamine from mast cells, whereas indirect degranulators exert their effects via alteration of arachidonic acid metabolism. Unfortunately, an etiology cannot be determined in more than 75% of cases of chronic urticaria, so the designation *idiopathic* is used [4•].

Diagnosis and Evaluation

Urticaria and angioedema are usually easily diagnosed. As mentioned previously, however, the etiology of chronic urticaria often remains obscure. Patients with acute urticaria often do not present for evaluation because the cause is readily apparent. The physician is often faced with the frustration of evaluating the patient with chronic urticaria. A detailed history will establish a pattern of occurrence, relationship to physical agents, medication usage, and concomitant infection or underlying disease. Physical examination may reveal the characteristic small wheals (1 to 2 mm) with large erythematous flares of cholinergic urticaria. These lesions usually develop with exercise. Simple provocative tests can be performed in patients suspected of having a physical urticaria [5] (Table 15-2 and Fig. 15-3). A recent report by Barlow and coworkers [6••] documents a high incidence (71%) of physical urticarias in patients with urticaria. One hundred and thirty-five chronic urticaria patients were specifically tested for immediate dermatographism, delayed-pressure urticaria and, when indicated by the history, for cholinergic and/or cold urticaria. Fifty patients (37%) had delayed-pressure urticaria, 30 (22%) had immediate dermatographism, 15

TABLE 15-2 PROVOCATIVE TESTING OF PHYSICAL URTICARIAS	
Urticaria	**Diagnostic test**
Dermatographism	Stroke skin with firm pressure
Pressure	Apply a 15-lb weight for 20 min, with inspection at 4–8 h
Solar	Perform phototesting with ultraviolet light and fluorescent light
Familial cold	Expose to cold air for 20–30 min (ice-cube test results are negative)
Acquired cold	Place a plastic-wrapped ice cube on the skin for 5 min
Cholinergic	Exercise; mecholyl skin test
Aquagenic	Apply 35°C water compress on the upper body skin for 30 min
Vibratory	Apply vortex vibration to forearm for 5 min

(11%) had cholinergic urticaria, and 3 (2%) had cold urticaria. Lin and Schwartz [7•] also report three patients seropositive for HIV antibody with cold urticaria. These patients had no AIDS-defining illness and two of them were taking zidovudine at the time of onset of urticaria. Skin biopsy is not helpful unless urticarial vasculitis is suspected (ie, if wheals last longer than 24 hours or resolve with purpura or hyperpigmentation). Laboratory testing should be directed by the history and physical examination findings, but most patients with chronic urticaria probably warrant a basic evaluation with a complete blood count and differential, measurement of the erythrocyte sedimentation rate, and urinalysis.

Treatment

The ideal treatment for urticaria is identification and elimination of its cause. However, because the etiology is often obscure, symptomatic treatment is usually necessary. Antihistamines are considered the mainstay of therapy. Although the classic (H_1) antihistamines are effective, their use is limited by central nervous system effects such as sedation, anticholinergic effects such as dry mouth, and inconvenient dosing. Most of these agents must be used every 4 to 6 hours. Representative H_1 antagonists include chlorpheniramine maleate (Chlor-Trimeton; Schering Plough, Liberty Corner, NJ), diphenhydramine hydrochloride (Benadryl; Parke Davis, Morris Plains, NJ), cyproheptadine hydrochloride (Periactin; Merck & Co., West Point, PA), hydroxyzine hydrochloride (Atarax; Roerig, New York, NY), and clemastine fumarate (Tavist; Sandoz, East Hanover, NJ). Cyproheptadine hydrochloride is said to be the drug of choice for acquired cold urticaria [5].

New second-generation H_1 antihistamines have recently been developed. These agents have the advantage of low affinity for brain H_1 receptors, producing less sedation and no potentiation of alcohol or benzodiazepines. Dosing schedules are also convenient, ie, daily to twice daily. Terfenadine (Seldane; Merrell Dow, Kansas City, MO), astemizole (Hismanal; Janssen, Titusville, NJ), and loratadine (Claritin; Schering, Kenilworth, NJ) are available in the United States, whereas cetirizine (Reactin; Pfizer, New York, NY) awaits Food and Drug Administration approval. Clinical efficacy studies have established the superiority of these agents to placebo and their comparability to the traditional H_1 antagonists [8,9•]. The safety profile for these agents is good, although astemizole and terfenadine may interact with ketoconazole, itraconazole, or erythromycin to produce cardiac side effects. These agents should also be avoided in patients with underlying hepatic dysfunction [8].

Histamine$_2$ antihistamines, such as cimetidine hydrochloride (Tagamet; SmithKline Beecham, Deerfield, IL) and ranitidine hydrochloride (Zantac; Glaxo, Research Triangle Park, NC), may also be beneficial in the treatment of urticaria when they are combined with an H_1 blocker. The tricyclic antidepressant doxepin hydrochloride (Sinequan; Roerig, New York, NY) has activity against both histamine receptors and may be initiated in doses of 10 to 25 mg twice daily. In general, systemic corticosteroids have no place in the regular therapy for chronic urticaria because of their unacceptable risk-to-benefit ratio. Finally, avoidance of aspirin, nonsteroidal anti-inflammatory drugs, narcotics, and benzoates may help control urticaria in some patients.

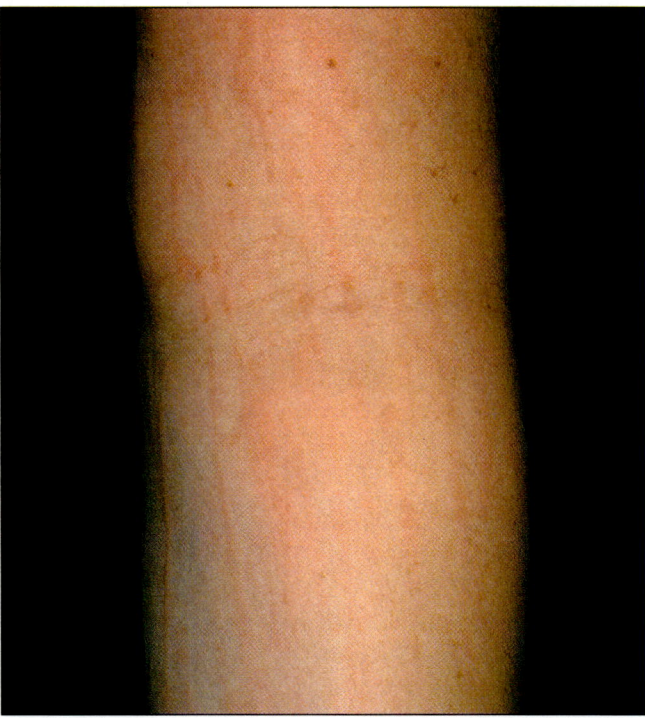

FIGURE 15-3 Dermatographism can be demonstrated by stroking the skin with firm pressure.

Erythema Multiforme

General Considerations

Erythema multiforme (EM) is a reactive hypersensitivity erythema that targets mucosal as well as cutaneous surfaces. The mucocutaneous syndrome can be broadly subdivided into EM minor and EM major (Stevens-Johnson syndrome). This discussion focuses on EM minor (80% of all EM cases); for Stevens-Johnson syndrome, *see* Liang-Federman and Kerdel, Life-Threatening Dermatoses.

Erythema multiforme is a benign, self-limited, and frequently recurrent host immune response to an antigenic stimulus. This hypersensitivity reaction develops 7 to 14 days after initial exposure and is probably both humoral and cell mediated [10,11]. Young adults are the primary target, although 20% of cases develop in children and teenagers [11].

Etiology

The possible etiologic agents of EM are innumerable, but they can be grouped into the categories of infections, medications, collagen vascular disease, and neoplasms. Table 15-3 lists the most common etiologic agents in each of these categories. In the United States, herpes simplex virus (HSV) infection (Fig. 15-4) and medications are the

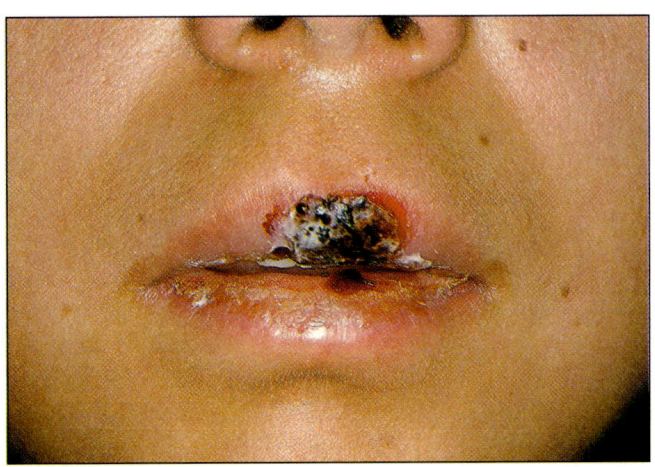

FIGURE 15-4 Herpes labialis of the upper lip with erythema multiforme erosions of the lower lip.

most common causes, with HSV infection probably responsible for more than 50% of all EM cases [10]. Use of the polymerase chain reaction technique has shown HSV to also be an overwhelming etiologic agent of childhood EM [12•].

Clinical Presentation

Erythema multiforme begins as an acral eruption characterized initially by fixed erythematous macules that may progress to papules and urticarial plaques, 1 to 2 cm in diameter (Figs. 15-5 and 15-6). The characteristic lesion with targetlike appearance (central blister and purpura or necrosis) is not always seen. The palms and soles are commonly involved (Fig. 15-7), and lesions often progress to involve the trunk over a 1-week period (Fig. 15-8). Resolution then proceeds over a 1- to 2-week period, with postinflammatory hyperpigmentation but no scarring typical. This eruption may be completely asymptomatic or

TABLE 15-3 SOME ETIOLOGIC AGENTS ASSOCIATED WITH ERYTHEMA MULTIFORME

Infections

Herpes simplex
Mycoplasma pneumoniae infection
Mononucleosis
Yersinia infections
Tuberculosis
Deep fungal infections (*eg*, histoplasmosis and coccidioidomycosis)

Medications

Penicillins
Sulfonamides
Phenytoin
Barbiturates

Neoplasms*

Lymphoproliferative disorders
Solid tumors
Dysproteinemias

Connective tissue disease*

Systemic lupus erythematosus
Rheumatoid arthritis

*These associations are rare.

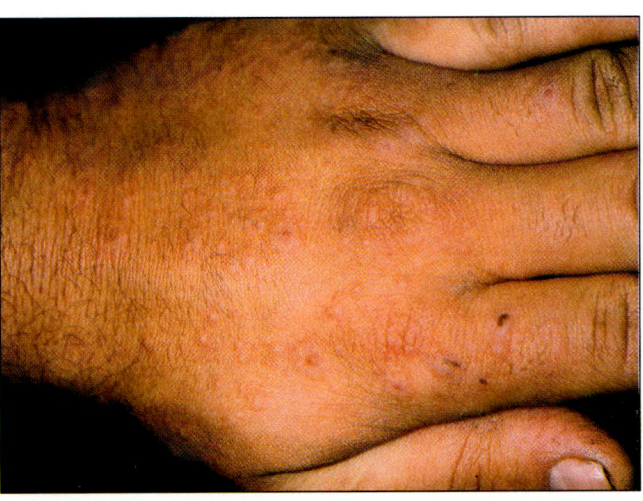

FIGURE 15-5 Urticarial papules and targetlike lesions on the dorsum of the hand, in a patient with erythema multiforme.

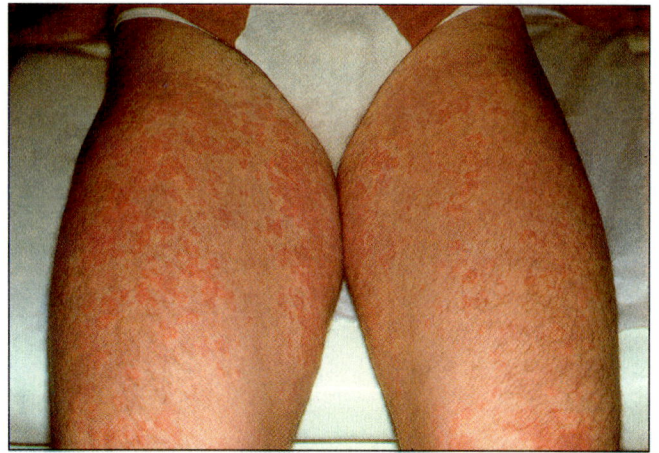

FIGURE 15-6 Urticarial papules and plaques on the thighs of a patient with erythema multiforme.

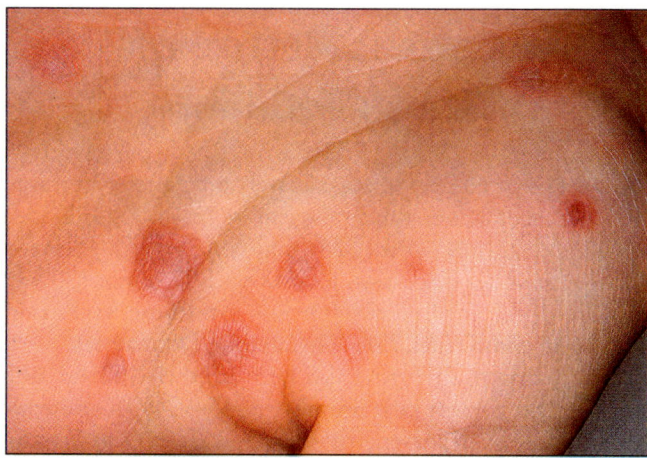

FIGURE 15-7 Classic target-like palmar lesions in a patient with erythema multiforme minor.

associated with itching and burning, and it has a tendency to develop in areas of trauma or ultraviolet exposure (isomorphic phenomenon) [11,13]. Mucosal involvement occurs in 20% to 45% of EM minor cases and is usually mild, with erosions of the oral mucosa as a common feature (Fig. 15-9) [11]. Constitutional symptoms are usually absent, and hospitalization is usually avoidable.

Evaluation

Evaluation of the EM patient centers on identification of the etiologic agent, which is often possible with a thorough history and physical examination, including a medication history and review of symptoms for infectious processes. No specific laboratory abnormality is present with EM minor, although an elevated erythrocyte sedimentation rate, mild leukocytosis, or both may be encountered. Laboratory testing is not always necessary if the etiologic agent is apparent from the history and physical examination findings. The choice of laboratory tests should be directed by

these findings. Table 15-4 provides a partial list of suggested tests. Skin biopsy often reveals the characteristic hydropic degeneration of basal keratinocytes with mixed dermal infiltrate [10,11] but is not helpful in pinpointing the etiology.

Treatment

Treatment of EM minor centers on the removal or treatment of the etiologic agent, or both, and on symptomatic care. Antihistamines, oatmeal baths, and emollients with menthol may help symptoms of itching. Topical corticosteroids may also help symptoms but have little other benefit [14]. Oral lesions may be treated with a 1:1 mixture of diphenhydramine elixir and attapulgite

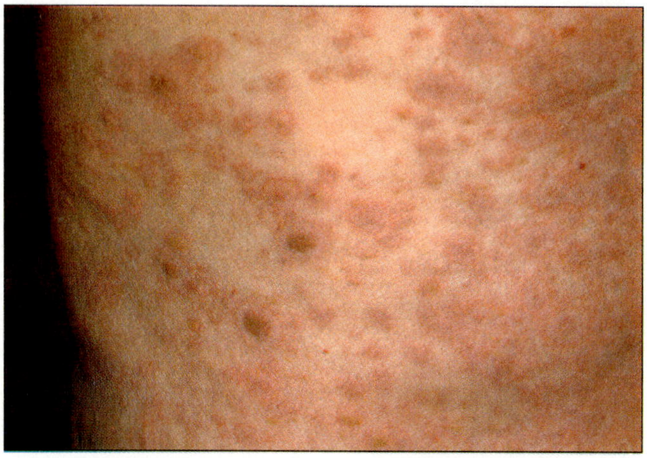

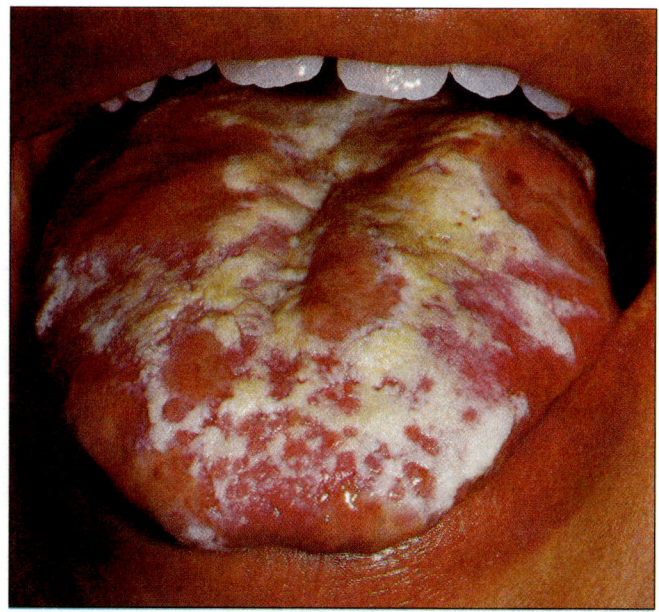

FIGURE 15-9 Oral mucosal erosions in a patient with erythema multiforme minor.

FIGURE 15-8 Trunk involvement in a patient with erythema multiforme.

TABLE 15-4 LABORATORY EVALUATION IN ERYTHEMA MULTIFORME
Complete blood count with differential
Liver function tests
Urinalysis
Erythrocyte sedimentation rate
Anti-streptolysin O titer
Chest roentgenography
Viral cultures or titers
Cold agglutinins

(Kaopectate; Upjohn, Kalamazoo, MI). The use of systemic corticosteroids, although common, is controversial. If the EM is HSV associated, the patient should be counseled about the risk of recurrent EM with future episodes of HSV infection. Sunscreens and sun avoidance should be recommended in herpes labialis-associated EM. Oral acyclovir (Zovirax; Burroughs Wellcome, Research Triangle Park, NC), given episodically for infrequent recurrences of HSV infection (200 mg five times a day for 5 days) or as a long-term suppressive regimen for frequent recurrences (400 mg twice daily), may prevent EM if the HSV episode can be aborted. Even without treatment, EM minor is benign and self-limited within 2 to 6 weeks.

ERYTHEMA NODOSUM

General Considerations

Erythema nodosum (EN) is a reactive hypersensitivity process in which the target of the inflammatory reaction is the subcutaneous fat (panniculitis). EN is the most common cause of inflammatory nodules on the lower extremities [15].

As with other reactive erythemas, EN develops as the host mounts an immune response to an antigenic stimulus. Both humoral and cell-mediated immune mechanisms probably play a role in the pathogenesis of EN. Circulating immune complexes (type III hypersensitivity) are postulated to participate in this process because patients often present with a serum sickness-like syndrome [16].

Etiology

Multiple agents may play an antigenic role in the development of EN. Table 15-5 summarizes the most common etiologic associations. Infections, sarcoidosis, medications, and pregnancy head the list in the United States today. In the 1950s, tuberculosis was the primary infectious trigger for EN, but infection with group A β-hemolytic streptococci is most common today. Yersinia infections remain an important etiologic agent in Europe [15]. Of the medica-

tions listed, oral contraceptives are the leading trigger, and often the physician neglects to obtain a history of their use in the female patient presenting with EN. Finally, with respect to inflammatory bowel disease, the patient with ulcerative colitis is much more likely to develop EN than the patient with Crohn's disease.

Clinical Presentation

The typical patient with EN is usually a woman who presents with the sudden development of multiple tender, red, warm nodules (1 to 5 cm in diameter) on the pretibial surfaces (Fig. 15-10). These nodules are not suppurative and do not ulcerate. After a 3- to 6-week course, the nodules eventuate into a bruise without scar formation. Atypical presentations include subcutaneous nodules on the trunk, arms, calves, or face. Patients may present with a serum sickness–like syndrome with associated findings of fever, chills, malaise, leukocytosis, and arthropathy.

Evaluation

As with any disease process, evaluation of the EN patient begins with a thorough history and physical examination to pinpoint a possible etiologic factor. A thorough medication history, including information on the use of oral contraceptives, must be obtained, and women need to be questioned about the possibility of pregnancy. A biopsy is not always necessary with the classic presentation, but if a biopsy is performed, an adequate specimen that includes subcutaneous fat is paramount. Usually this requires an incisional wedge biopsy. Histopathologic changes include septal inflammation of the subcutaneous

TABLE 15-5 ETIOLOGIC AGENTS OF ERYTHEMA NODOSUM
Infections
Group A β-hemolytic streptococcus infections
Chlamydial infections
Deep fungal infections
Tuberculosis
Yersinia infections
Medications
Oral contraceptives
Sulfonamides
Bromides
Systemic conditions
Sarcoidosis
Inflammatory bowel disease
Behçet's syndrome
Lymphoreticular malignancy
Reiter's disease
Pregnancy

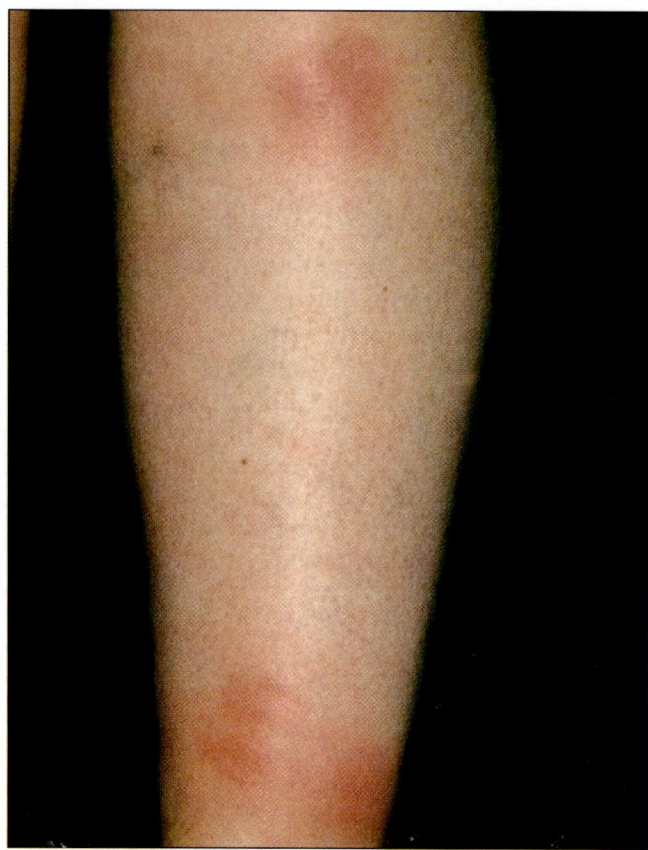

FIGURE 15-10 Tender subcutaneous inflammatory nodules of the pretibium that are typical of erythema nodosum.

tissue with possible granuloma formation. Vasculitis and fat necrosis are not seen [16]. The selection of laboratory tests should be directed by the history and physical examination findings. Table 15-6 provides a partial listing of suggested tests.

Treatment

Treatment of EN centers on the removal or treatment of the etiologic agent, or both. Supportive therapy includes bed rest, the use of an elastic support bandage, leg eleva-

TABLE 15-6 LABORATORY EVALUATION IN ERYTHEMA NODOSUM
Chest roentgenography
Urinalysis
Throat culture
Complete blood count with differential
Erythrocyte sedimentation rate
Anti-streptolysin O titer or anti-DNAase titer
Pregnancy test
Plus/minus intradermal tests for tuberculosis, histoplasmosis, or coccidioidomycosis

tion, and the use of nonsteroidal anti-inflammatory agents. Many clinicians favor the use of aspirin (650 mg three times a day) or indomethacin (50 mg two to three times a day). The use of potassium iodide (300 mg three times a day) or supersaturated potassium iodide (0.3 mL three times a day) is often beneficial [17], as may be colchicine (0.6 mg twice a day). Patients should be warned of possible gastrointestinal side effects with all of these agents. Finally, some physicians advocate a 2-week systemic corticosteroid taper. In patients given systemic corticosteroids, the physician needs to exclude underlying fungal or mycobacterial disease before administration of these agents is started.

ACKNOWLEDGMENTS

I thank Dr. Jeffrey P. Callen for supplying the clinical photographs for this manuscript and also for his editorial suggestions. I also thank Ms. Sandy Lingle for her secretarial assistance.

REFERENCES AND RECOMMENDED READING

Recently published papers of particular interest have been highlighted as:
• Of interest
•• Of outstanding interest

1. Jorizzo JL: Urticaria. In *Dermatological Signs of Internal Disease.* Edited by Callen JP and Jorizzo JL. Philadelphia: WB Saunders; 1988:59–69.

2.•• Soter NA: Urticaria: current therapy. *J Allergy Clin Immunol* 1990, 86:1009–1014.

3.•• Kulp-Shorten CL, Callen JP: Urticaria and angioedema. In *Conn's Current Therapy.* Edited by Rakel RE. Philadelphia: WB Saunders; 1993:827–828.

4.• Sibbald RG, Cheema AS, Lozinski A, *et al.*: Chronic urticaria: evaluation of the role of physical, immunologic, and other contributory factors. *Int J Dermatol* 1991, 30:381–386.

5. Casale TB, Sampson HA, Hanifin J, *et al.*: Guide to physical urticarias. *J Allergy Clin Immunol* 1988, 82:758–763.

6.•• Barlow RJ, Warburton F, Watson K, *et al.*: Diagnosis and incidence of delayed pressure urticaria in patients with chronic urticaria. *J Am Acad Dermatol* 1993, 29:954–958.

7.• Lin RY, Schwartz RA: Cold urticaria and HIV infection. *Br J Dermatol* 1993, 129:465–467.

8. Monroe EW: Chronic urticaria: Review of nonsedating H$_1$ antihistamines in treatment. *J Am Acad Dermatol* 1988, 19:842–849.

9.• Sharpe GR, Shuster S: The effect of cetirizine on symptoms and wealing in dermographic urticaria. *Br J Dermatol* 1993, 129:580–583.

10. Huff JC: Erythema multiforme. *Dermatol Clin* 1985, 3:141–152.

11. Ledesma GN, McCormack PC: Erythema multiforme. *Clin Dermatol* 1986, 4:70–80.

12.• Weston WL, Brice SL, Jester JD, *et al.*:Herpes simplex virus in childhood erythema multiforme. *Pediatrics* 1992, 89:32–34.

13. Fitzpatrick JE, Thompson PB, Aeling JL, *et al.*: Photosensitive recurrent erythema multiforme. *J Am Acad Dermatol* 1983, 9:419–423.

14. Tonnesen MG: Erythema multiforme. In *Conn's Current Therapy*. Edited by Rakel RE. Philadelphia: WB Saunders; 1993:812–814.

15. White JW: Erythema nodosum. *Dermatol Clin* 1985, 3:119–127.

16. Jorizzo JL: Erythema nodosum. In *Dermatological Signs of Internal Disease*. Edited by Callen JP, Jorizzo JL. Philadelphia: WB Saunders; 1988:76–79.

17. Horio T, Danno K, Okamoto H, *et al.*: Potassium iodide in erythema nodosum and other erythematous dermatoses. *J Am Acad Dermatol* 1983, 9:77–81.

SELECT BIBLIOGRAPHY

Champion RH: Urticaria: then and now. *Br J Dermatol* 1988, 119:427–436.

Chan H-L, Stern RS, Arndt KA, *et al.*: The incidence of erythema multiforme, Stevens-Johnson syndrome, and toxic epidermal necrolysis. *Arch Dermatol* 1990, 126:43–47.

Kalivas J, Breneman D, Tharp M, *et al.*: Urticaria: clinical efficacy of cetirizine in comparison with hydroxyzine and placebo. *J Allergy Clin Immunol* 1990, 86:1014–1018.

Monroe EW: The role of antihistamines in the treatment of chronic urticaria. *J Allergy Clin Immunol* 1990, 86:662–665.

Simons FER: Recent advances in H1-receptor antagonist treatment. *J Allergy Clin Immunol* 1990, 86:995–999.

16 Small Vessel Vasculitis and Neutrophilic Dermatoses

Jamie A. Alpert
Joseph L. Jorizzo

Key Points

- Necrotizing venulitis is characterized by palpable purpura clinically and by leukocytoclastic vasculitis pathologically.

- Patients evaluation can involve histopathologic confirmation of the diagnosis, determination of the extent of disease, and attempting to uncover and underlying etiology.

- Sweet's syndrome is characterized by inflammatory cutaneous plaques with a neutrophilic vascular reaction pathologically.

- Behçet's disease is characterized by oral aphthae and various combinations of genital aphthae, synovitis, cutaneous pustular vasculitis, and meningoencephalitis.

- Pyoderma gangrenosum belongs in this category of disease because the histopathologic findings in early lesions (controversial) may represent a neutrophilic vascular reaction.

NECROTIZING VENULITIS

Clinical Features

The hallmark of necrotizing venulitis is the palpable purpuric papule. However, there is a spectrum of clinical presentation [1]. Lesions begin as erythematous macules and progress to palpable purpura. They usually occur in crops on dependent sites (Fig. 16-1). The papules are usually less than 1 cm in diameter, and they often become confluent to form plaques, which may ulcerate. They are often asymptomatic but may be pruritic or painful. Frequently, patients have associated serum sickness–like symptoms, such as arthralgias, arthritis, myalgias, and fever.

Patients may have internal involvement, presumably resulting from circulating immune complex–mediated vessel damage [2]. Systemic involvement may include involvement of the renal glomeruli, resulting in proteinuria or hematuria; involvement of the neurologic system with focal, diffuse, central, or peripheral neurologic impairment: synovial involvement with polyarthritis; involvement of the gastrointestinal tract with associated abdominal pain or gastrointestinal bleeding; and involvement of the cardiovascular system or the respiratory tract with pericarditis or pleuritis [2,3••]. An algorithm for patient evaluation is shown in Figure 16-2.

Histopathology

Leukocytoclastic vasculitis is a disease that affects postcapillary venules in the dermis. Its histopathologic features include 1) endothelial swelling, 2) invasion of neutrophils into blood vessels, 3) leukocytoclasia, 4) extravasation of erythrocytes, and 5) fibrinoid necrosis of blood vessel walls [4]. Positive direct immunofluores-

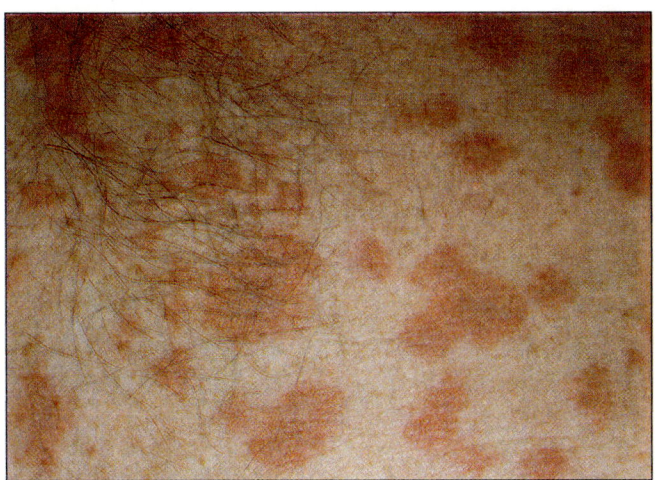

FIGURE 16-1 Necrotizing venulitis. Note the typical palpable purpura.

cence has been identified for IgG, IgM, IgA, C3, C4, C1q, and fibrin. However, results are inconsistent and are usually positive only in early lesions [5,6].

Prognosis and Therapy

The prognosis depends on the presence and severity of internal involvement. The course may be acute, chronic, or relapsing [7]. There have been reports of death associated with diffuse or proliferative glomerulonephritis, as well as from pulmonary, neurologic, and gastrointestinal bleeding [2]. The course of the underlying disease may also affect prognosis (eg, collagen vascular disease).

No treatment of necrotizing vasculitis has ever been subjected to the scrutiny of a double-blind, prospective trial. The course can be variable, further complicating the assessment of therapies. In patients in whom there is a recognized cause, removal of that cause can eradicate the disease (eg, drug-induced, or herpes simplex virus infection).

Systemic corticosteroids are used if there is systemic involvement or severe progressive cutaneous ulcerating lesions. Prednisone (1 mg/kg/d) given as a single morning dose is the most commonly enforced regimen. Split dosing increases the effectiveness, but it also increases the side effects. Every-other-day dosing is suboptimal for treating immune complex–mediated disease.

Corticosteroids should be tapered slowly because rebound may occur if tapering is done too quickly. Pulse therapy (1 g/d) of methylprednisolone sodium succinate (Solu-Medrol; Upjohn, Kalamazoo, MI) over 3 to 5 days has been reported to be beneficial, and this treatment can be used in life-threatening cases [2]. It is necessary to monitor for cardiac arrhythmias and sudden electrolyte

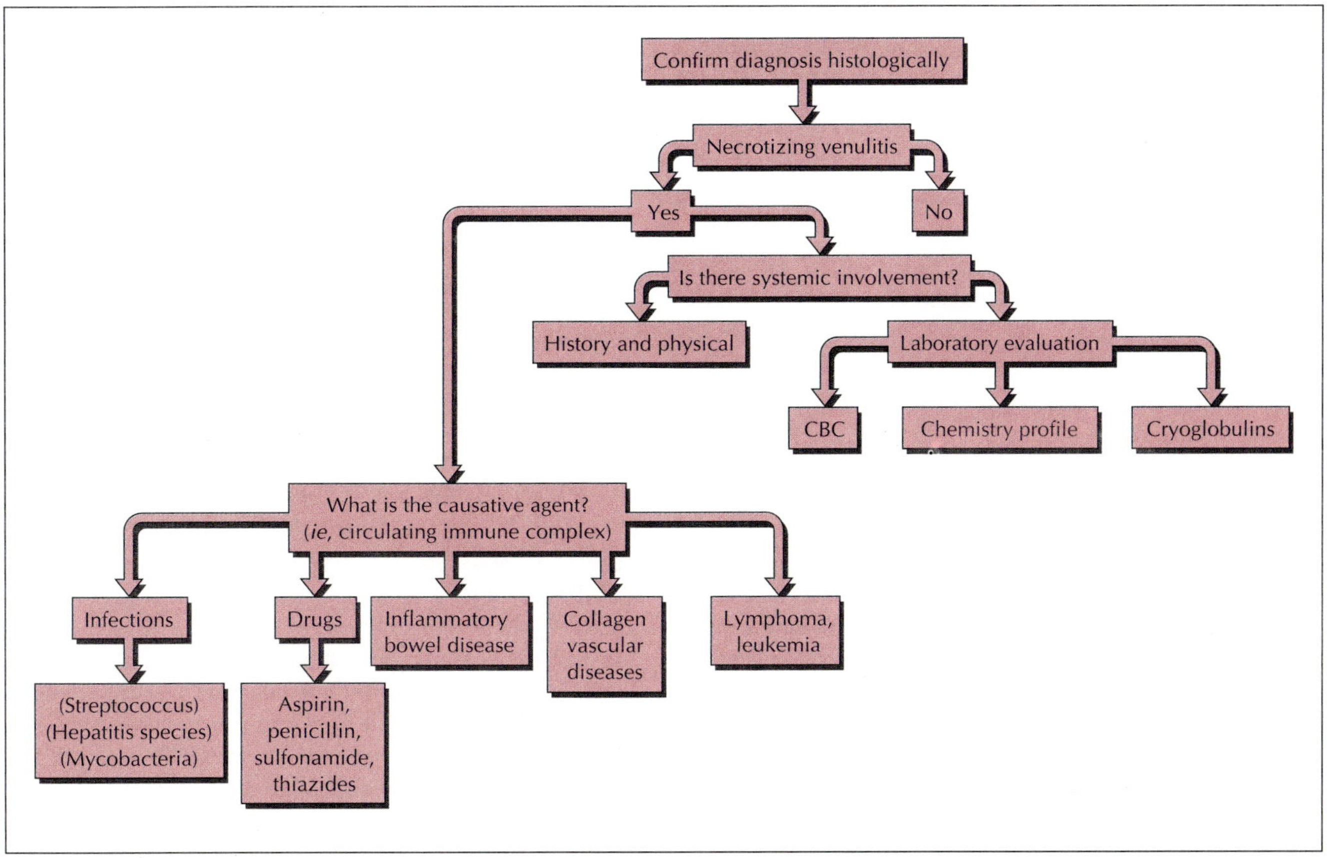

FIGURE 16-2 Patient evaluation procedure for necrotizing vasculitis. CBC—complete blood count.

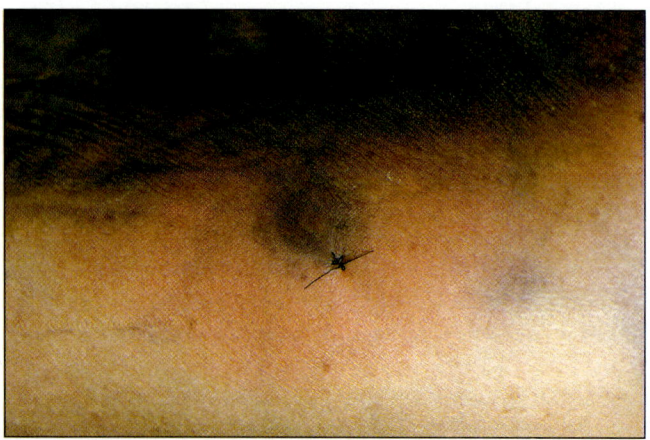

FIGURE 16-3 Sweet's syndrome: an erythematous plaque on a patient who has no underlying disease after an extensive work-up.

shifts if pulse therapy is used [2]. Cyclophosphamide and azathioprine, which have been successfully used in large vessel vasculitis, are usually not necessary for small vessel necrotizing vasculitis [2]. Low-dose weekly methotrexate may have a role in treating this disease.

Patients with cutaneous lesions only may not require therapy. Antihistamines have been used but are not helpful in our opinion [2]. Oral colchicine has been reported to be effective in doses of 0.6 mg orally two or three times daily [2]. Nonsteroidal anti-inflammatory drugs may be beneficial in treating serum sickness–like symptoms, but they do little for the cutaneous lesions. Oral dapsone therapy may also be helpful [2].

SWEET'S SYNDROME

Clinical Features

Sweet's syndrome is characterized by recurrent episodes of inflammatory cutaneous plaques, fevers, arthralgias, and neutrophilia and by histologic evidence of neutrophilic dermal inflammation occurring in the absence of infection. Cutaneous findings include erythematous, well-marginated inflammatory plaques varying from 1 to 3 cm in diameter (Fig. 16-3). Usually no epidermal change is seen; however, some vesicle or pustule formation can occur, as can postinflammatory desquamation. Occasionally, there is associated epidermal necrosis. Lesions can occur anywhere on the body but are usually limited to the trunk, face, and upper extremities. Usually, lesions occur in crops over a 1- to 2-month period. Signs and symptoms associated with this syndrome include fever, myalgia, arthralgia, headache, dyspepsia, and conjunctivitis. Mucosal involvement is unusual. Systemic involvement often lags behind the cutaneous eruption by 7 to 10 days.

Sweet's syndrome is often associated with other systemic diseases, such as acute myelogenous leukemia, ulcerative colitis, or even leukemia and lymphoma. There are no specific laboratory abnormalities, but there is often neutrophilia, an increased white blood cell count (> 20,000 cells/mL), and an elevated erythrocyte sedimentation rate (50 to 100 mm/h).

Histopathology

The characteristic histopathologic findings in specimens from patients with Sweet's syndrome are a dense, diffuse neutrophilic infiltrate with leukocytoclasia; dermal edema; and endothelial swelling. However, no fibrinoid necrosis is seen. There have been reports of involvement of the panniculus, but this is unusual [7,8].

Patient Evaluation

It is important to distinguish Sweet's syndrome from diseases such as erythema multiforme, erythema annulare centrifugum, erythema elevatum diutinum, granuloma facile, erythema nodosum, bromoderma, and pustular vasculitis associated with Behçet's disease. Infection should be excluded clinically and histologically. In addition, associated diseases (*eg*, leukemia and other myeloproliferative disorders, malignancy, ulcerative colitis, Sjögren syndrome, rheumatoid arthritis, and systemic lupus erythematosus) should be excluded.

Prognosis and Therapy

The lesions of Sweet's syndrome normally remit spontaneously in several weeks to months. Usually 50% of patients have at least one recurrence [6]. The most effective treatment is the use of systemic corticosteroids, but these agents are often not required. No prospective, double-blind assessment of this or any other treatment has been performed. The usual doses required range from 30 to 80 mg of prednisone per day, which is then tapered over several weeks [9••,10]. Other therapies have been tried, including indomethacin, potassium iodide, colchicine, dapsone, and oral isotretinoin. The effect of these drugs on neutrophil migration may at least partially explain their benefit [8,11].

PUSTULAR VASCULITIS: BEHÇET'S DISEASE

Behçet's disease is a multisystem disease named after and first described by a Turkish dermatologist. It is characterized by oral aphthae and two of the following systemic or mucocutaneous findings: 1) genital aphthae, 2) synovitis, 3) posterior uveitis, 4) cutaneous pustular vasculitis, and 5) meningoencephalitis. It is important to exclude inflammatory bowel disease and other autoimmune disease [12,13]. There are no pathognomonic laboratory tests; the diagnosis is made on clinical criteria only [13]. Behçet's disease is common in the Middle East and Japan and rare in the United States and Northern Europe. The disease usually affects young adults and rarely children [13].

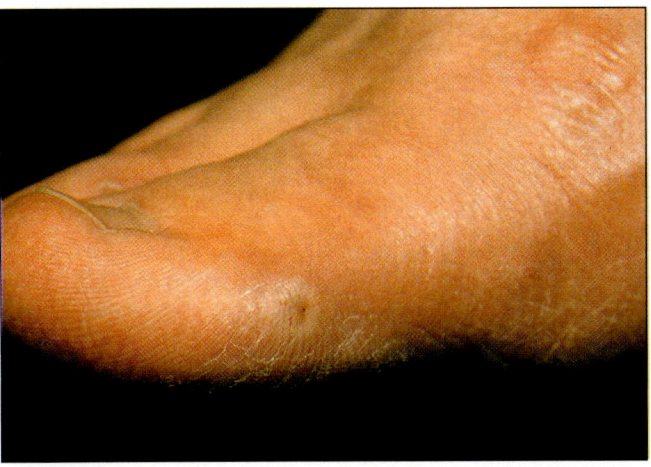

FIGURE 16-4 Behçet's disease: pustular vasculitis. An indistinguishable lesion can be seen in bowel bypass syndrome.

TABLE 16-1 TREATMENT OF BEHÇET'S DISEASE
Mucosal lesions only Topical corticosteroids Intralesional corticosteroids Viscous lidocaine
Mucocutaneous disease or more severe mucosal disease Oral colchicine, 0.6 mg orally, two to three times daily. (monitor for neutropenia) Oral dapsone Oral thalidomide Oral corticosteroids (limited because of long-term side effects) Possible low-dose weekly methotrexate

Mucocutaneous disease and ocular or neurologic symptoms
Oral corticosteroids
Immunosuppressive therapy
   Azathioprine
   Methotrexate
   Cyclosporine

Clinical Features

Behçet's disease has an extremely variable course. Morbidity depends on the development of ocular manifestations. Death is rare and usually occurs from neurologic or large vessel vascular disease. The cutaneous findings are varied. However, only pustular vasculitis and erythema nodosum–like nodules should be accepted as diagnostic criteria (Fig. 16-4). Follicular-based or acneiform lesions should not be included [13].

Behçet's disease has a number of ocular manifestations [13]. However, posterior uveitis is the principal ophthalmic cause of major morbidity. The posterior uveitis represents a retinal vasculitis that may result in blindness [6]. The associated arthritis is asymmetric, nonerosive, and oligoarthritic [13,14]. Meningoencephalitis is the principal neurologic manifestation [13]. There are a multitude of diffuse, focal, central, and peripheral neurologic associations [2]. Neurologic involvement usually occurs later in the disease process. Vascular involvement includes aneurysm, arterial occlusion, venous occlusion, and varices and can be fatal [15]. The vascular lesions are not always vasculitis and do not always respond to medical therapy.

Histopathology

Biopsy specimens from aphthae or from pustular vasculitis lesions show fully developed leukocytoclastic vasculitis or a neutrophilic vascular reaction.

Patient Evaluation

It is important to remember that 20% of the normal population has oral aphthae [16]. Clinical criteria for Behçet's disease must be met, and inflammatory bowel disease must be excluded. It is essential to exclude herpes virus infection by culture, histologic examination, or polymerase chain reaction from mucocutaneous lesions in patients suspected of having Behçet's disease. Periodic ophthalmologic examination is also required. Rheumatologic and neurologic consultations are often appropriate as well.

Prognosis and Therapy

The clinical course is variable. The mucocutaneous and arthritic manifestations usually precede any neurologic manifestations [2]. There is chronic morbidity due to mucosal ulcerations and joint aches, but the mortality rate is low in patients without ophthalmic or neurologic involvement [13]. Death is usually due to central nervous system complications, vascular disease, or less frequently, bowel perforation or cardiopulmonary disease [17].

Palliative therapies are delineated in Table 16-1 [18,19,20•].

PYODERMA GANGRENOSUM

Clinical Features

Pyoderma gangrenosum is a cutaneous ulcerative disease of unknown etiology. The lesions start as tender papules or pustules and evolve into ulcers with raised, characteristic, undermined borders with a dusty purple hue (Fig. 16-5 and 16-6). There is destruction of the skin down to subcutaneous fat, with associated granulation tissue and necrotic purulent material at the base of the ulcer. One lesion or many lesions may be present. The lesions demonstrate pathergy and may expand in an explosive fashion if the

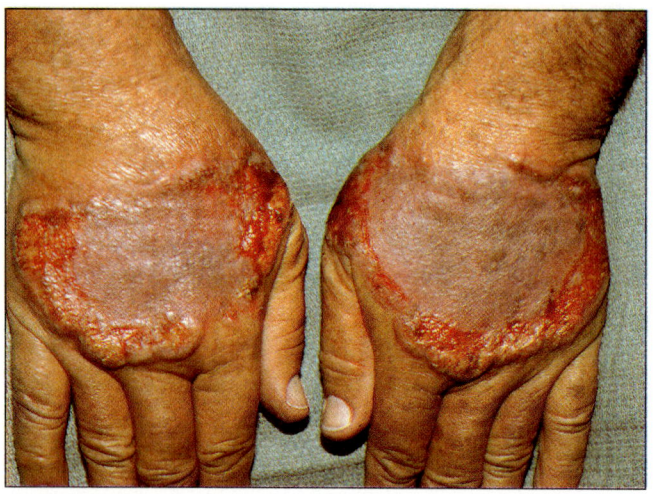

FIGURE 16-5 Bullous pyoderma gangrenosum: atypical lesions are common in patients with myleodysplastic syndrome.

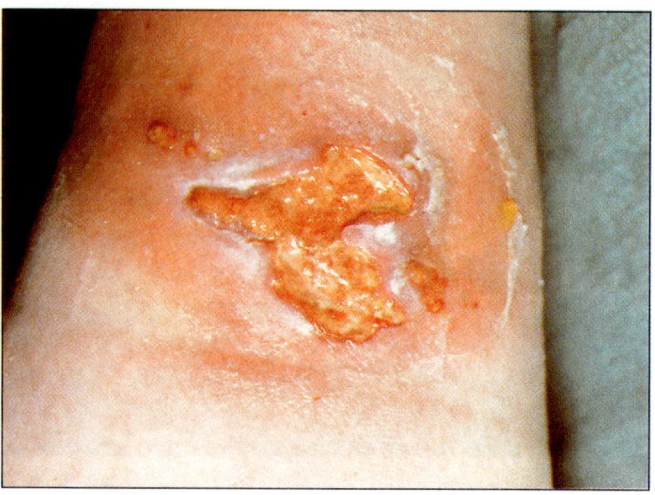

FIGURE 16-6 Pyoderma gangrenosum: typical clinical presentation.

borders are traumatized by débridement or by mechanical manipulation [5]. Pyoderma gangrenosum is a diagnosis of exclusion [21] (Table 16-2).

Histopathology

The classic histopathologic findings in specimens from pyoderma gangrenosum lesions are controversial. Findings are usually nonspecific, with specimens showing chronic inflammatory changes. The debate focuses on whether early lesions show a neutrophilic infiltrate or primarily a lymphocytic infiltrate [22]. The degree of vessel involvement may range from none to endothelial swelling to fibrinoid necrosis. The histopathologic findings obviously depend on the stage of the ulcer. Findings from early lesions of pyoderma gangrenosum resemble those from lesions of pustular vasculitis associated with Behçet's disease and show a neutrophilic vascular reaction [6].

Bullous pyoderma gangrenosum and Sweet's variant associated with myeloproliferative disease show predominantly a neutrophilic inflammatory infiltrate. More fully developed lesions show extensive tissue necrosis with surrounding mild inflammatory cell infiltrate with associated foreign body giant cells [22,23].

Patient Evaluation

It is essential to exclude other dermatoses, as outlined in the clinical section. This may be accomplished with a deep incisional biopsy specimen with routine histology, with special stains for mycobacteria, bacteria, and fungi, and with a second biopsy specimen for culture of these organisms. It is important to evaluate the patient for the following underlying conditions: ulcerative colitis, regional enteritis, hepatitis (chronic persistent or chronic active), paraproteinemia, myeloproliferative disease, and rheumatoid and seronegative arthritis [23,24].

Prognosis and Therapy

The most important aspect of treatment and prognosis is to identify the disease process correctly. The spread of the disease may be rapid, with significant local tissue destruction. Local care may consist of preventing bacterial overgrowth and gentle débridement. Aggressive déebridement will lead to extension and flaring of existing ulcers (ie, pathergy). Intralesional corticosteroids have been used for mild localized disease. However, debate surrounds the effectiveness of this approach [25]. Systemic corticosteroids are the treatment of choice for most patients. Initially, very aggressive

TABLE 16-2 ETIOLOGIES OF ULCERS THAT CAN RESEMBLE PYODERMA GANGRENOSUM
Infections
Bacterial
Fungal
Mycobacterial
Rheumatologic disease
Systemic lupus erythematosus
Rheumatoid vasculitis
Behçet's disease
Wegener's granulomatosis
Factitial ulceration
Bromoderma or iododerma
Malignant neoplasm
Squamous cell carcinoma

therapy with 1 mg/kg/d is usually necessary. If there is continued expansion of lesions, a doubling of the dosage may be necessary. Pulse corticosteroids (1 g/d) are effective but require close monitoring [22]. Maintenance therapy is often required. Rebound may occur if corticosteroids are tapered too quickly. Dapsone and sulfapyridine have also been used, in dosages of 100 to 300 mg/d and 3 g/d, respectively, for maintenance therapy [25]. Azathioprine, cyclophosphamide, clofazimine, and antibiotics such as rifampin and minocycline have also had some beneficial effect.

BOWEL-ASSOCIATED DERMATOSIS-ARTHRITIS SYNDROME

Bowel bypass syndrome consists of cutaneous lesions that are pustular vasculitis associated with signs and symptoms similar to those of serum sickness. This syndrome has also been reported in people who have not had bypass surgery, such as those with inflammatory bowel disease or a blind loop due to another surgical procedure [2].

Clinical Features

The lesions associated with bowel bypass syndrome begin as small macules; they then evolve into papules and blossom into pustules on purpuric bases. They can range in size from 0.5 to 1.5 cm. Usually, they are located on the upper body, not the legs. Pathergy may be important in clinical distribution. Each cycle of lesions lasts for more than 2 weeks, and often recovery occurs over a 1- to 7-month period [26]. The lesions may be associated with fevers, myalgias, flulike syndromes, or gastrointestinal upset. Patients may have arthralgias and a nonerosive polyarthritis.

Histopathology

The histopathologic changes seen in specimens from the early lesions of pustular vasculitis associated with bowel-associated dermatosis-arthritis syndrome have been described as identical to the vessel changes associated with Behçet's disease and as similar to those seen in Sweet's syndrome [26,27].

Patient Evaluation

Patients with pustular vasculitis lesions with histologically confirmed neutrophilic vascular reactions must be distinguished from those with Behçet's disease, disseminated gonococcemia, or meningococcemia [2].

A complete history taking and physical examination are essential. It is important to exclude blind loops of bowel and inflammatory bowel disease with appropriate radiologic assessments, endoscopic evaluation; or both. If bowel disease has been excluded, Behçet's disease must also be eliminated.

Prognosis and Therapy

The bowel bypass syndrome usually resolves with correction of bowel anatomy. If the underlying condition is inflammatory bowel disease, progress depends on the prognosis of the underlying bowel disease. Therapy has included the use of multiple antibiotics, such as tetracycline, metronidazole, and erythromycin [26]. Systemic corticosteroids have been used in patients with refractory conditioning and thalidomide has been useful [18].

REFERENCES AND RECOMMENDED READING

Recently published papers of particular interest have been highlighted as:
• Of interest
•• Of outstanding interest

1. Sams WM Jr, Thorne EG, Small P, et al.: Leukocytoclastic vasculitis. Arch Dermatol 1976, 112:219–226.

2. Jorizzo JL, Solomon AR, Zanolli MD: Neutrophilic vascular reaction. J Am Acad Dermatol 1988, 19:983–1005.

3.•• Jorizzo JL: Classification of vasculitis. J Invest Dermatol 1993, 100:106F–100F.

4. Winklemann RK, Ditto WB: Cutaneous and visceral syndromes of necrotizing or "allergic" angiitis: A study of 38 cases. Medicine 1964, 43:59–89.

5. Schroeter AL, Copeman PWM, Jordon RE, et al.: Immunofluorescence of cutaneous vasculitis associated with systemic disease. Arch Dermatol 1971, 104:254–259.

6. Dambuyant C, Thivolet J: Antigenic similarities within circulating immune complexes in patients suffering from cutaneous vasculitis. Dermatologica 1981, 162:429–437.

7. Ekenstam EA, Callen JP: Cutaneous leukocytoclastic vasculitis: clinical and laboratory features of 82 patients seen in private practice. Arch Dermatol 1984, 120:484–489.

8. Su WPD, Liu HNH: Diagnostic criteria for Sweet's syndrome. Cutis 1987, 37:167–174.

9.•• Vondendriesch P: Sweets syndrome acute neutrophilic dermatosis. J Am Acad Dermatol 1994, 31:535–560.

10. Storer JS, Nesbitt LT, Galen WK, DeLeo VA: Sweet's syndrome. Int J Dermatol 1983, 22:8–12.

11. Hoffman GS: Treatment of Sweet's syndrome (acute febrile neutrophilic dermatosis) with indomethacin. J Rheumatol 1977, 4:201–206.

12. Jorizzo JL, Hudson RD, Schmalstieg FC: Bowel associated syndrome, immune regulation, circulating immune complexes, neutrophil migration and colchicine therapy. J Am Acad Dermatol 1984, 10:205–214.

13. Jorizzo JL, Rogers RS: Behçet's disease: an update based on the International Conference held in Rochester, Minnesota. J Am Acad Dermatol 1989, 23:738–741.

14. Yurkakul S, Yuzici H, Tuzan Y, et al.: The arthritis of Behçet's disease: a prospective study. Ann Rheum Dis 1983, 42:1505–1515.

15. Shimizu T, Ehrlich GE, Goro I, et al.: Behçet's disease. Semin Arthritis Rheum 1979, 8:223–260.

16. Rogers RS III: Recurrent aphthous ulcers: clinical characteristics and evidence for immunopathogenesis. J Invest Dermatol 1977, 69:499–509.

17. Schreiner DT, Jorizzo JL: Behçet's disease and complex aphthosis. Dermatol Clin 1987, 4:769–778.

18. Jorizzo JL, Schmalstieg FS, Solomon AR: Thalidomide effects in Behçet's syndrome and pustular vasculitis. Arch Intern Med 1986, 146:878–881.

19. Nassenblatt RB, Palestine AG, Chan CC, *et al.*: Effectiveness of cyclosporin therapy for Behçet's disease. *Arthritis Rheum* 1985, 28:671–679.

20•. Jorizzo JL: Behçet's disease: and update based on international conference, Paris. *J Eur Acad Dermatol Veneral* 1994, 3:215–223.

21. Spiers EM, Hendricks SL, Jorizzo JL, Solomon AR: Sporotrichosis masquerading as pyoderma gangrenosum. *Arch Dermatol* 1986, 122:691–694.

22. Su WP, Schroeter AL, Perry HO, Powell FC: Histopathologic and immunopathologic study of pyoderma gangrenosum. *J Cutan Pathol* 1986, 13:323–330.

23. Stathel GM, Abbott LG, McGuiness AE: Pyoderma gangrenosum in association with regional enteritis. *Arch Dermatol* 1987, 95:375–380.

24. Green LK, Herbert AA, Jorizzo JL, Solomon AR: Pyoderma gangrenosum and chronic persistent hepatitis. *J Am Acad Dermatol* 1985, 13:892–897.

25. Johnson RB, Lazarus GS: Pulse Therapy: Therapeutic efficacy in treatment of pyoderma gangrenosum. *Arch Dermatol* 1982, 118:76–84.

26. Ely PH: The bowel bypass syndrome: A response to bacterial peptidoglycans. *J Am Acad Dermatol* 1980, 2:473–487.

27. Jorizzo JL, Schmalstieg FC, Dinehart SM, *et al.*: Bowel associated dermatosis-arthritis syndrome: Immune complex-mediated vessel damage and increased neutrophil migration. *Arch Intern Med* 1984, 144:738–740.

Drug Eruptions 17

Paul I. Oh
Neil H. Shear

Key Points

- Rashes are a common adverse effect of drug therapy.
- Clinical features of the rash may suggest a drug reaction.
- Drugs are not the only cause of such rashes, and a stepwise clinical approach is needed.
- The propensity to develop severe reactions may be based on genetic differences in drug metabolism.

It is well known that drugs are a common cause of skin rashes. In the Boston Collaborative Drug Surveillance Program [1], the frequency of cutaneous adverse reactions varied from 0% to 5.1%, depending on the drug in question. In clinical practice the situation is somewhat more enigmatic as patients present with a rash, and one or more drugs are considered in the differential etiology. The clinician therefore requires a systematic approach to the following aspects of the problem: 1) rashes in general, 2) adverse drug reactions, 3) determination of causation, and 4) current and future management of the patient. An overview of types of drug eruptions is given in Figure 17-1.

TYPES OF DRUG ERUPTIONS

Exanthematous Eruptions

Exanthematous eruptions are the most common rashes seen by physicians and are known by the synonyms *morbilliform*, scarlatiniform and toxic erythema [2••,3–5]. The term maculopapular is used widely, but should be discouraged because of a lack of specificity. Any drug may cause these reactions. Repeated administration of the same drug in the future will most likely cause a similar syndrome, rather than a more accelerated or severe reaction. The major differential diagnosis for these rashes, particularly in children, are viral exanthems. Exanthematous eruptions start as erythematous macules and papules on the trunk, become confluent, and later spread symmetrically to the face and limbs.

Simple eruptions (Fig. 17-2) usually occur within 1 week of beginning therapy, especially if the patient has been previously sensitized, and resolve within 7 to 14 days. A common scenario is the occurrence of a generalized rash in almost all patients with infectious mononucleosis who are treated with ampicillin. A similar reaction occurs in approximately 50% of HIV-infected patients who are exposed to aromatic amines such as sulfonamide antibiotics [6•]. Many other antibiotics, with or without concurrent viral infections, have been associated with simple rashes.

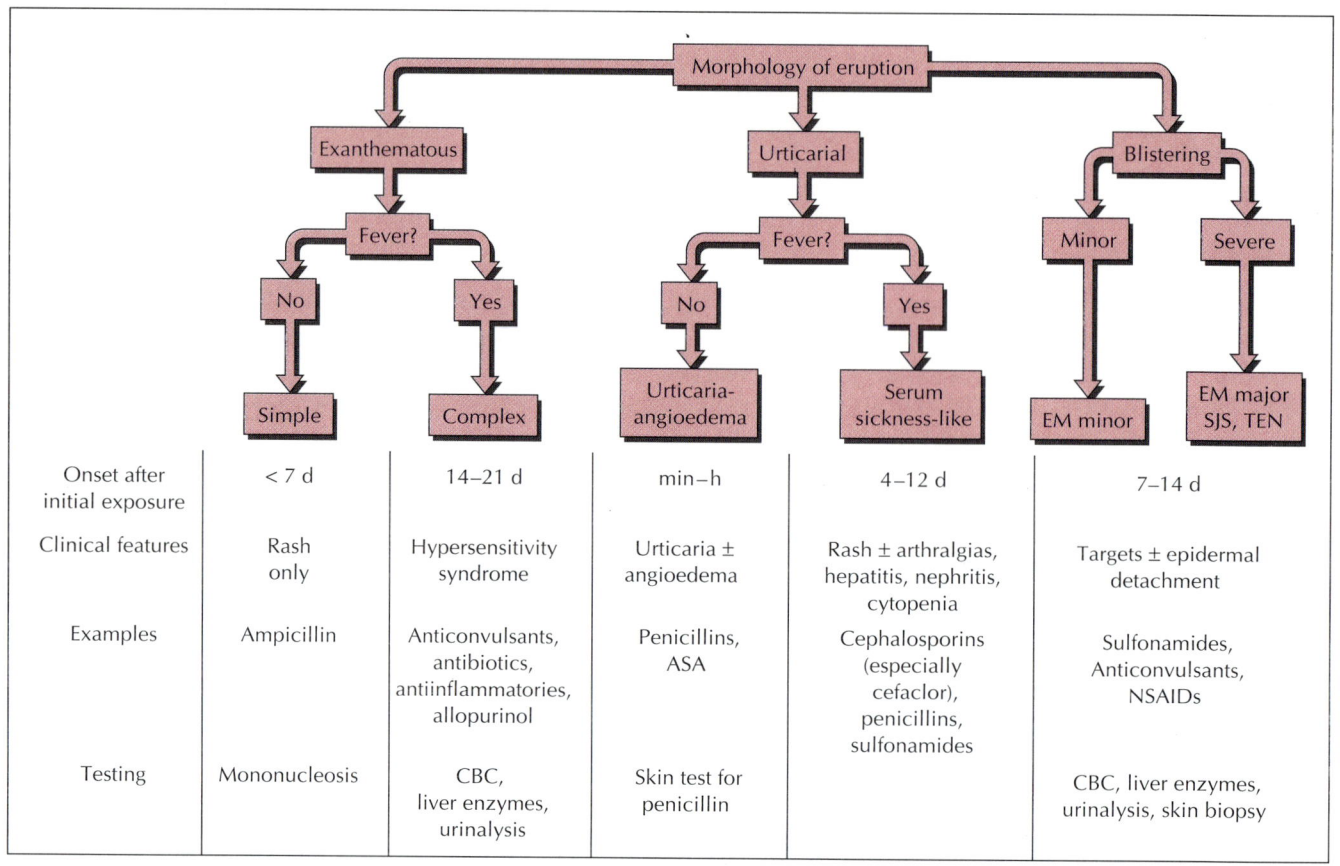

	Exanthematous		Urticarial		Blistering	
	Simple	Complex	Urticaria-angioedema	Serum sickness-like	EM minor	EM major SJS, TEN
Onset after initial exposure	< 7 d	14–21 d	min–h	4–12 d	7–14 d	
Clinical features	Rash only	Hypersensitivity syndrome	Urticaria ± angioedema	Rash ± arthralgias, hepatitis, nephritis, cytopenia	Targets ± epidermal detachment	
Examples	Ampicillin	Anticonvulsants, antibiotics, antiinflammatories, allopurinol	Penicillins, ASA	Cephalosporins (especially cefaclor), penicillins, sulfonamides	Sulfonamides, Anticonvulsants, NSAIDs	
Testing	Mononucleosis	CBC, liver enzymes, urinalysis	Skin test for penicillin		CBC, liver enzymes, urinalysis, skin biopsy	

Figure 17-1 Algorithm to aid the clinical diagnosis of drug rashes. ASA—acetylsalicyclic acid; CBC—complete blood count; EM—erythema multiforme; NSAIDs—nonsteroidal anti-inflamma-tory drugs; SJS—Stevens-Johnson syndrome; TEN—toxic epidermal necrolysis.

Complex rashes (Fig. 17-3) occur as a part of a *hypersensitivity syndrome* that is characterized by delayed onset of an exanthema (with or without pruritus) in association with fever, lymphadenopathy, and possibly hepatitis, nephritis, thyroiditis, and hematologic abnormalities [7]. The frequencies of these other findings is shown in Table 17-1. The syndrome usually begins with fever at 2 to 3 weeks from initial drug exposure, but an onset as long as 3 months into therapy has been reported. The major groups of drugs associated with hypersensitivity syndromes are the anticonvulsants (phenytoin, carbamazepine, and phenobarbital), antibiotics (sulfonamides), anti-inflammatories (gold and nonsteroidal anti-inflammatory drugs [NSAIDs] such as piroxicam), and allopurinol. There may be cross reactivity among different medications, and patients should therefore be advised about potentially hazardous drugs for the future. For example, in the case of anticonvulsants, 80% of patients who have had a hypersensitivity response to any one of phenytoin, phenobarbital, or carbamazepine will react to the other two in a similar way if exposed. The preferred choice for future treatment would then be an agent such as valproic acid. The propensity to develop a reaction is inherited. Genetic differences in drug-metabolizing enzymes result in insufficient clearance of toxic intermediates. Direct relatives of a patient who has had

a hypersensitivity reaction may have a dramatically increased risk of having a similar response when compared with the general population. Thus, counseling of family members is a crucial part of the assessment.

Urticarial Eruptions

Urticarial rashes are characterized by pruritic red wheals of varying sizes that can occur with any medication. When deep dermal and subcutaneous tissues are also swollen, the

TABLE 17-1 MANIFESTATIONS OF ANTICONVULSANT HYPERSENSITIVITY SYNDROME

Symptom	Incidence, %
Fever	100
Skin rash	87
Hepatitis	51
Eosinophilia	30
Nephritis	11
Pneumonitis	9
Atypical lymphocytosis	6

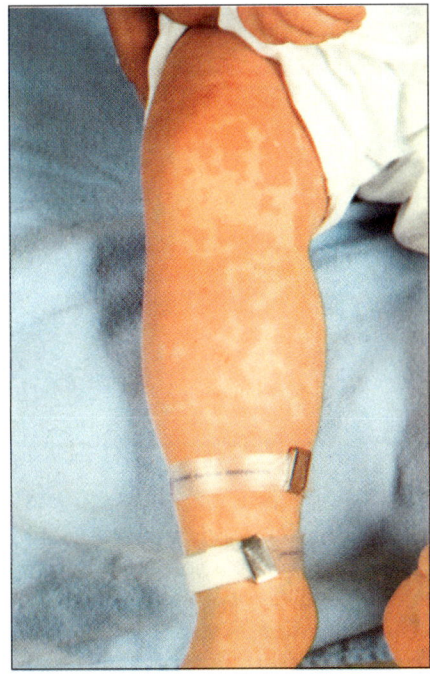

FIGURE 17-2 Exanthematous eruption caused by amoxicillin. There were no systemic symptoms, and no evidence of Epstein–Barr virus infection.

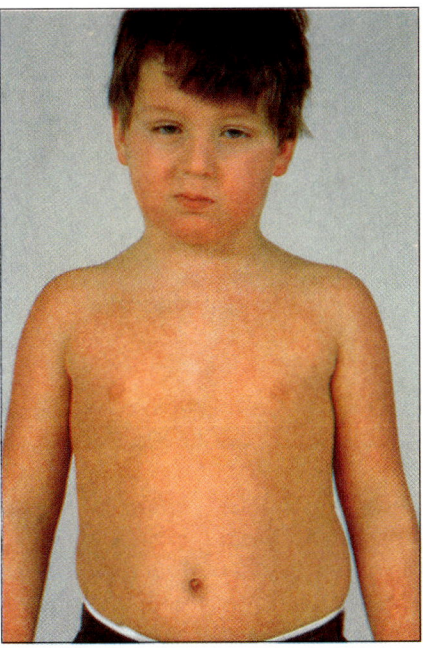

FIGURE 17-3 Generalized erythematous eruption associated with fever, lymphadenopathy, and nephritis. Hypersensitivity syndrome to phenobarbital was confirmed by *in vitro* testing.

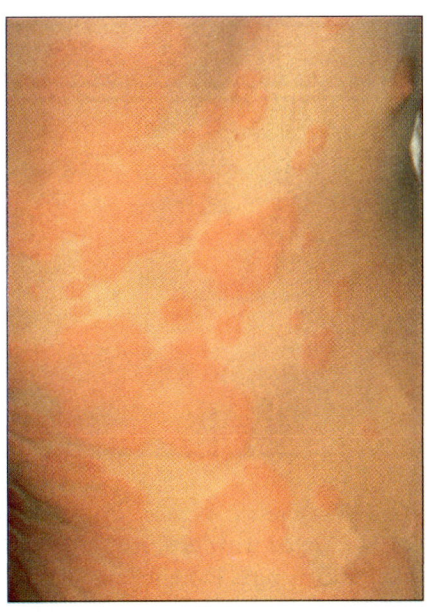

FIGURE 17-4 Itchy, red raised plaques that last for less than 24 hours are characteristic of urticaria. The annular morphology is commonly seen and often misdiagnosed as erythema multiforme. This reaction was caused by cloxacillin and confirmed by skin testing to penicillin.

reaction is known as angioedema. Angioedema may involve mucous membranes and be part of an anaphylactic reaction. There are several mechanisms for urticarial eruptions that are distinguished by their time course and accompanying features [2••,3–5].

Immunoglobulin E-dependent *urticaria* occurs within minutes to hours of drug exposure and is typified by immediate reactions to penicillins or acetylsalicylic acid (ASA) (Fig. 17-4). Combinations of the drug or metabolite with IgE bound to the surfaces of cutaneous mast cells lead to activation, degranulation, and release of vasoactive mediators such as histamine, leukotrienes, and prostaglandins. The resulting vasodilatation and increased vascular permeability lead to hive formation. *Angioedema* may occur in the absence of urticaria, but the two are often seen together in drug reactions. Idiopathic chronic recurrent urticaria can be confused with drug reactions unless the timing of reactions (*eg* occurrence of hives independent of drug exposure) is examined carefully. True urticaria usually resolves within 24 hours.

Immune complex disease, such as serum sickness reactions, are characterized by urticarial rashes, palpable purpura, or ulcerations, in association with fever, arthralgias, and possibly a combination of hepatitis, nephritis, hematologic or neurologic abnormalities that occur 4 to 12 days after exposure. Penicillins, cephalosporins, sulfonamides, animal-derived sera such as antivenom and antilymphocyte globulins, and streptokinase are common causative agents. Circulating immune complexes that

subsequently cause complement activation are thought to be one of the major pathogenic factors in these reactions. Circulating immune complexes have not been demonstrated in all the associated drugs (*eg*, antibiotics). The term *serum sickness–like reaction* (Fig. 17-5) has therefore been

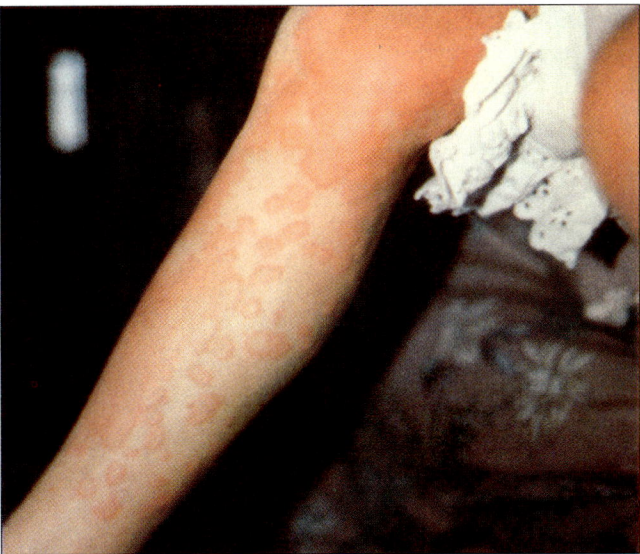

FIGURE 17-5 Annular urticarial plaques that last for more than 24 hours and are associated with fever and arthralgias are characteristic of serum sickness–like reactions. This patient had received cefaclor therapy for pharyngitis.

Classification	EM minor	EM major	SJS	TEN
Epidermal detachment, *% of body surface area*	<10	<10	<10	>30
Typical targets	Yes	No	No	No
Atypical targets	Raised	Flat	Flat	Flat
Macules	No	No	Yes	Yes
Mucous membrane involvement	No	Yes	Yes	Yes
Severity	+	++	+++	++++
Likelihood of drug etiology	+	++	+++	++++

EM—erythema multiforme; SJS—Stevens-Johnson syndrome; TEN—toxic epidermal necrolysis; +—low; ++++—high.

used in reference to these drug reactions. These reactions are associated with urticarial plaques, arthralgia, and fever. Nephritis is rare. Patients usually improve with supportive care in 5 to 7 days. Cefaclor is a common cause.

Urticarial reactions may also result from nonimmunologic activation of inflammatory mediators. Drugs such as ASA, NSAIDs, radiographic dyes, and opiates may directly cause release of histamine from mast cells independent of IgE, or activate complement and arachidonic acid pathways.

There are few laboratory tests that are helpful in the diagnosis of drug-induced urticaria or angioedema. Radioallergosorbent testing (RAST), if available, may help define the IgE-dependence of the reaction. At present, skin testing is of value for investigating suspected immediate hypersensitivity reactions to penicillins, but for other drugs no well-verified tests are available.

Blistering Eruptions

Eruptions associated with blisters or bullae encompass a spectrum from erythema multiforme (EM) to more serious reactions such as Stevens-Johnson syndrome (SJS) and toxic

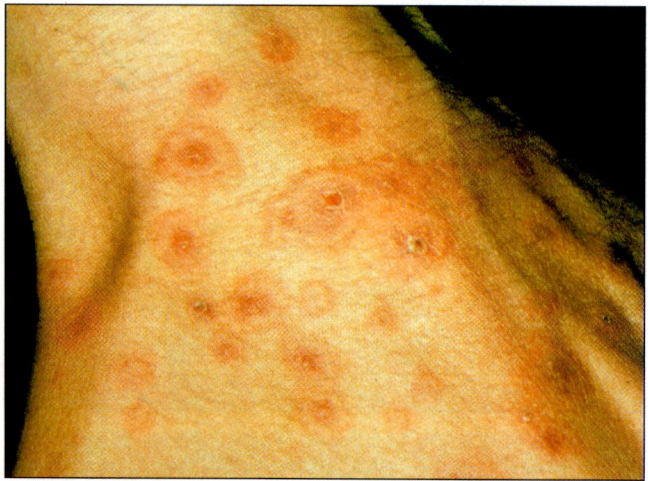

FIGURE 17-6 Typical target lesions with three concentric rings. This patient had a preceding mycoplasma infection.

epidermal necrolysis (TEN). These reactions can all be caused by drugs, but whereas TEN is almost always related to a drug exposure, EM and SJS have also been associated with infectious diseases such as *Mycoplasma pneumoniae* and herpes simplex. A recent international consensus conference [8•] proposed a standardized classification system for these eruptions, based on the presence or absence of target lesions and percentage of epidermal detachment as shown in Table 17-2. Classification may be further aided by the use of a photographic atlas illustrating the various types of lesions.

Bullous EM is characterized by both typical targets (red or bluish lesions with a regular round shape, well-defined border, and at least three different concentric zones, usually occurring on the limbs; Fig. 17-6) and atypical targets (round edematous, palpable lesions with only two zones and a poorly defined border; Fig. 17-7). Sulfonamide-induced EM is the best characterized of the drug eruptions in this category (Fig. 17-8). The reaction to this drug occurs 7 to 14 days after initiation of therapy and may be associated with fever or other constitutional symptoms. Other drugs that have been associated with EM include penicillins, phenytoin, carbamazepine, phenobarbital, rifampin, thiazides, and NSAIDs such as phenylbutazone. The same drugs may cause the more severe SJS, in which hemorrhagic bullae, erosions, and crusts appear in the mouth, on the lips and other mucous membranes, and where more prominent systemic features such as myalgias and arthralgias occur. A very severe disease course is associated with ocular involvement and possibly respiratory and renal pathology. Complete blood counts, liver enzymes, chest x-ray, and urinalysis should be performed to evaluate internal organ involvement. A skin biopsy may also be of value. Treatment is supportive, and the use of corticosteroids is still controversial.

Toxic epidermal necrolysis or Lyell's syndrome is the most serious cutaneous drug reaction (Fig. 17-9). The onset is generally acute and, in adults, drugs such as sulfonamides, barbiturates, NSAIDs (phenylbutazone, piroxicam), allopurinol, carbamazapine, and phenytoin are the most frequent cause of the reaction. It is important to emphasize that the scalded skin syndrome that occurs in children secondary to group 2 staphylococcal infections is a

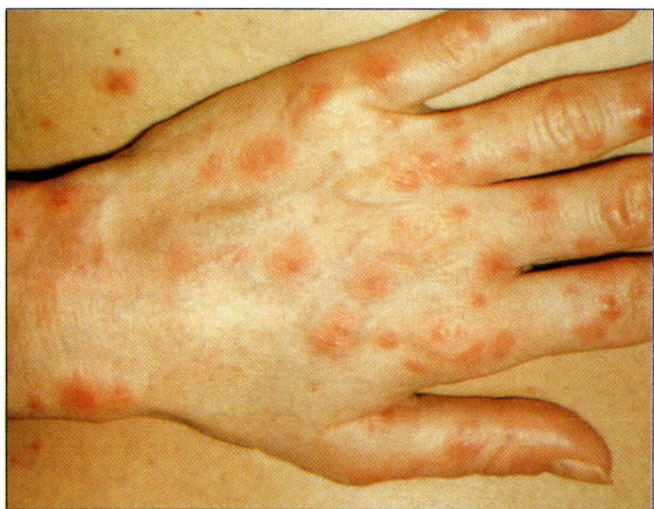

FIGURE 17-7 Inflammatory papules and blisters with surrounding erythema are characteristic of atypical targets. These lesions are usually found in severe blistering reactions to drugs, including erythema multiforme, Stevens-Johnson syndrome, and toxic epidermal necrolysis.

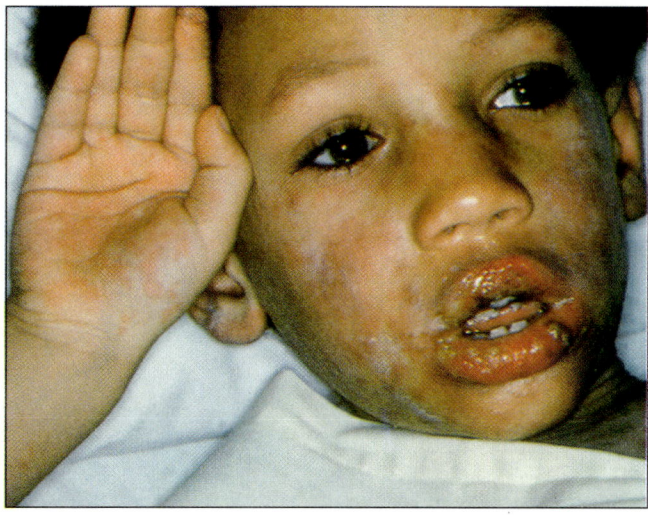

FIGURE 17-8 Mucosal erosions and atypical targets characteristic of a bullous drug eruption. The minor amount of blistering on the skin suggests a diagnosis of erythema multiforme rather than Stevens-Johnson syndrome. The diagnosis of drug reaction was not confirmed for this patient, and the differential diagnosis included both a sulfonamide reaction and post-mycoplasma erythema multiforme.

distinct entity and is not drug metabolizing. The clinical features, pathology, etiology, and prognosis are quite different. True TEN does occur in children as a potentially lethal drug-induced disease. The typical course consists of generalized tender erythema of the skin followed by extensive epidermal necrosis and sloughing of any area of skin or mucous membranes. This widespread denudation leads to a marked loss of fluids and electrolytes and also predisposes to pneumonia and septicemia. Mortality as high as 30% has been reported as a result of these complications. Investigations should include assessment for internal organ involvement (liver, kidney, or hematologic) as in hypersensitivity syndromes, and skin biopsies may be helpful. Treatment should take place in a specialized burn unit and be mainly supportive, but if the patient survives the acute phase of the illness the prognosis is generally favorable, with complete regeneration of the epidermal surfaces within a few weeks.

Photosensitivity

Photosensitive eruptions are produced by an interaction with the drug or its metabolite, and light energy. The drug itself may have been administered topically or orally, and the rash usually appears in sun-exposed areas such as the face, neck, arms, back of hands, and anterior thighs. Three major mechanisms can be considered in the pathogenesis of these reactions (Fig. 17-10) [2••,3–5], and the most common drugs are listed in Table 17-3.

Phototoxic reactions are the most frequent of the photosensitivity responses (Fig. 17-11). Reactions are not immunologic, and may occur on first exposure to the drug if an adequate dose of both drug and light are present. These reactions resemble sunburns and are caused by a lowered sun-sensitivity threshold. Ultraviolet light activates the drug

and the energy that is subsequently emitted damages adjacent tissue. The most commonly implicated medications include chlorpromazine, tetracyclines, psoralens, NSAIDs such as piroxicam and benoxaprofen, sulfonamides, and amiodarone. Appropriate sun protection such as clothing, hats, and use of sunscreens may be preventative.

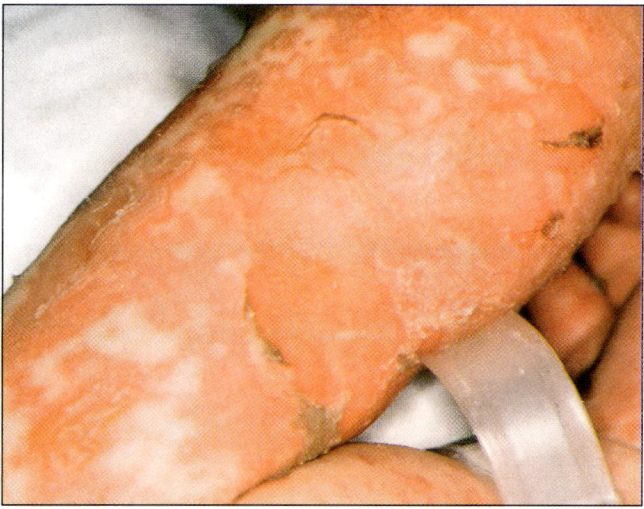

FIGURE 17-9 Painful erythema, blistering, and sloughing skin are caused by toxic epidermal necrolysis. This patient reacted to phenobarbital given for febrile seizures. The skin disease was associated with neutropenia, fever, lymphadenopathy, and pulmonary infiltrates. Supportive treatment was provided in a burn unit. The patient survived, but developed extensive postinflammatory hyperpigmentation.

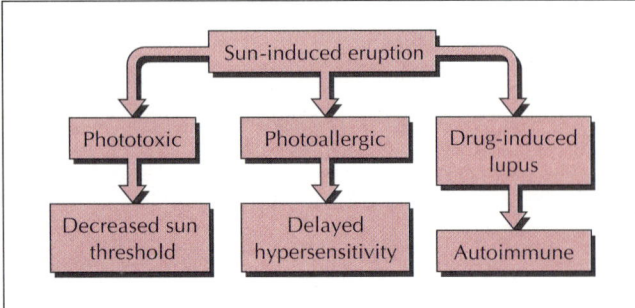

FIGURE 17-10 Algorithm of photosensitive eruptions.

TABLE 17-3 DRUGS CAUSING PHOTOSENSITIVITY		
Drug	**Incidence**	**Main reaction**
Amiodarone	High	Phototoxic
Chlorpromazine	Medium	Photoallergic
Nalidixic acid	High	Phototoxic
NSAIDs (*eg*, ketoprofen, naproxen, piroxicam, tiaprofenic acid)	Low	Phototoxic
Protriptyline	High	Phototoxic
Psoralens	High	Phototoxic
Sulfonamides (both antibi- otics and sulfonylureas)	Low	Photoallergic
Tetracyclines		
Doxycycline	Medium	Phototoxic
Tetracycline	Low	Phototoxic
Thiazide diuretics	Medium	Photoallergic

NSAIDs—nonsteroidal anti-inflammatory drugs.

Photoallergic eruptions are delayed hypersensitivity responses similar to contact dermatitis, and therefore occur only after initial sensitization. Light acts on the drug or drug metabolite to form a hapten that binds with a tissue antigen. Upon repeat light exposure, a cellular reaction with lymphocytic infiltration results that manifests with a variety of possible morphologies ranging from lichenoid papules to eczema. Hydrochlorothiazide, NSAIDs, and sulfonamides are the drugs most frequently involved.

Drug-induced lupus erythematosus is occasionally seen during treatment with hydralazine, procainamide, isoniazid, alphamethyldopa, and β-blockers such as acebutolol. Patients may develop facial rashes, as seen in systemic lupus erythematosus, but other organ involvement such as nephritis is less common. There may be a genetic predisposition to this condition, as is the case with the slow-acetylator phenotype and isoniazid.

Fixed-Drug Eruptions

Fixed-drug eruptions consist of a solitary or a few sharply demarcated erythematous lesions, usually involving the face or genitalia (Fig. 17-12). As the name would imply, drugs are the only known etiologic agent, but the pathogenesis remains unknown. They recur in the same location with repeat drug exposures and are associated with burning or pruritus. Once the acute inflammation resolves over 2 to 3 weeks, there is often residual local hyperpigmentation. Pathology of the lesion may be reported as showing features of erythema multiforme, but the two conditions should not be confused. Many drugs have been implicated but the most frequently reported ones are listed in Table 17-4 [2••,3–5].

Contact Dermatitis

For certain drug preparations, topical application leads to local sensitization [2••,3–5]. Upon repeat exposure, redness, pruritus, and a papular eruption, followed by edema and vesiculation, may develop as a result of lymphocytic infiltration. Systemic exposure in the future might lead to flare-ups at the sites of previous reactivity, but more generalized eruptions might also be induced. In sensitized persons, the reaction usually becomes evident 6 to 48 hours after contact.

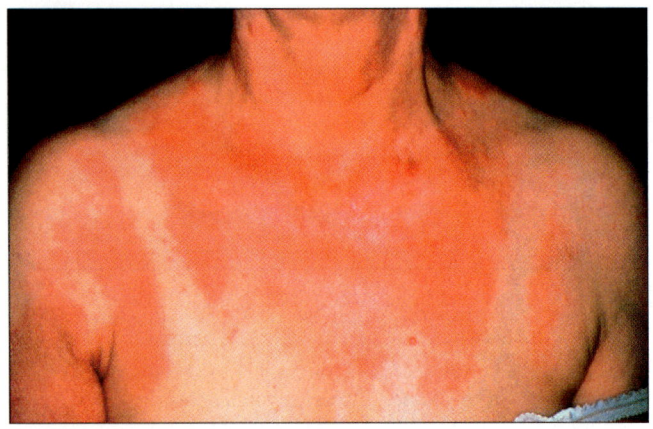

FIGURE 17-11 Erythema and scaling in sun-exposed areas. The patient was taking chlorpromazine.

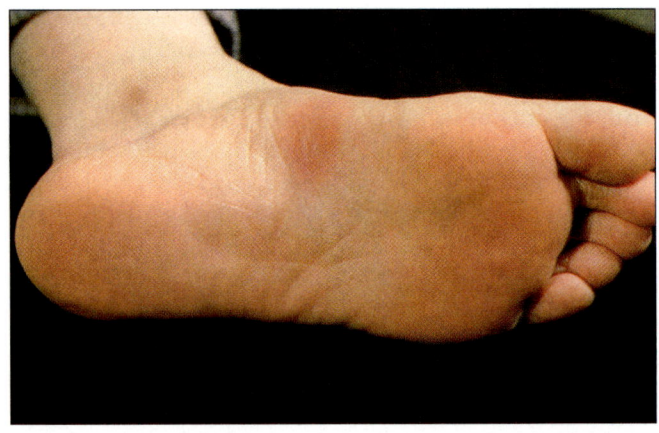

FIGURE 17-12 Well-demarcated red oval of fixed drug eruption, caused by phenolphthalein.

TABLE 17-4 DRUGS CAUSING FIXED DRUG ERUPTIONS

Antibiotics	Benzodiazepines
Sulfonamides	Chloral hydrate
Tetracyclines	
Penicillins	**NSAIDs and analgesics**
Erythromycin	Acetylsalicylic acid
Nystatin	Phenylbutazone
Metronidazole	Ibuprofen
	Acetominophen
Sedatives and hypnotics	
Barbiturates	**Phenolphthalein**
Opiates	

NSAIDs—nonsteroidal anti-inflammatory drugs.

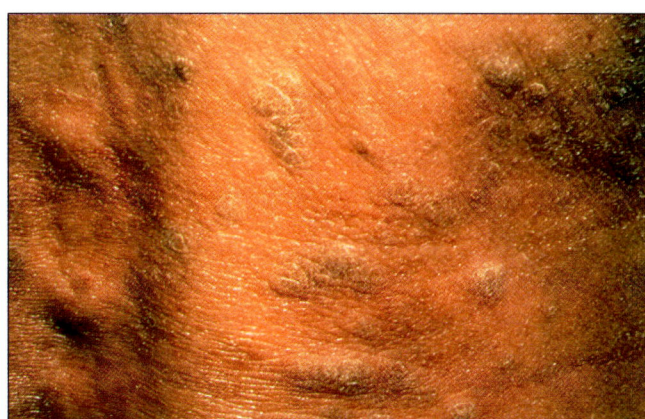

FIGURE 17-13 Purple-red plaques with striated surface show pathologic features of lichen planus-like drug eruption. Drug-induced etiology can be inferred from the pathological features. The patient was receiving intramuscular gold therapy for rheumatoid arthritis.

The most commonly implicated drugs for contact dermatitis include topically applied local anesthetics, antihistamines, antibiotics (*eg,* penicillin, sulfonamides, and neomycin), and corticosteroids. Sometimes the reaction is induced by other components of the cream or lotion rather than the drug itself. The differential diagnosis includes primary irritant contact dermatitis that is nonimmunologic and other forms of dermatitis (*eg,* nummular).

The causal agent of contact dermatitis can often be identified through a careful history, but skin testing may be of benefit when there is uncertainty. In patch testing, components of the topical agent including the drug itself, preservatives such as paraben esters, fragrances, and any other excipients are each applied separately to a small area of skin and left in place for 48 hours. Development of a typical lesion of contact dermatitis is considered positive and confirms the diagnosis [9].

Other Eruptions

Lichenoid cutaneous reactions (Fig. 17-13) that are identical to lichen planus have been reported in association with gold, antimalarials, β-blockers, and captopril. The mechanism by which these agents produce this reaction is unknown.

Erythema nodosum is a panniculitis that is characterized by tender subcutaneous erythematous nodules, usually located over the anterior portion of the lower extremities. It has occasionally been associated with medications such as oral contraceptives, sulfonamides, salicylates, bromides, iodides, and gold, but is most commonly related to infections such as streptococcus, fungi, and tuberculosis, or to chronic granulomatous diseases such as sarcoidosis. The pathogenesis is unknown.

Vasculitis may be confined to the skin or be part of a more generalized multiorgan process such as polyarteritis nodosa. Cutaneous necrotizing vasculitis presents with palpable purpuric lesions, usually over the lower extremities. Although it is believed that immune mechanisms such as immune complex formation are involved in drug-induced vasculitis, the exact pathogenesis is unknown. The following drugs have been associated with vasculitic reactions: sulfonamides, NSAIDs such as phenylbutazone and indomethacin, propylthiouracil, and phenytoin. In addition, almost all antibiotics have been linked to a case of vasculitis.

Drug-induced bullous pemphigoid and pemphigus are occasionally seen, and are similar in appearance to the idiopathic conditions. Bullous pemphigoid has been reported with a number of drugs, many of which have in common the presence of a sulfur group (*eg,* frusemide, penicillamine, and sulfasalazine). Pemphigus has been seen with medications containing a thiol group in the molecule in over 80% of cases (*eg,* penicillamine, captopril, and gold sodium thiomalate), as well as with antibiotics such as penicillin and cephalosporins.

APPROACH AND MANAGEMENT

The approach to diagnosing drug eruptions is the same as that used for adverse drug reactions in general (Table 17-5) [10•]. Drug reactions occur in complicated clinical scenarios that often entail exposures to multiple agents, but a systematic, stepwise approach that examines each component of the reaction in turn can lead the clinician to the correct diagnosis. Accurate recognition of the rash may require the aid of a dermatologist and possibly a skin biopsy. References such as *A Guide to Drug Eruptions* [2••] provide a quick cross-index between rashes and particular medications as well as a listing of relevant literature. Figure 17-3 illustrates a simple algorithm to follow in order to differentiate among the various types of eruptions, which highlights distinguishing clinical features and key investigations.

TABLE 17-5 STEPS IN THE APPROACH TO A SUSPECTED ADVERSE DRUG REACTION

- Clinical diagnosis of the adverse event (a dermatology consult is often helpful)
- Analysis of drug exposure (timing, consideration of multiple drugs, patient factors, underlying or coexisting diseases)
- Differential diagnosis of skin rash
- Literature search (a clinical pharmacist can be of great help)
- Confirmation (*in vivo* or *in vitro* testing or challenge, where possible)
- Advice to patient (which drug, likelihood of reaction, future risks, safe medications for future use, possible genetic predisposition)
- Reporting to state or federal regulators and drug manufacturer of severe or unusual reactions

Treatment of drug eruptions may simply involve stopping and avoiding the offending agent. Symptomatic care could include topical corticosteroids and oral antihistamines for pruritus. In some of the more severe hypersensitivity reactions, such as SJS, TEN, or vasculitis, systemic corticosteroids or other immunosuppressive therapy might be indicated. It might also be helpful to determine serum concentrations of a drug to confirm exposure and possibly establish a dose–response relationship. Most other testing is either experimental, not readily available, or of limited utility. There are decision aids in the form of questionnaires or computerized spreadsheets with databases to work through the problems of adverse reactions [11•], but these are also not generally available. Physicians should follow a thoughtful, comprehensive, clinical approach to the diagnosis and management of adverse cutaneous drug reactions.

REFERENCES AND RECOMMENDED READING

Recently published papers of particular interest have been highlighted as:

- Of interest
- •• Of outstanding interest

1. Bigby M, Jick S, Jick H, *et al.*: Drug-induced cutaneous reactions. A report from the Boston Collaborative Drug Surveillance Program on 15 438 consecutive inpatients, 1975 to 1982. *JAMA* 1986, 256:3358–3363.

2.•• Bruinsma W: *A Guide to Drug Eruptions*, edn 5. Oosthuizen: The File of Medicines; 1990.

3. Wintroub BU, Stern R: Cutaneous drug reactions: pathogenesis and clinical classification. *J Am Acad Dermatol* 1985, 13:167–179.

4. Kaplan AP: Drug-induced skin disease. *J Allergy Clin Immunol* 1984, 74:573–579.

5. Breathnach SM, Hintner H: *Adverse drug reactions and the skin.* Oxford: Blackwell Scientific Publications; 1992.

6.• Coopman SA, Johnson RA, Platt R, Stern RS: Cutaneous disease and drug reactions in HIV infection. *N Engl J Med* 1993, 328:1670–1674.

7. Shear NH, Spielberg SP: Anticonvulsant hypersensitivity syndrome. *J Clin Invest* 1988, 89:1826–1832.

8.• Bastuji-Garin S, Rzany B, Stern RS, *et al.*: Clinical classification of cases of toxic epidermal necrolysis, Stevens-Johnson syndrome, and erythema multiforme. *Arch Dermatol* 1993, 129:92–96.

9. Bruynzeel DP, van Ketel WG: Patch testing in drug eruptions. *Seminar Dermatol* 1989, 8:196–203.

10.• Shear NH: Diagnosing cutaneous adverse reactions to drugs. *Arch Dermatol* 1990, 126:94–97.

11.• Naranjo CA, Shear NH, Lanctot KL: Advances in the diagnosis of adverse drug reactions. *J Clin Pharmacol* 1992, 32:897–904.

SELECT BIBLIOGRAPHY

Breathnach SM, Hintner H: Adverse drug reactions and the skin. Oxford: Blackwell Scientific Publications; 1992.

Prussick R, Knowles S, Shear NH: Cutaneous drug reactions. *Current Prob Dermatol* 1994, 6:81-124.

Life-Threatening Dermatoses 18

Grace S. Liang-Federman
Francisco A. Kerdel

Key Points

- Dermatologic disorders with manifestations that usually remain confined to the skin may on rare occasions become so widespread that they result in systemic complications.
- Conditions such as psoriasis, pemphigus, and erythematous drug reactions must be managed aggressively to limit morbidity and reduce associated mortality.
- Systemic diseases such as streptococcal or staphylococcal infections, rickettsial and meningococcal infections, and coagulopathies leading to purpura fulminans can first be recognized by changes in the skin.
- Rapid intervention with systemic therapies must be combined with treatment of the skin to reverse systemic disease processes.

The skin is an ideal organ for the direct examination and rapid availability of tissue samples, allowing us easy access to diagnostic clues for various disorders. Although true dermatologic emergencies are fortunately rare, when they do arise, prompt recognition and immediate intervention can be life saving. The life-threatening dermatoses can be divided into two categories: disorders that are primary skin conditions with potential systemic complications, and systemic disorders that have prominent manifestations in the skin. Immunocompromised patients represent a subset of patients who are susceptible to a host of other unusual skin conditions, especially those that are infectious (Table 18-1). In these patients the clinical presentation can be greatly modified by unpredictable inflammatory responses, making skin findings atypical or nonspecific.

PRIMARY SKIN DISORDERS WITH POTENTIAL SYSTEMIC COMPLICATIONS

Toxic Epidermal Necrolysis

Toxic epidermal necrolysis (TEN), or acute disseminated epidermal necrosis, is a fulminant desquamating process that begins as a generalized morbilliform or confluent erythema and rapidly progresses to extensive bullae formation with exfoliation (Fig. 18-1). The skin lesions are typically painful, and mucosal involvement can be extensive. Loss of nails is not uncommon, but the scalp is usually spared. Patients are often febrile, and the acute phase may be associated with multiple complications, including fluid and electrolyte imbalances, and sepsis. These latter complications result in a mortality rate of 25% to 70%.

The majority of TEN cases have been associated with the intake of various drugs; antibiotics, antiseizure medications, nonsteroidal antiinflammatory drugs, and allopurinol are commonly implicated. Skin lesions appear between 2 to 21 days after the ingestion of a given agent and become generalized within 24 to 48

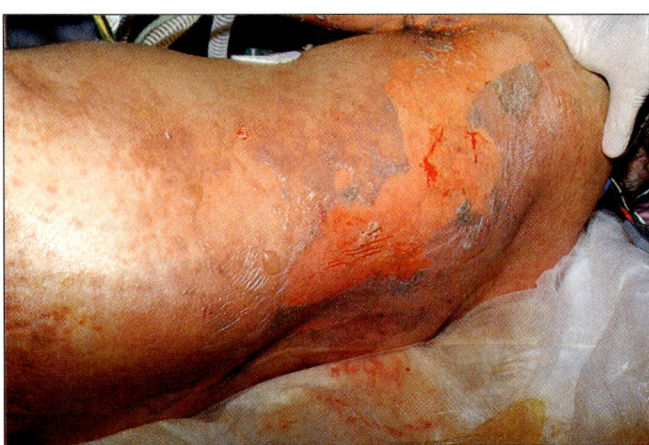

FIGURE 18-1 Toxic epidermal necrolysis: widespread areas of desquamation on the back with erythema.

hours. Laboratory tests may yield findings such as prerenal azotemia, elevated liver enzyme levels, disseminated intravascular coagulation, and, rarely, pancreatitis. Neutropenia, lymphopenia, anemia, and thrombocytopenia portend a poor prognosis. Histopathologic analyses of skin biopsy specimens show full-thickness epidermal necrosis with a minimal-to-absent dermal mononuclear cell infiltrate.

The management of TEN should ideally be undertaken in a burn unit or intensive care setting where fluid and electrolyte levels can be closely monitored, and careful attention can be paid to nutritional support. Ophthalmologic consultation is essential to prevent long-term sequelae, including xerophthalmia, visual impairment, and even blindness from conjunctival, corneal, and lacrimal duct damage. Skin care should be aimed at rapid healing and prevention of infection. Areas not affected should be handled carefully to minimize progression. Some authors advocate stripping the necrotic epidermis and placing xenografts, homografts, or skin substitutes while the patient is receiving general anesthesia. Silver nitrate irrigation, 0.5%, or frequent dressing changes may be as effective. Corticosteroids should not be administered because they may increase the frequency of medical complications, mask signs of impending sepsis, and impair wound healing. Likewise, prophylactic antibiotic use is not recommended, although careful monitoring for secondary skin infection and vigorous pulmonary toilet are essential. *Staphylococcus aureus* is a common skin pathogen found early in the course of the disease whereas *Pseudomonas aeruginosa* infection may develop at later stages. The role of other treatment modalities such as plasmapheresis, cyclophosphamide therapy, and hyperbaric oxygen application have yet to be defined [1••,2].

Erythema Multiforme Major

Erythema multiforme (EM) is considered by some authors to be related to TEN in that the entities may represent ends of a spectrum of hypersensitivity disorders [3]. EM minor accounts for 80% of EM cases and is characterized by targetlike plaques with dusky centers and "multiform" urticarial, annular, solid, and bullous plaques often involving the palms, soles, and distal extremities. EM minor is commonly associated with an antecedent history of herpes simplex virus infection. In EM major or Stevens-Johnson syndrome, which constitutes the other 20% of EM cases, skin involvement is extensive and is associated with involvement of at least two mucosal surfaces as well as prominent systemic symptoms (Fig. 18-2). Most cases are sporadic, lasting 3 to 6 weeks, but recurrent cases have been reported. EM major is commonly associated with drugs or infection with *Mycoplasma pneumoniae*, and less often with herpes simplex virus infection. The treatment of EM major depends on the severity of disease and on the underlying condition. If involvement is extensive, TEN-like management may be required [4••].

Staphylococcal Scalded Skin Syndrome

Toxic epidermal necrolysis must be distinguished from another disease characterized by extensive sloughing of the

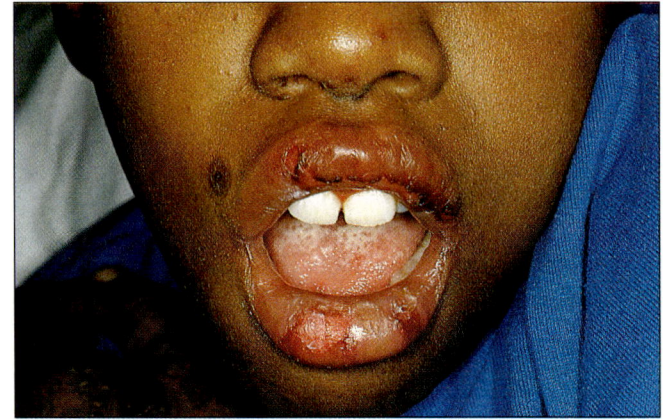

FIGURE 18-2 Erythema multiforme major (Stevens-Johnson syndrome) with severe involvement of the oral mucosa.

TABLE 18-2 CONDITIONS ASSOCIATED WITH EXFOLIATIVE ERYTHRODERMA	
Condition	**Diagnostic clues**
Psoriasis	Family history, skin biopsy
Dermatitis: atopic, contact, seborrheic	Eosinophilia, increased IgE
Drug induced	History
Cutaneous T-cell lymphoma (mycosis fungoides)	Skin biopsy: atypical lymphocytes
Lymphoma, leukemia	Skin or lymph node biopsy, CBC, chest radiograph
Pityriasis rubra pilaris	Clinical presentation, skin biopsy
Underlying malignancy	Radiographic studies, tissue biopsy
Icthyosis	Family history, skin biopsy
CBC—complete blood count.	

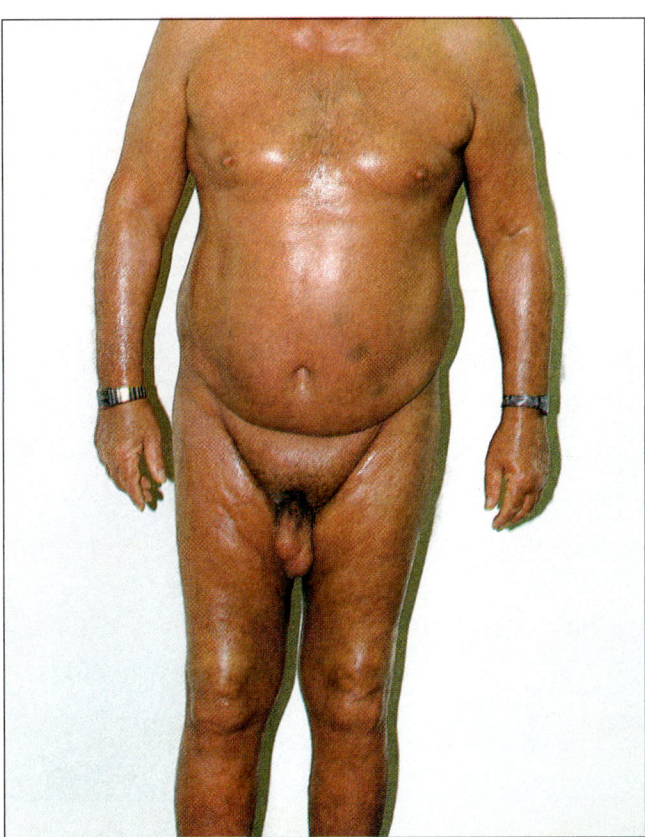

FIGURE 18-3 Diffuse erythroderma secondary to psoriasis.

skin, staphylococcal scalded skin syndrome (SSSS) [5•]. Most patients with SSSS are children under 5 years of age; in this setting the condition runs a benign course. However, when SSSS occurs in adults, especially those with impaired renal function, the condition has a worse prognosis. Patients present with a faint, scarlatiniform erythema and superficial desquamation, often with periorificial and flexural accentuation. Mucous membrane involvement is not prominent, but an occult focus of staphylococcal infection may be present in the nose, conjunctiva, or umbilicus.

Staphylococcal scalded skin syndrome is the result of an exfoliating toxin produced by *S. aureus* phage II; therefore, the skin lesions of SSSS are usually sterile. Frozen-section examinations of the blister roof or skin biopsy specimens can be used to distinguish SSSS from the more serious TEN. In SSSS, the split occurs subcorneally within the stratum granulosum, whereas a subepidermal split is seen in TEN. Cytodiagnosis (Tzanck smear) can also be helpful. In SSSS there are broad epithelial cells with small nuclei, whereas in TEN there are cuboidal cells with large nuclei and inflammatory cells. A prompt diagnosis allows rapid treatment of the staphylococcal focus with antibiotics to reduce the amount of toxin present. Careful attention to skin hygiene and abundant application of emollients are also indicated.

Exfoliative Erythrodermas

Exfoliative erythroderma is a generalized erythematous scaling eruption that may be secondary to a variety of conditions (Table 18-2). Despite attempts to determine the cause of the erythroderma, approximately 40% of cases remain of idiopathic origin. Patients may have associated peripheral edema, alopecia, nail dystrophy, lymphadenopathy, hepatosplenomegaly, and impaired temperature regulation.

A diagnostic evaluation should include multiple skin biopsies, with particular attention paid to the possibility of cutaneous T-cell lymphoma. In these cases, examinations for malignant cells in the circulation (Sézary cells) and for lymph node or systemic involvement are essential. Patients with psoriasis (Figs. 18-3 and 18-4) may have family histo-

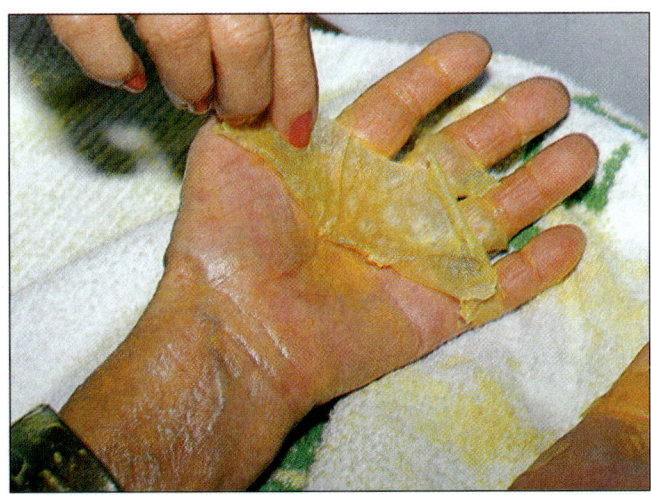

FIGURE 18-4 Desquamation of a thick keratoderma of the palm in a patient with psoriasis.

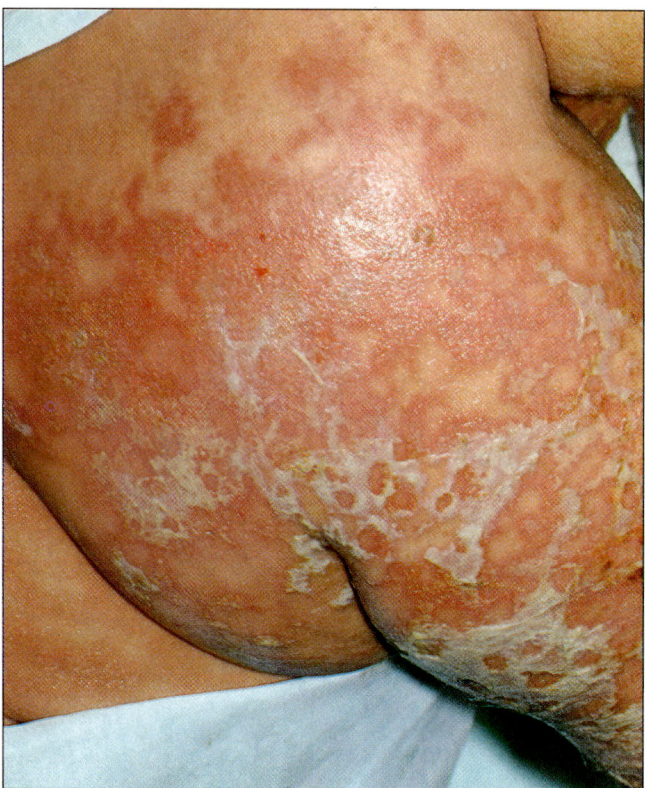

FIGURE 18-5 Generalized pustular psoriasis (Von Zumbusch type): "lakes of pus" with moist red plaques on the shoulder and back.

Treatment begins with hospitalization and conservative measures such as bedrest and sedation, topical emollient application, and maintenance of fluid and electrolyte balance. Provocative agents such as lithium, β-blockers, antimalarials, and salicylates should be discontinued. The discontinuation of systemic corticosteroid therapy or discontinuation of the widespread use of potent topical steroids under occlusion have precipitated generalized pustular psoriasis; therefore, their use in patients with psoriasis should be avoided. Phototherapy, the topical application of coal tar, and anthralin use are relatively contraindicated, and PUVA (psoralens and ultraviolet A light therapy) should be used only with extreme caution. Systemic agents such as methotrexate, etretinate, dapsone, hydroxyurea, and cyclosporin-A should be given according to the severity of the disease. In the case of impetigo herpetiformis, systemic steroid administration and general supportive measures are recommended. (*See* Simpson and Lowe, *Psoriasis*.)

Pemphigus and Pemphigoid

Severe cases of pemphigus vulgaris (and less often, bullous pemphigoid) can lead to extensive cutaneous denudation. Before corticosteroids were available for treatment use, the disease carried a mortality rate in excess of 50%. Paraneoplastic pemphigus is a recently described entity associated with antibodies against desmoplakin-I [8]. This disease is associated most often with reticuloendothelial malignancies and has a particularly poor prognosis.

SYSTEMIC DISORDERS WITH PROMINENT CUTANEOUS MANIFESTATIONS

Toxic Shock and Associated Syndromes

Toxic Shock Syndrome (TSS) has an incidence rate of 3 to 14 per 100,000 women of menstrual age and a mortality rate of 2%. It is most often seen in association with menstruation, and 98% of affected women have reported having used tampons at the onset of the disease. The incidence of this disease appears to be decreasing with the discontinued use of some super-absorbency tampons. Postoperative wound infections, superficial skin infections, and postpartum complications are less common predisposing causes of TSS [9,10].

Clinical features of TSS include fever (>40°C), hypotension, and a diffuse nontender erythroderma that appears within the first 24 hours and leads to a generalized desquamation after 7 to 10 days, most prominently on the hands and feet. Mucosal involvement may manifest as a strawberry tongue or as conjunctival, oropharyngeal, or vaginal hyperemia. The patient can have a sore throat, myalgias, gastrointestinal symptoms, and renal failure, and central nervous system changes such as headaches, dizziness, confusion, and agitation.

ries of psoriasis or classic nail changes. Patients with atopic dermatitis may have severe pruritus and lichenification, peripheral eosinophilia, and elevated serum IgE levels. The erythroderma of pityriasis rubra pilaris usually has a distinct salmon-pink hue with islands of spared skin and a yellowish keratoderma of the palms and soles. Histories of drug or contact allergy should be sought.

Patients with erythroderma should be treated according to the underlying process. In cases with no discernible cause, conservative measures are recommended, including whirlpool baths, emollient application, mid-potency topical steroid administration, and occlusive dressings [6•].

Pustular Psoriasis

Patients with the Von Zumbusch type of pustular psoriasis present with fulminant widespread erythema, with crops of sterile subcorneal pustules that coalesce into "lakes of pus" (Fig. 18-5). The oral mucosa and tongue may be involved, and the patient is usually febrile. The condition may be associated with hypocalcemia, hypoalbuminemia, and leukocytosis. Fluid and protein loss, cardiac failure, and sepsis are not unusual complications [7•]. A similar generalized form of pustular psoriasis can occur during pregnancy (impetigo herpetiformis), typically appearing before the sixth month of pregnancy and often recurring in subsequent pregnancies.

TSS is thought to be caused by exotoxins (*eg*, TSST-1) produced by a phage group I strain of *Staphylococcus aureus*. Blood cultures, however, are only rarely positive for staphylococcal organisms, and there may not be actual infection but only colonization of the responsible strain as a part of the patient's local flora. Failure to eradicate the organisms or lack of development of antibodies against the endotoxin may cause recurrences of TSS at rates of as high as 30%.

Prompt recognition and early intervention are essential. Tampon removal, drainage of pus, and debridement or irrigation of wounds serve to reduce bacterial load. Aggressive fluid replacement, and if necessary, the administration of systemic adrenergic agents, should be undertaken to maintain adequate blood pressure. The use of antistaphylococcal antibiotics is recommended to eliminate the focus of staphylococcal organisms, but these agents do not actually alter the immediate course of TSS. The antibiotics of choice are penicillinase-resistant penicillins (oxacillin or nafcillin), or first-generation cephalosporins, vancomycin, or clindamycin in penicillin-allergic patients.

Staphylococcal-induced TSS must be differentiated from streptococcal toxic shock–like syndrome (TSLS), or "toxic strep syndrome," which is caused by pyrogenic exotoxins (M types 1 and 3) produced by group A *Streptococcus*. TSLS is a fulminant disease that can be seen in association with cellulitis or other soft-tissue infections. Clinical features include fever, hypotension, mental status changes, toxin-induced renal impairment (distinct from poststreptococcal glomerulonephritis), and a variety of cutaneous changes such as swelling, erythema, bullae, scarletiniform rash, and desquamation. Unlike in TSS, blood cultures are often positive for streptococcal organisms [11•,12].

The recommended treatment for TSLS is similar to that for TSS. Fluid and electrolyte support, surgical debridement, and antibiotic therapy (high-dose penicillin or clindamycin) must be initiated promptly.

Kawasaki Syndrome

Kawasaki syndrome or mucocutaneous lymph node syndrome is an idiopathic, acute disease resembling toxic shock syndrome [13,14•,15]. It primarily affects children and adolescents, with 95% of patients being less than 5 years of age. Clinical criteria for diagnosis include fever lasting 5 or more days; bilateral conjunctivitis; oropharyngeal mucous membrane inflammation manifested by diffuse erythema, fissured lips, or strawberry tongue; edema and erythema of distal extremities with periungual desquamation; a diffuse erythematous rash that may be scarlatiniform, morbilliform, or macular; and cervical lymphadenopathy measuring greater than 1.5 cm (Table 18-3). Early histopathologic changes show vasculitis involving arterioles, venules, and capillaries.

Although the initial febrile course is self-limited, approximately 1.5% of patients die of late cardiac complications, especially coronary artery aneurysm and myocardial infarction. Treatment to prevent coronary artery

TABLE 18-3 CLINICAL CRITERIA FOR THE DIAGNOSIS OF KAWASAKI SYNDROME
Fever lasting ≥5 d
Bilateral conjunctivitis
Oropharyngeal mucous membrane inflammation
Distal extremity edema, erythema, desquamation
Diffuse erythematous rash
Cervical lymphadenopathy >1.5 cm

lesions and to reduce systemic inflammation entails giving aspirin (100 mg/kg/d for 14 days, then 3–5 mg/kg/d) with intravenous gammaglobulin in a single infusion of 2 g/kg over 10 hours [16].

Purpura Fulminans

Disseminated intravascular coagulation (DIC) can result in the sudden onset of extensive petechiae, purpura, hemorrhagic bullae, and severe skin necrosis due to generalized cutaneous thromboses (Fig. 18-6). Patients have various signs of hemolysis, bleeding, and thromboembolism. Most cases of purpura fulminans are fatal within 2 to 3 days of onset and can be seen in association with severe infections (especially gram-negative septicemia, streptococcal and staphylococcal sepsis, and acute varicella infections), obstetric complications, malignancies, trauma, snake bites, and giant hemangiomas (Kasabach-Merritt syndrome). Patients with congenital or acquired protein C and protein S deficiencies may be particularly predisposed to developing purpura fulminans.

Characteristic laboratory findings show consumption of platelets and clotting factors with decreased fibrinogen and increased fibrin degradation products. Skin biopsy specimens show intravascular thrombi, hemorrhage, and necrosis.

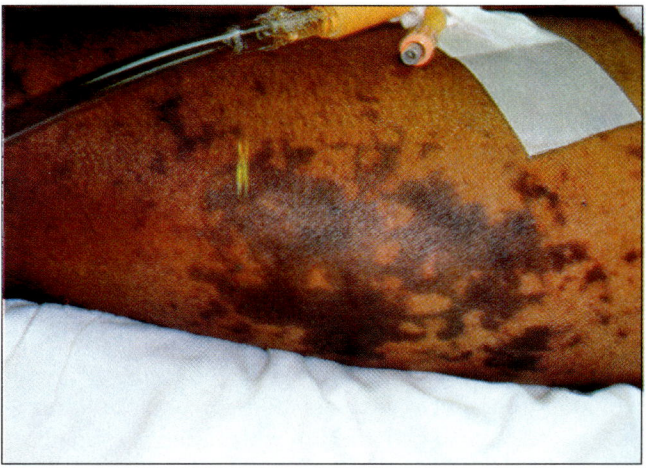

FIGURE 18-6 Purpura fulminans in a patient with acute meningococcemia: large areas of purpura and petechiae on the lateral trunk. (*Courtesy of* A. Blauvelt, MD).

The first objective of therapy is to treat the underlying condition and transfuse with blood, platelets, and fresh frozen plasma as indicated. Extensive cutaneous necrosis can be treated with skin debridement and grafting. Debate over the role of heparin and other agents such as aspirin, dipyridamole, and ϵ-aminocaproic acid in controlling consumption coagulopathy is still controversial [17••].

Meningococcemia

Septicemia and meningitis from *Neisseria meningitidis* (especially types A, B, and C) carry an overall mortality rate of 10% to 50%. Severe meningococcal infection is most common in children, but epidemics can occur in adults living in close contact—such as in military barracks. Cutaneous eruptions may be the first clue to early diagnosis, although in about 25% of cases there will be no skin findings. Early skin lesions are morbilliform, urticarial, or discrete macules and papules. Characteristic petechiae and purpura appear later and are caused by organisms within capillary walls and by DIC. Late purpuric lesions are the result of immune complex–mediated vasculitis. Nodules, bullae, ulcers, and even full-blown purpura fulminans may develop.

The diagnosis is confirmed by the detection of *N. meningitidis* organisms in blood cultures or cerebrospinal fluid. Treatment should begin promptly with the intravenous administration of high-dose benzyl penicillin, chloramphenicol, or ceftriaxone. Exposed persons in close contact with the patient should be given prophylactic treatment with rifampin [18,19].

Rocky Mountain Spotted Fever

The recognition of the most severe rickettsial infection, Rocky Mountain spotted fever (RMSF), is imperative because untreated cases carry a reported mortality rate of up to 80%. The disease is caused by *Rickettsia rickettsii* and is transmitted by the wood tick, *Dermacentor andersoni*, in the western United States, and mainly by *D. variabilis* in the eastern United States [20•].

Approximately 3 to 12 days after a tick bite, patients have the sudden onset of fevers, chills, malaise, headache, myalgias, and arthralgias. Two to six days later a maculopapular eruption characteristically appears on the wrists, ankles, and forearms, spreads to the palms and soles, and then extends centrally to the trunk and face. The rash soon becomes petechial and more confluent. Large ecchymoses and acral gangrene are not unusual. Patients appear severely ill and can have myocarditis, hepatitis, renal failure, and neurologic changes. The diagnosis can be established with skin biopsy specimens demonstrating vasculitis and organisms in the vascular endothelium when using immunofluorescent staining. Serologic studies are valuable in confirming the diagnosis of RMSF, but results do not become reliably positive for 6 to 10 days after the onset of clinical symptoms. Tetracycline, doxycycline, and chloramphenicol are effective when administered early. The use of sulfon-

TABLE 18-4 OTHER SYSTEMIC DISEASES WITH PROMINENT CUTANEOUS MANIFESTATIONS
Angioedema (hereditary and allergic)
Systemic lupus erythematosus or neonatal lupus
Dermatomyositis
Relapsing polychondritis
Vasculitis
Behçet's disease
Cholesterol emboli
Systemic mastocytosis
Histiocytosis X
Graft-versus-host disease

amides is contraindicated because they may actually enhance rickettsial infection. Other life-threatening disorders that have prominent manifestations in the skin are listed in Table 18-4.

CONCLUSION

Life-threatening skin conditions can have multiple morphologic patterns, and the differential diagnosis is often extensive. Establishing a diagnosis may be difficult, but it is important for the clinician to be familiar with these entities because the skin may offer the first clues to recognition of a severe systemic illness. Important information can be rapidly obtained through the performance of skin biopsies and other tests such as Tzanck smears and tissue cultures. Prompt intervention with systemic therapy and local skin care is imperative in such cases.

REFERENCES AND RECOMMENDED READING

Recently published papers of particular interest have been highlighted as:
• Of interest
•• Of outstanding interest

1.•• Roujeau JC, Chosidon O, Saiag P, Guillaume JC: Toxic epidermal necrolysis (Lyell syndrome). *J Am Acad Dermatol* 1990, 23:1039–1058.

2. Avakian R, Flowers FP, Araujo OE, Ramos-Caro FA: Toxic epidermal necrolysis: a review. *J Am Acad Dermatol* 1991, 25:69–79.

3. Bastuji-Garin S, Rzany B, Stern RS, *et al.*: Clinical classification of cases of toxic epidermal necrolysis, Stevens-Johnson syndrome, and erythema multiforme. *Arch Dermatol* 1993, 129:92–96.

4.•• Brice SL, Huff JC, Weston WL: Erythema multiforme. In *Current Problems in Dermatology*, edn 2. Edited by Weston WL. Chicago: Year Book; 1990:5–25.

5.• Resnick SD: Staphylococcal toxin-mediated syndromes in childhood. *Semin Dermatol* 1992, 11:11–18.

6.• Wilson DC, Jester JD, King LE: Erythroderma and exfoliative dermatitis. *Clin Dermatol* 1993, 11:67–72.

7.• Zelickson BD, Muller SA: Generalized pustular psoriasis: a review of 63 cases. *Arch Dermatol* 1991, 127:1339–1345.

8. Anhalt GJ, Kim SC, Stanley JR, *et al.*: Paraneoplastic pemphigus: an autoimmune mucocutaneous disease associated with neoplasia. *N Engl J Med* 1990, 323:1729–1735.

9. Reingold AL, Hargrett NT, Dan BB, *et al.*: Nonmenstrual toxic shock syndrome: a review of 130 cases. *Ann Intern Med* 1982, 96:871–874.

10. Reingold AL: Toxic shock syndrome: an update. *Am J Obstet Gynecol* 1991, 165:1236–1239.

11.• The Working Group on Severe Streptococcal Infections: Defining the group A streptococcal toxic shock syndrome. *JAMA* 1993, 269:390–391.

12. Wood TF, Potter MA, Jonasson O: Streptococcal toxic shock-like syndrome: the importance of surgical intervention. *Ann Surg* 1993, 217:109–114.

13. Gersony WM: Diagnosis and management of Kawasaki disease. *JAMA* 1991, 265:2699–2703.

14.• Wortmann DW: Kawasaki syndrome. *Semin Dermatol* 1992, 11:37–47.

15. Leung DYM, Meissner HC, Fulton DR, *et al.*: Toxic shock syndrome toxin-secreting *Staphylococcus aureus* in Kawasaki syndrome. *Lancet* 1993, 342:1385–1388.

16. Newburger JW, Takahashi M, Beiser AS, *et al.*: A single intravenous infusion of gamma globulin as compared with four infusions in the treatment of acute Kawasaki syndrome. *N Engl J Med* 1991, 324:1633–1639.

17.•• Francis RB. Acquired purpura fulminans. *Semin Thromb Hemostasis* 1990, 16:310–325.

18. Wong VK, Hitchcock W, Mason WH: Meningococcal infections in children: a review of 100 cases. *Pediatr Infect Dis J* 1989, 8:224–1227.

19. Klein NJ, Heyderman RS, Levin M: Management of meningococcal infections. *Br J Hosp Med* 1993, 50:42–49.

20.• Weber DJ, Walker DH: Rocky Mountain spotted fever. *Infect Dis Clin North Am* 1991, 5:19–35.

SELECT BIBLIOGRAPHY

Frieden IJ, Resnick SD: Childhood exanthems, old and new. *Pediatr Clin North Am* 1991, 38:859–887.

Kerdel FA: Life-threatening dermatoses. In *The Dermatological Signs of Internal Disease*, edn 2. Edited by Callen JP, Jorizzo J, Greer KE, *et al.* Philadelphia: WB Saunders; In press.

Krusinski PA, Flowers FP, eds: *Life Threatening Dermatoses*. Chicago: Year Book; 1987.

Levine N: Management of life-threatening dermatoses. *Emerg Med Clin North Am* 1985, 3:747–763.

Phillips TJ, Dover JS: Recent advances in dermatology. *N Engl J Med* 1992, 326:167–178.

19 Cutaneous Manifestations of Internal Malignancy

Philip R. Cohen

Key Points

- Cutaneous metastases are directly related to the tumor.
- Genodermatoses with malignant potential are a clinical feature of a cancer-associated inherited disorder.
- Cutaneous paraneoplastic syndromes are indirectly secondary to the neoplasm.
- Mucocutaneous reactions to antineoplastic agents are caused by treatment of the malignancy.
- Appropriate evaluation and treatment of an individual should be undertaken when a mucosal or skin lesion that may be a dermatologic manifestation of an internal malignancy is discovered.

Lesions of the skin and mucosa may be manifestations of internal malignancy. Systemic neoplasms may initially present with cutaneous metastases; alternatively, metastatic tumor involvement of the skin may reflect progressive or recurrent cancer. There are several inherited dermatoses in which patients may subsequently develop disease-related neoplasms. The mucocutaneous manifestations of these conditions may suggest or establish the diagnosis of a genodermatosis with malignant potential. There are also several dermatologic conditions that may precede, occur concurrently with, or follow the discovery of an associated internal malignancy. The identification of a cutaneous paraneoplastic syndrome should prompt an appropriate investigation for an asymptomatic neoplasm in a previously cancer-free individual, or a diligent search for a progressing or a recurring malignancy in an oncology patient. Once the diagnosis of an internal malignancy has been established, patients are often treated with systemic chemotherapeutic drugs. Therefore, adverse mucocutaneous reactions to antineoplastic agents may occur in these individuals. This chapter provides a brief overview of cutaneous manifestations of internal malignancy: cutaneous metastases, genodermatoses with malignant potential, cutaneous paraneoplastic syndromes, and mucocutaneous reactions to antineoplastic agents.

CUTANEOUS METASTASES

Cutaneous metastases may be the initial manifestation of an undiagnosed malignancy in a previously cancer-free individual or the cutaneous stigmata of tumor progression or recurrence in an oncology patient [1••]. However, a recently published retrospective study noted cutaneous involvement of internal malignancy at the time of presentation in merely 1.3% of 7316 patients; in fact, skin involvement was the first sign of cancer in only 59 patients (0.8%) [2•].

Solid Tumors

The malignancies that occur most frequently in the general population account for the cancers that most commonly metastasize to the skin. These include pulmonary and colon carcinoma, melanoma, and tumors of the oral cavity, kidney, and stomach in men. In women, carcinomas of the breast, colon, lung, and ovary, followed by melanoma, are the malignancies that most often have skin metastases [1••].

The morphology, pattern, and distribution of these lesions can be variable. The clinical presentation can range from bound-down, indurated sclerodermoid skin changes (Fig. 19-1) to dermal papules or subcutaneous nodules (with or without ulceration) (Fig. 19-2) or to inflammatory patches or plaques of erythema (Fig. 19-3). Carcinoma metastatic to the skin often presents with skin lesions that overlie the site of the underlying neoplasm. The scalp and the umbilical region (Sister Joseph's nodule) are two of the more frequent sites of distant metastases. Less commonly, metastatic carcinoma may occur in a subungual location and mimic an acute paronychia [3] or may present in a dermatomal distribution and mimic a varicella-zoster virus infection [4]. When the possibility of a cutaneous metastasis is suspected, a biopsy of the lesion for microscopic evaluation should be considered in order to confirm the diagnosis.

Patients with solid tumors, as well as leukemias, lymphomas, and sarcomas, may present with or develop skin lesions. This particularly affects patients with Stewart-Treves syndrome, which is characterized by lymphangiosarcomas that appear in the lymphedematous upper extremity of patients approximately 10 years after they have been treated for breast cancer by means of radical mastectomy with or without local radiotherapy.

Leukemia Cutis

Leukemia cutis is characterized by the infiltration of leukemic cells into the skin; the lesions may also be referred to as either chloromas (because the presence of granulocyte myeloperoxidase may result in a green appearance of the gross specimen) or granulocytic sarcomas (when the cutaneous leukemic infiltrate is composed of immature cells of the granulocytic series) (Fig. 19-4) [5]. Although leukemia cutis may present as gingival hypertrophy in acute monocytic leukemia and acute myelomonocytic leukemia, or as erythroderma or bullous lesions in chronic lymphocytic leukemia, it most commonly appears as papules and nodules. The onset of leukemia cutis is generally a poor prognostic sign: 37 of 42 patients in one series died within 1 year after their leukemic infiltrates had been detected.

Lymphoma Cutis

Lymphoma cutis may be either cutaneous T-cell lymphoma (mycosis fungoides), Hodgkin's lymphoma, or non-Hodgkin's (cutaneous B-cell) lymphoma. **Cutaneous T-cell lymphoma** typically presents as either erythematous

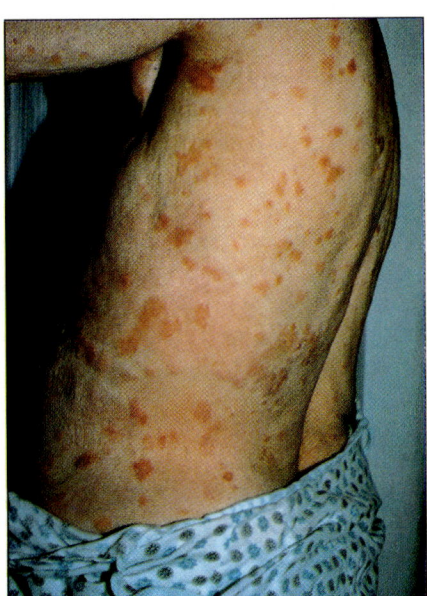

FIGURE 19-1 Carcinoma en cuirasse is characterized by the erythematous area of confluent induration secondary to neoplasm on the left flank; red tumor nodules and plaques of metastatic breast carcinoma are also present. (*From* Cohen [1••]; with permission.)

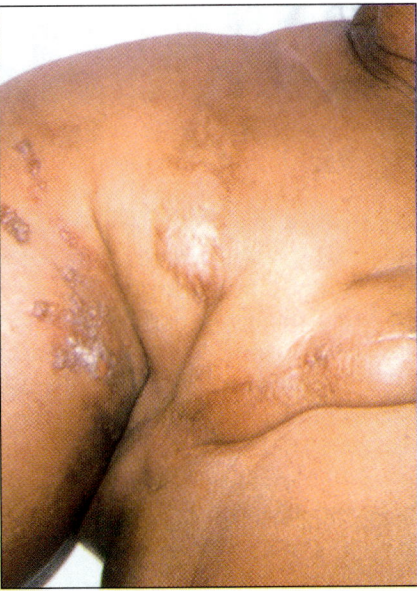

FIGURE 19-2 Papules in the mastectomy scar and ipsilateral edematous arm of a woman with recurrent breast carcinoma. (*From* Cohen [1••]; with permission.)

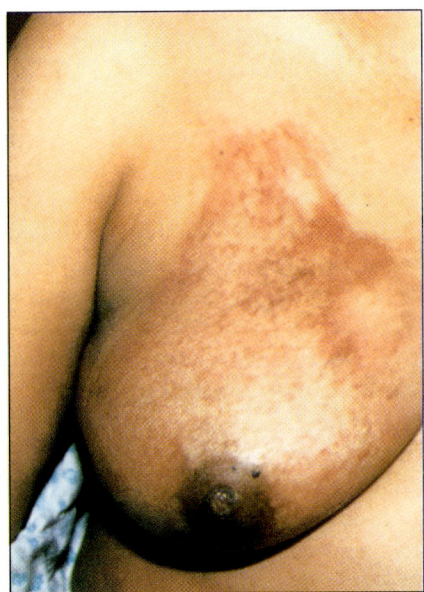

FIGURE 19-3 Carcinoma erysipelatoides is a morphologic pattern of metastatic carcinoma (often involving the lymph vessels) that appears as sharply demarcated areas of erythema that mimic an erysipelas infection. (*From* Cohen [1••]; with permission.)

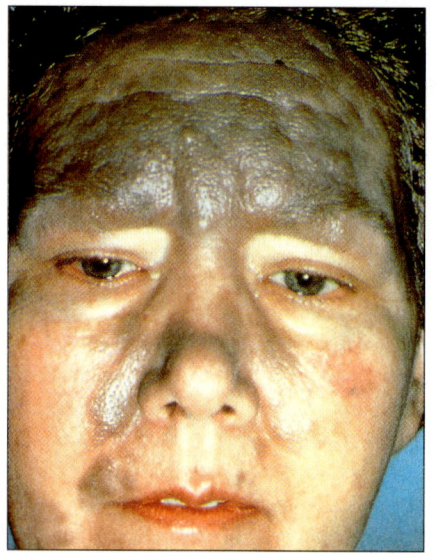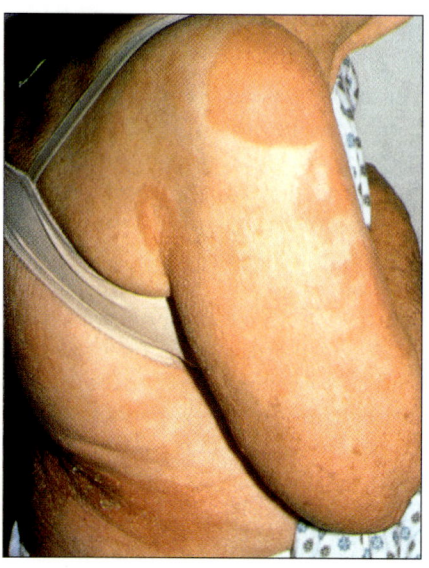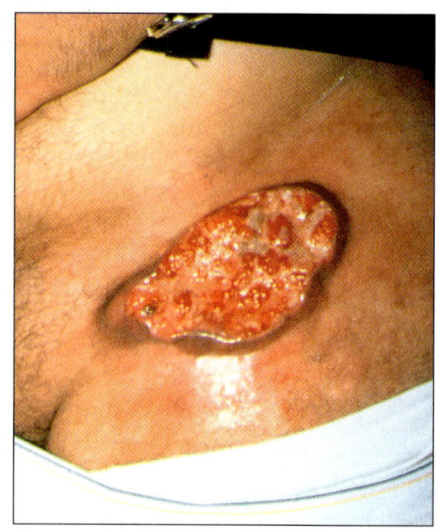

FIGURE 19-4 Leukemia cutis on the face of a 52-year-old white woman with chronic myelomonocytic leukemia that presented as extensive asymptomatic blue-gray to purple infiltrated plaques. (*From* Cohen and coworkers [5]; with permission.)

FIGURE 19-5 Cutaneous T-cell lymphoma appearing as erythematous patches and plaques, which have been present for several years, on the right shoulder, arm, and back of an elderly white woman. (*From* Cohen [1••]; with permission.)

FIGURE 19-6 A large ulcer with a granulation tissue–like base and advancing, indurated borders and surrounding erythema on the left inguinal area that demonstrated recurrent Hodgkin's disease on microscopic evaluation of a lesional biopsy. (*From* Cohen [1••]; with permission.)

patches (Fig. 19-5), lichenoid plaques, or tumor nodules; Sézary syndrome refers to cutaneous T-cell lymphoma with pruritus, exfoliative erythroderma, and abnormal mononuclear cells (mycosis cells or Sézary cells) circulating in the blood. Depending on the extent of disease, patients with cutaneous T-cell lymphoma often receive, either sequentially or concurrently, several of the available treatment modalities: conventional or electron-beam radiotherapy, extracorporeal or routine photochemotherapy, interferon alpha, retinoids (oral isotretinoin or etretinate), and systemic or topical chemotherapy [1••].

Cutaneous involvement of **Hodgkin's disease** is uncommon. The skin lesions usually appear as papules or nodules; dermal infiltration, erythroderma, plaques, tumors, and ulcers are other clinical morphologies (Fig. 19-6). Although the specific skin lesions often respond to systemic chemotherapy, local radiotherapy, or both, the prognosis for the patient is generally poor because cutaneous Hodgkin's disease usually reflects hematogenous dissemination in patients with advanced disease [1••].

Non-Hodgkin's lymphomas of the skin are also uncommon and can either present with the skin as the primary site of involvement (often in patients with an early clinical stage of lymphoma, and therefore, a prolonged disease-free survival) or develop in the skin as a secondary site of dissemination (in patients with advanced clinical stages of disease associated with a poor prognosis). Cutaneous lesions of non-Hodgkin's lymphoma typically appear as a solitary nodule or a few nonulcerating tumors on the head and neck. When the disease is limited to the skin, local treatment (excision or

radiotherapy) may be curative; if the lymphoma is extracutaneous, systemic polychemotherapy (with or without adjuvant local treatment) is necessary [1••].

GENODERMATOSES WITH MALIGNANT POTENTIAL

Inherited disorders with dermatologic manifestations are referred to as genodermatoses [6••]. Some genodermatoses are associated with the potential for subsequent development of a disease-related malignancy (Table 19-1) [6••,7•,8,9]. The individual genodermatoses with malignant potential may be inherited in an autosomal dominant, an autosomal recessive, or an X-linked pattern. The detection of disease-associated cutaneous features should enable the physician to suspect the systemic condition. Once the diagnosis of a genodermatosis with malignant potential has been confirmed, the patient should be appropriately screened and periodically followed up for disease-associated neoplasms. In addition, the members of the patient's family should be evaluated for the genodermatosis. Both the patient and the patient's family should receive genetic counseling, as well. The cutaneous features of some of the autosomal dominant genodermatoses with malignant potential are briefly summarized in the following section.

Nevoid Basal Cell Carcinoma Syndrome
Cutaneous findings that may be present in patients with nevoid basal cell carcinoma syndrome are basal cell carci-

TABLE 19-1 GENODERMATOSES WITH MALIGNANT POTENTIAL

Genodermatosis	Inheritance	Predominant malignancies
Ataxia telangiectasia	AR	Lymphoma, leukemia
Bloom's syndrome	AR	Leukemia
Bruton's sex-linked agammaglobulinemia	XL	Leukemia, lymphoma
Chédiak-Higashi syndrome	AR	Lymphoma
Cowden's syndrome (multiple hamartoma syndrome)	AD	Breast carcinoma, thyroid carcinoma
Dyskeratosis congenita	XL	Squamous cell carcinoma of the skin, mucosa, and esophagus; pancreatic carcinoma; Hodgkin's lymphoma; leukemia
Fanconi's anemia	AR	Leukemia
Gardner's syndrome	AD	Colon adenocarcinoma
Hemochromatosis	AR	Hepatocellular carcinoma
Howel-Evans syndrome (tylosis)	AD	Esophageal carcinoma
Muir-Torre syndrome	AD	Colorectal carcinoma, genitourinary carcinoma
Multiple endocrine neoplasias IIB or III (multiple mucosal neuroma syndrome)	AD	Medullary carcinoma of thyroid, pheochromocytoma
Neurofibromatosis 1 (von Recklinghausen's disease)	AD	Neurofibrosarcomas, brain tumors, neuroblastomas, pheochromocytoma, medullary thyroid carcinoma, melanoma, Wilms' tumor, rhabdomyosarcoma, leukemia
Nevoid basal cell carcinoma syndrome (Gorlin's syndrome)	AD	Basal cell carcinomas, medulloblastoma, fibrosarcoma of the jaw
Peutz-Jeghers syndrome	AD	Reproductive organ neoplasms, colon adenocarcinoma
Porphyria cutanea tarda	AD	Hepatocellular carcinoma
Tuberous sclerosis (Bourneville's disease)	AD	Cardiac rhabdomyoma, astrocytoma, glioblastoma
von Hippel-Lindau	AD	Cerebellar and spinal hemangioblastomas, pheochromocytoma, hypernephroma
Werner's syndrome (adult progeria)	AR	Sarcomas, meningiomas
Wiskott-Aldrich syndrome	XL	Leukemia, lymphoma

AD—autosomal dominant; AR—autosomal recessive; XL—X-linked. *From* Cohen [6••]; with permission.

nomas, café au lait macules, dermal calcinosis, epithelial cysts, fibromas, lipomas, milia, and palmoplantar pits (Fig. 19-7). The basal cell carcinomas often mimic the appearance of benign nevi and continue to develop throughout the patient's life. In addition to calcification of the falx cerebri and odontogenic keratocysts of the jaw, several skeletal anomalies (most commonly involving the ribs and vertebrae) are also present in these patients (Fig. 19-8) [6••].

Gardner's Syndrome

The presence of colonic polyposis in individuals with multiple epidermoid cysts, desmoid tumors, fibromas, or osteomas characterizes Gardner's syndrome (Fig. 19-9). Dental anomalies, ocular pigmentation of the fundi, and polyps of the small intestine and stomach are additional features of this syndrome. Because malignant transformation of the colonic polyps occurs in all patients with Gardner's syndrome, prophylactic colectomy is recommended [6••].

Howel-Evans Syndrome

Howel-Evans syndrome is the association of hereditary palmar and plantar hyperkeratosis (tylosis) with the development of esophageal carcinoma. Since the original description of this syndrome in 1958, only a small number of additional families with this condition have been reported. Nonfamilial, acquired keratosis of the palms and soles, however, has been observed in several individuals with an associated bronchial, esophageal, or pulmonary malignancy [6••].

Muir-Torre Syndrome

The association of sebaceous tumors (adenomas, epitheliomas, and carcinomas) and an internal malignancy (most commonly colorectal carcinomas proximal to the splenic flexure and genitourinary neoplasms) is defined as the Muir-Torre syndrome (Fig. 19-10) [7•,10]. Because these sebaceous lesions are rare, the detection of even one Muir-Torre syndrome–associated cutaneous tumor warrants an

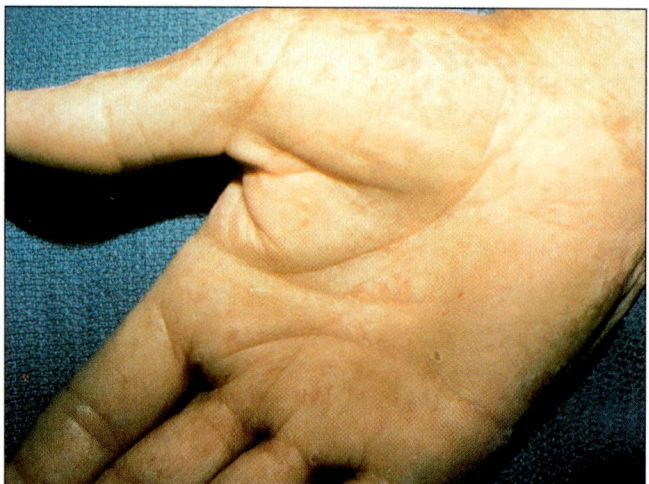

FIGURE 19-7 Pits in the palm of a patient with nevoid basal cell carcinoma syndrome. (*From* Cohen [6••]; with permission.)

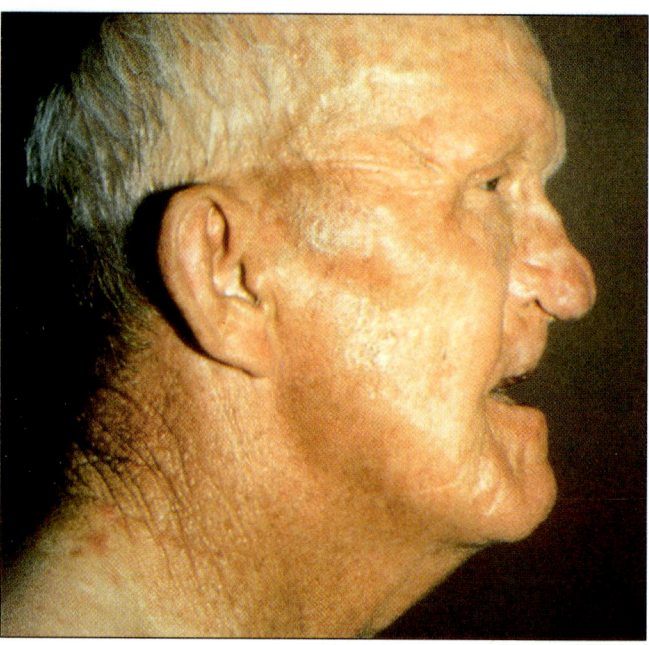

FIGURE 19-8 Frontal bossing, hypertelorism, and prognathism are nevoid basal cell carcinoma syndrome–associated skeletal anomalies that can be observed on the lateral view of this patient; multiple prior surgical sites from which basal cell carcinoma was removed are also demonstrated. (*From* Cohen [6••]; with permission.)

initial evaluation and periodic assessment for malignancy in that individual [8]. Keratoacanthoma is another skin lesion that has been observed in at least 20% of patients with this syndrome.

Neurofibromatosis Type 1

The gene responsible for neurofibromatosis type 1 (*NF1*) has recently been mapped to band 11.2 of the long arm of chromosome 17. The phenotypic expression of this disease is variable; some individuals with NF1 are severely affected, whereas others have minimal skin or systemic stigmata. Café au lait macules (Fig. 19-11*A*), axillary or inguinal "frecking" (referred to as Crowe's sign) (Fig. 19-11*B*, and neurofibromas (Fig. 19-11*C*) are cutaneous manifestations of neurofibromatosis type 1 [9]. Other diagnostic criteria for neurofibromatosis type 1 are disease-specific osseous lesions, optic

gliomas, pigmented hamartomas of the iris (Lisch nodules), and a first-degree relative with the condition [6••].

Peutz-Jeghers Syndrome

Macular hyperpigmentation and polyposis of the gastrointestinal tract (stomach, small intestine, colon, and rectum) defines Peutz-Jeghers syndrome. The pigmented macules either are present at birth or appear in childhood. They may

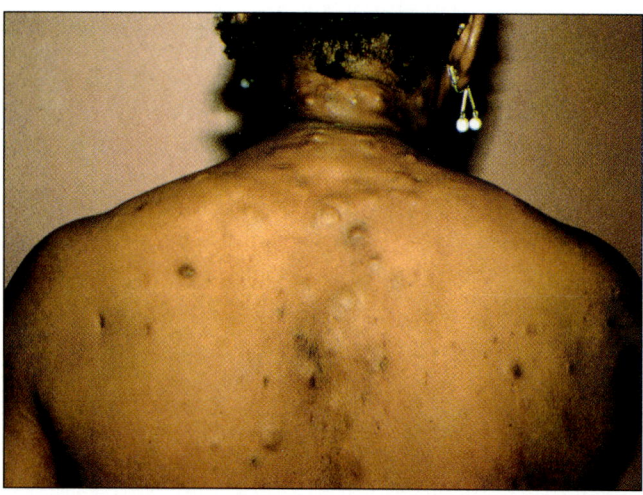

FIGURE 19-9 Multiple epidermoid cysts on the back of a black woman with Gardner's syndrome. (*From* Cohen [6••]; with permission.)

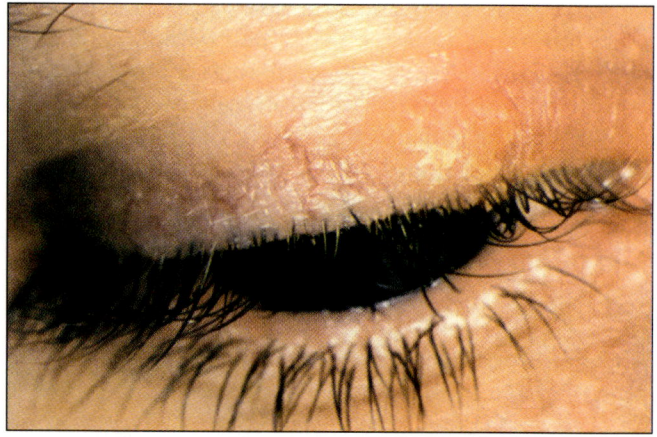

FIGURE 19-10 A diagnosis of the Muir-Torre syndrome was made when a sebaceous carcinoma (the hyperkeratotic nodule on the medial upper eyelid) was discovered in a young man who had previously been successfully treated for Hodgkin's lymphoma. (*From* Cohen [10]; with permission.)

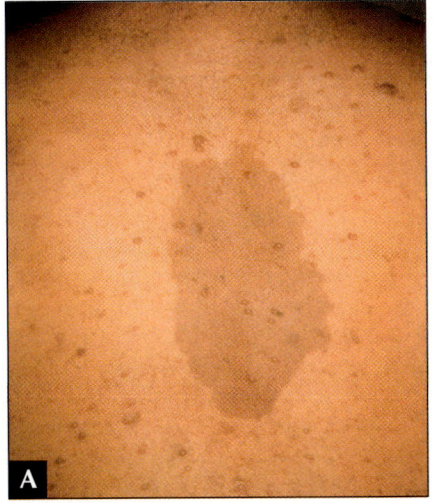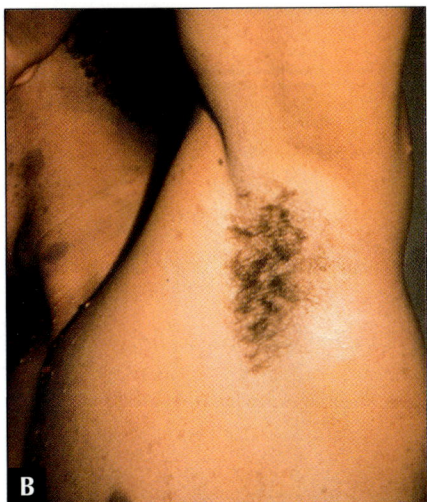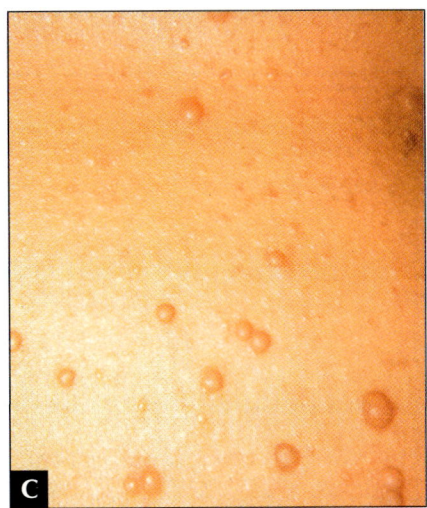

FIGURE 19-11 Café au lait macules (*panel A*), Crowe's sign (freckling in the axilla) *panel B*) and neurofibromas (*panel C*) are cutaneous features of neurofibromatosis type 1. (*From* Cohen [6••]; with permission.)

be located on the acral skin, buccal mucosa, face, gums, hard palate, and lips; they are most frequently periorificial. Whereas the facial lesions may fade as the patient becomes older, the mucosal pigmentations persist [6••].

CUTANEOUS PARANEOPLASTIC SYNDROMES

Cutaneous paraneoplastic syndromes are a group of dermatoses that appear either before, concurrent with, or after an associated malignancy [11••]; the syndromes, their clinical characteristics, and their associated malignancies are summarized in Table 19-2 (Figs. 19-12 through 19-17) [11••,12,13•,14,15,16•,17,18•,19•]. In addition, some of these dermatoses may be observed in cancer-free individuals, either in association with a systemic disease or as an isolated dermatologic condition.

Criteria for Defining Cutaneous Paraneoplastic Syndromes

The criteria for establishing a causal relationship between a dermatosis and a malignant internal disease were initially proposed by Curth in 1976 [11••]. They included:

- The two conditions begin simultaneously (*ie*, dermatomyositis)
- The two conditions follow a parallel course (*eg*, malignant acanthosis nigricans)
- In certain syndromes, neither the course nor the onset of one of the two conditions is dependent on the course or onset of the other condition because the two conditions are part of a genetic syndrome (*eg*, Gardner's syndrome)
- A specific tumor (*ie*, adenocarcinoma in malignant acanthosis nigricans) occurs in connection with a specific dermatosis
- The dermatosis is usually not common (*ie*, erythema gyratum repens)

- The associated tumor is found in a high percentage of cases of the dermatosis

The criteria for defining a cutaneous paraneoplastic syndrome have been modified since Curth's original description. For example, the last three criteria are not essential for a mucocutaneous condition to be a paraneoplastic syndrome [11••]. In addition, the third criterion (genetic syndromes that may be associated with an internal malignancy) is more appropriately classified as "genodermatoses with malignant potential" [6••].

Evaluation for Associated Malignancy

Although a cutaneous paraneoplastic syndrome may initially appear in an individual with an established diagnosis of cancer (and thereby may be the heralding sign of recurrent neoplastic disease), it often precedes or coincides with the clinical detection of the related neoplasm. Therefore, once the diagnosis of a potential cutaneous paraneoplastic syndrome is confirmed, an appropriate systemic evaluation for an underlying neoplasm should be considered in a cancer-free individual and a search for possible recurrent or metastatic disease should be performed in a patient with a known history of malignancy. The initial work-up should include a detailed medical history, a complete physical examination, and routine screening laboratory tests. Subsequent studies should then be directed by the abnormalities discovered during the patient's preliminary evaluation, with an emphasis placed on detecting malignancies that are especially prevalent in association with that individual's specific cutaneous paraneoplastic syndrome [11••].

Etiology

The etiology of many of these dermatoses remains undetermined. However, recent studies have suggested that the cutaneous paraneoplastic syndromes are likely to be caused

Cutaneous paraneoplastic syndrome	Clinical characteristics	Site or type of associated malignancies
Acanthosis nigricians (*see* Fig. 19-12)	Flexural (axillae and posterior neck) verrucous, velvety-textured, hyperpigmented epidermal hyperplasia	Intraabdominal (stomach)
Acquired ichthyosis	Diffuse rhomboid scales with free edges	Hodgkin's lymphoma
Amyloidosis	Purpura; macroglossia, tongue papules, or both; periocular purpura, waxy papules, or both	Myeloma, Hodgkin's lymphoma, kidney
Bazex's syndrome (acrokeratosis paraneoplastica)	Erythematous, scaling papulosquamous lesions on the fingers, toes, ears, and nose; nail dystrophy; palmoplantar keratoderma	Squamous cell carcinomas of the upper aerorespiratory tract or a neoplasm with cervical lymph node metastases in white men older than 40 y
Bowen's disease	Erythematous plaque on a photodistributed or non–sun-exposed site	Controversial (age-associated neoplasms)
Bullous pemphigoid	Erythematous-based, subepidermal tense bullae on flexor thighs and forearms	Controversial (lung, larynx, breast, gallbladder, kidney, bladder, ovary, uterus, rectum, prostate, cervix, thyroid, stomach)
Dermatitis herpetiformis	Pruritic papulovesicles on the elbows and knees, upper back, and buttocks	Lymphoma (gastrointestinal and nongastrointestinal), lung, small intestine, bladder
Dermatomyositis	Periocular heliotrope rash, Gottron's papules, periungual telangiectasias, poikiloderma	Age-associated neoplasms
Epidermolysis bullosa acquisita	Adult-onset, subepidermal blisters at trauma sites	Controversial (myeloma, lung, lymphoma, chronic lymphocytic leukemia)
Erythema annulare centrifugum	Expanding, annular erythema with a raised edge, peripheral scale, and central clearing	Lung, lymphoma (Hodgkin's and non-Hodgkin's), histiocytosis, prostate
Erythema gyratum repens	Advancing erythematous rings with "wood grain" or striped appearance	Lung, esophagus, uterus, cervix, breast, stomach
Erythroderma and exfoliative dermatitis	Generalized erythema with or without scaling	Lymphoma (cutaneous T-cell and Hodgkin's), chronic lymphocytic leukemia, acute and chronic myelogenous leukemia, uterus, lung, stomach, prostate, thyroid, liver, larynx
Erythromelalgia [12,13•]	Severe burning pain, erythema, and warmth of the distal extremities relieved by cold exposure, elevation of the extremity, or both	Polycythemia vera, essential thrombocythemia, agnogenic myeloid metaplasia, chronic myelogenous leukemia
Extramammary Paget's disease (*see* Fig. 19-13)	Erythematous, exudative plaque located on the vulva, perianal area, penis, scrotum, or groin	Cutaneous adnexal carcinoma; internal malignancies: breast, uterus, rectum, bladder, vagina, or prostate
Florid cutaneous papillomatosis	Verrucous papillomas on the trunk and the extremities	Intraabdominal (stomach, bladder, bile ducts, ovary, uterus)
Glucagonoma syndrome	Necrolytic migratory erythematous patch, glossitis, angular stomatitis	α-Cell pancreatic carcinoma (glucagonoma)
Hypertrichosis lanuginosa acquisita	Generalized pale, fine-textured hair growth	Lung, colorectal, breast, uterus, bladder, lymphoma
Hypertrophic pulmonary osteoarthropathy [14] (*see* Fig. 19-14)	Clubbing of fingers and toes with tender swelling of the distal arms, legs, and adjacent joints	Lung, mediastinal tumors, sarcomas
Multicentric reticulohistiocytosis	Papules, nodules, and rapidly progressive, debilitating polyarthritis	Breast, lymphoma, cervix, stomach, ovary, colon, lung, pleura, acute myelogenous leukemia

Paraneoplastic pemphigus	Polymorphous pruritic papules and blisters; cutaneous and painful mucosal erosions	Lymphoma, chronic lymphocytic leukemia, sarcoma, lung, thymoma
Pemphigus vulgaris	Intraepidermal bullae of the skin, oral blisters and erosions	Lymphoreticular (Kaposi's sarcoma), thymus, breast, skin
Pityriasis rotunda	Noninflammatory, geometrically perfect circular patches of scales	Liver
Porphyria cutanea tarda	Early: photodistributed subepidermal vesicles, skin fragility, facial hypertrichosis, and hyperpigmentation	Controversial (liver)
	Late: scarring, milia, sclerodermoid changes, calcinosis cutis, alopecia	
Pruritus (*see* Fig. 19-15)	Excoriations, prurigo nodularis, lichen simplex chronicus	Lymphoma (Hodgkin's and cutaneous T-cell), polycythemia vera
Pyoderma gangrenosum (*see* Fig. 19-16)	Papulopustule that develops into a nodule that ulcerates with an irregular, violaceous, undermined border	Hematologic malignancies
Sign of Leser-Trélat	Seborrheic keratoses (may be pruritic)	Stomach, lymphoma, breast, lung
Sweet's syndrome (acute febrile neutrophilic dermatosis) [15,16•]	Tender, erythematous pseudovesicular plaques on the arms, head, and neck	Acute myelogenous leukemia
Tripe palms [17,18•,20] (*see* Fig. 19-17)	Thickened, velvet- or moss-textured, honeycombed or cobbled palms with pronounced dermatoglyphics	Lung, stomach
Trousseau's syndrome	Thrombophlebitis (often superficial and migratory)	Pancreas, lung, stomach
Vasculitis [19•]	Palpable, nonblanchable purpura; erythematous nodules	Leukemia (hairy cell and myelogenous), myeloma, lymphoma, myelodysplastic syndrome

From Cohen [11••]; with permission.

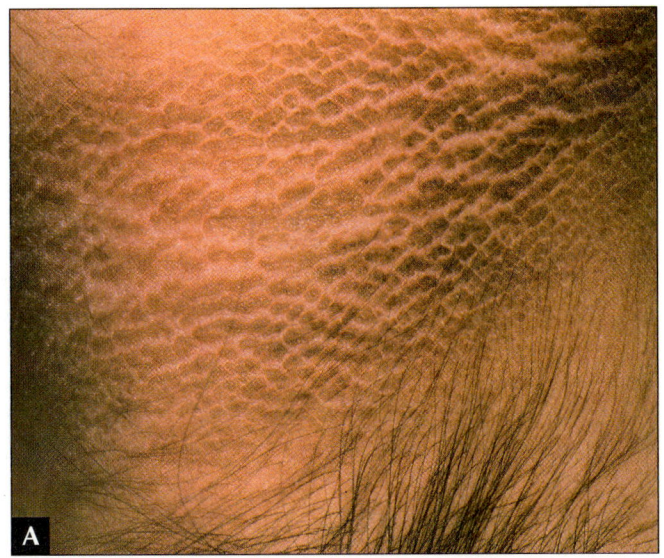
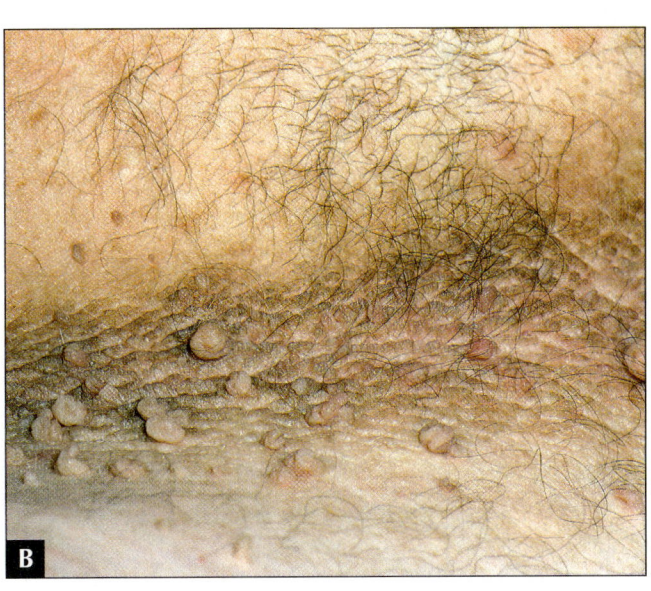
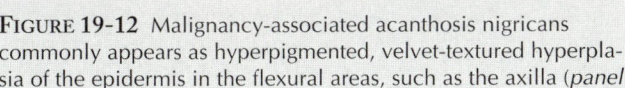

FIGURE 19-12 Malignancy-associated acanthosis nigricans commonly appears as hyperpigmented, velvet-textured hyperplasia of the epidermis in the flexural areas, such as the axilla (*panel A*), and the posterior neck (*panel B*), of patients with intraabdominal neoplasms. (*Panel A courtesy of* D. Hazelrigg, Evansville, IN; *Panel B courtesy of* K. Greer, Charlottesville, VA.)

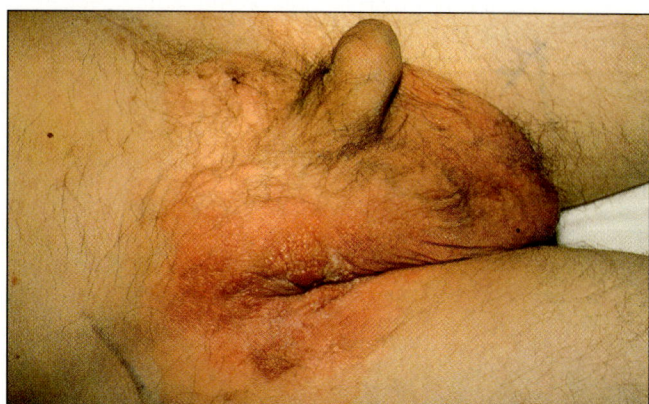

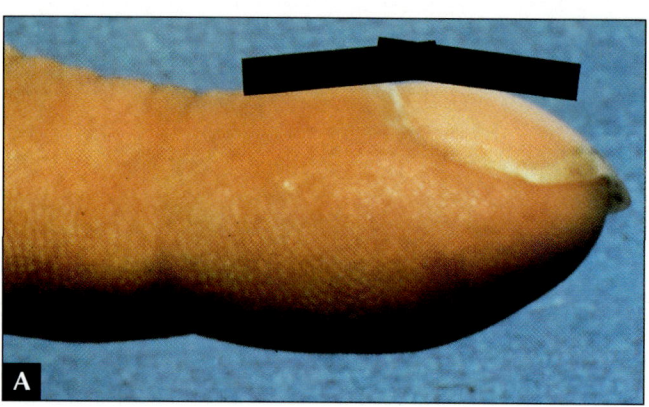

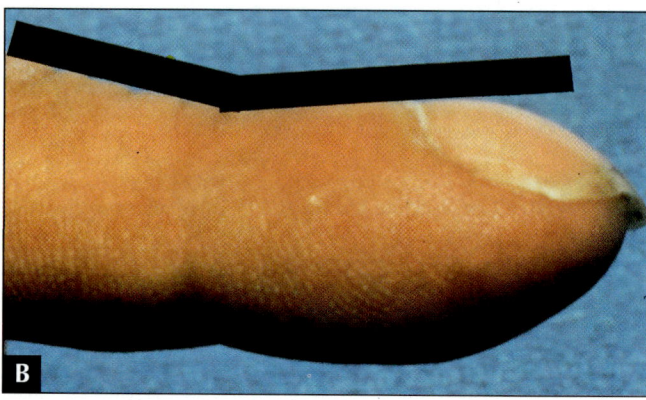

FIGURE 19-13 Extramammary Paget's disease, a cutaneous adenocarcinoma that appears as a pruritic, erythematous, dermatitis-like plaque, is often associated with an underlying adnexal carcinoma or an underlying internal malignancy, frequently of the digestive system (when perianal in location) or the genitourinary organs (when at a penile, scrotal, or groin location). (*From* Cohen [11••]; with permission.)

FIGURE 19-14 Clinical indicators of clubbing are Lovibond's profile sign (*panel A*) and Curth's modified profile sign (*panel B*). Clubbing is present when the angle between the curved nail plate and the proximal nail fold (which is normally less than or equal to 160°) exceeds 180° (*panel A*) or the angle between the middle and the terminal phalanx at the interphalangeal joint (which is normally about 180°) is reduced to less than 160° (*panel B*). (*From* Cohen [11••]; with permission.)

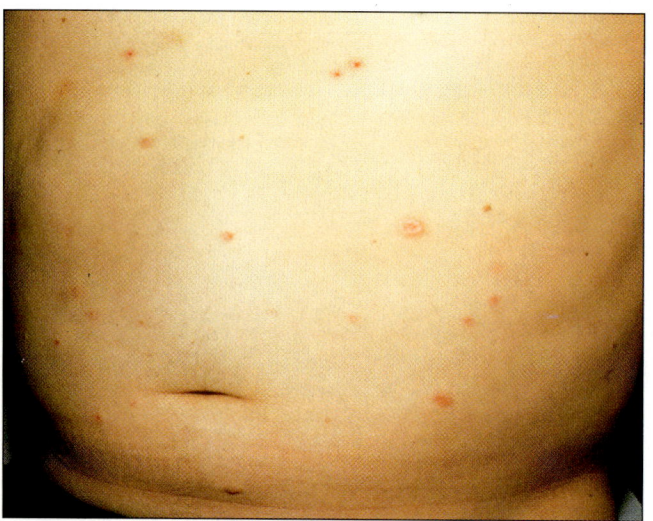

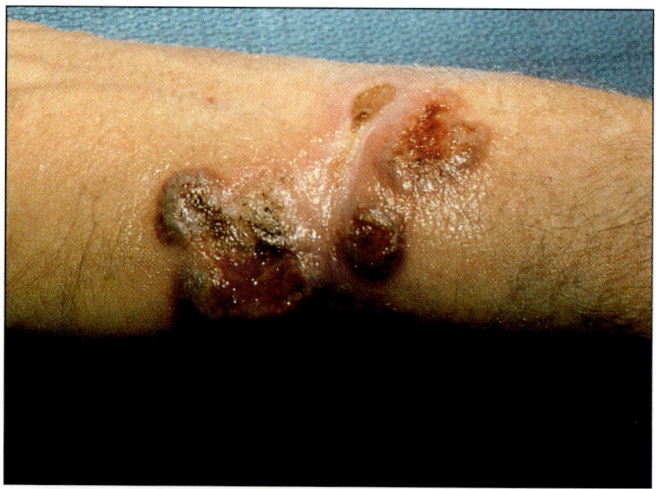

FIGURE 19-15 Although paraneoplastic pruritus (which may appear as excoriated papules and prurigo nodules) has most frequently been associated with Hodgkin's disease, it is also a common symptom in patients who have either cutaneous T-cell lymphoma or polycythema vera. (*From* Cohen [11••]; with permission.)

FIGURE 19-16 Hematologic malignancies, and rarely solid tumors, may be associated with "atypical" or "bullous" pyoderma gangrenosum, which often begins as a painful erythematous papule or pustule and subsequently develops into a bullous nodule that frequently breaks down and forms an ulcer with violaceous, irregular, undermined borders and a boggy, necrotic base. (*From* Cohen [11••]; with permission.)

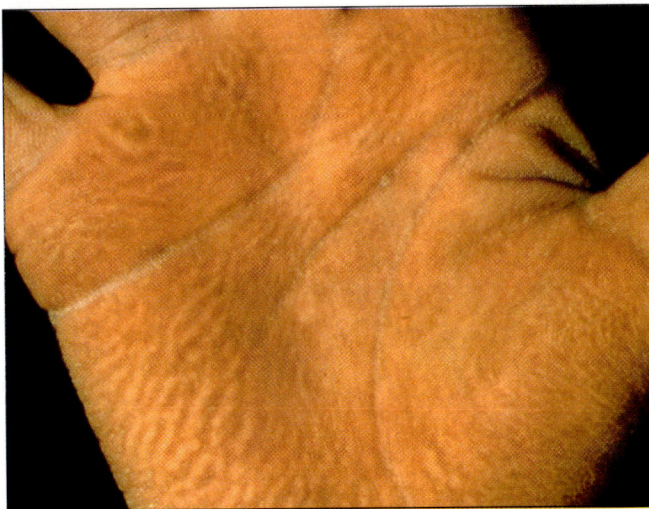

FIGURE 19-17 Pulmonary and gastric carcinomas are the most common neoplasms in patients with malignancy-associated tripe palms, which can appear as thickening of the palms with moss-like, velvet-textured exaggeration of the palmar dermatoglyphics. (*From* Cohen and coworkers [20]; with permission.)

directly by a cytokine secreted by the tumor; alternatively, the tumor may participate indirectly by inducing accessory cells to secrete the causative factor. The investigation of patients with these malignancy-associated dermatoses may provide additional insight not only into the biologic behavior of their underlying neoplasms but also into the pathogenesis of these conditions when they occur in a paraneoplastic setting or as an idiopathic disorder [11••].

MUCOCUTANEOUS REACTIONS TO ANTINEOPLASTIC AGENTS

Mucocutaneous reactions may be observed in patients receiving cancer chemotherapy (Tables 19-3 and 19-4) [21••,22,23]. Some of these reactions are primarily associated with a specific malignancy or the administration of a specific agent. Most of these reactions, however, are related neither to a specific neoplasm nor to a particular medication. The severity of these reactions can range from an incidental asymptomatic clinical observation to a life-threatening or drug-limiting toxicity. Certain reactions are dose dependent (either single or cumulative dose), whereas others represent hypersensitivity reactions that are not influenced by the quantity administered. Some of these reactions can be adequately managed symptomatically and will resolve after chemotherapy has been completed; alternatively, other reactions require either reduction of the dose of the chemotherapeutic agent or discontinuation of the drug.

Alopecia

One of the most frequently observed cutaneous reactions to the use of chemotherapeutic agents is alopecia (Fig. 19-18).

Because the antineoplastic drugs affect actively proliferating hair follicles, an anagen effluvium occurs; the hair loss is dose dependent and reversible once the chemotherapy has been discontinued. The most common site of involvement is the scalp; the chemotherapy-induced alopecia is often only partial because 10% to 15% of the hairs on the scalp are not in the proliferating (anagen) stage at any specific time. With long-term therapy, patients may also experience loss of axillary, facial, and pubic hair [21••,22].

Stomatitis

Stomatitis or mucositis is also a common adverse mucocutaneous side effect of antineoplastic therapy. Symptoms can range from mild to dose limiting (Fig. 19-19) [22]. The rapid replication rate of the mucosal epithelium of the conjunctiva, gastrointestinal tract, oral cavity, perianal region, urethra, and vagina makes these tissues extremely susceptible to the direct cytotoxic effect, the immunosuppressive (infectious) effects, and the myelosuppressive (bleeding) effects of the chemotherapeutic drugs. Symptoms (burning and reddening) often begin shortly after administration of the agent, and erosions or ulcerations appear within 1 to 5 days. Within 2 weeks after stopping the drug, healing has usually occurred. Supportive treatment is the mainstay of therapy. Often, symptomatic relief can be provided by "swishing and swallowing" 5 to 15 mL of the following solution (Powell's mouthwash) three to four times daily: tetracycline (7500 mg), hydrocortisone powder (1500 mg), nystatin oral suspension (100,000 U/mL x 180 mL), and diphenhydramine cough syrup with minimal alcohol (to a total volume of 3750 mL or 1 gal) [21••].

TABLE 19-3 MUCOCUTANEOUS REACTIONS TO CANCER CHEMOTHERAPY
Common
Alopecia
Stomatitis
Less common
Acral erythema
Extravasation injuries
Hyperpigmentation (*see* Table 19-4)
Inflammation of actinic keratoses
Radiation interactions
Rare
Hypersensitivity reactions
Neutrophilic eccrine hidradenitis
Reactive erythemas
Vasculitis
From Cohen [21••]; with permission.

Pattern of hyperpigmentation	Associated chemotherapeutic agent
Generalized (nonspecific)	
Mucous membranes	Busulfan, doxorubicin
Nails	Bleomycin, cyclophosphamide, daunorubicin, doxorubicin, fluorouracil
Skin	Bleomycin, busulfan, carmustine (topical), cyclophosphamide, daunorubicin, doxorubicin, fluorouracil, hydroxyurea, mechlorethamine (topical), methotrexate, mithramycin, mitomycin, thiotepa
Teeth	Cyclophosphamide
Specific	
Flag sign of chemotherapy (hair)	Methotrexate
Flagellate hyperpigmentation (see Fig. 19-21)	Bleomycin
Serpentine supravenous hyperpigmentation	Fluorouracil, fotemustine

From Cohen [21••]; with permission.

Less Common Reactions to Chemotherapy

Less common reactions to chemotherapeutics are listed in Table 19-3 [21••,22,23]. Chemotherapy-induced acral erythema (also referred to as hand-foot syndrome or palmar-plantar erythrodysesthesia) is most frequently associated with the administration of either cytarabine, doxorubicin, or fluorouracil. It presents as painful macular reddening primarily involving the palms and soles and may progress to blister formation before superficial desquamation and reepithelialization of the involved skin (Fig. 19-20) [23]. Extravasation injuries, which may be caused by several of the antineoplastic drugs, can range in severity from phlebitis to chemical cellulitis with or without tissue necrosis. Generalized and specific patterns of mucocutaneous hyperpigmentation secondary to chemotherapeutic agents are summarized in Table 19-4 and illustrated in Figure 19-21 [21••,22]. Inflammation of previously asymptomatic actinic keratoses may follow the systemic administration of several different chemotherapeutic drugs (Fig. 19-22); this reaction neither requires discontinuation of the agent nor contraindicates future use of the medication. Photosensitivity, radiation enhancement (drugs act synergistically with radiation), radiation recall (inflammatory response in tissues previously irradiated), and reactivation of ultraviolet light–induced erythema (in patients who have received either intramuscular, intravenous, or oral methotrexate) are four types of interactions that have been observed between chemotherapeutic agents and either ionizing or ultraviolet radiation [21••,22].

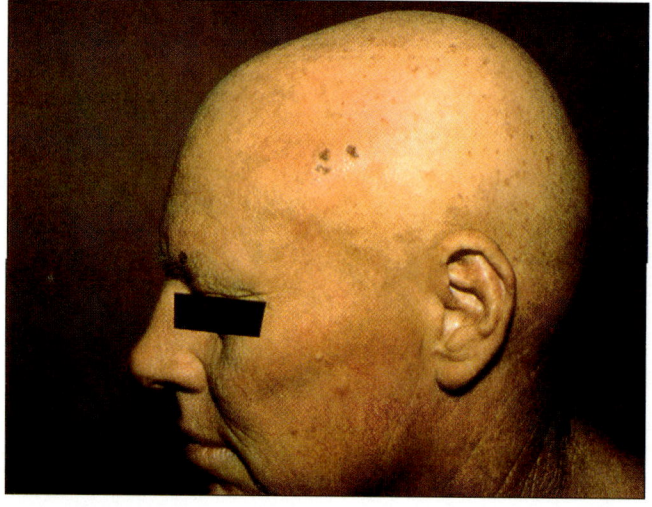

FIGURE 19-18 Alopecia of the scalp following treatment with systemic chemotherapy; cutaneous lesions of a concurrent disseminated varicella-zoster virus infection appear as erythematous-based crusted erosions. (*From* Cohen [21••]; with permission.)

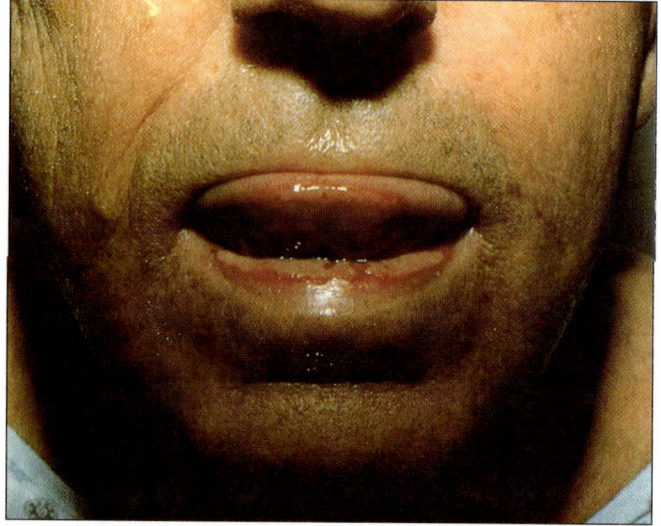

FIGURE 19-19 The mucosal erosions of the tongue and lower lip are secondary to treatment of this man's metastatic colon carcinoma with fluorouracil. (*From* Cohen [21••]; with permission.)

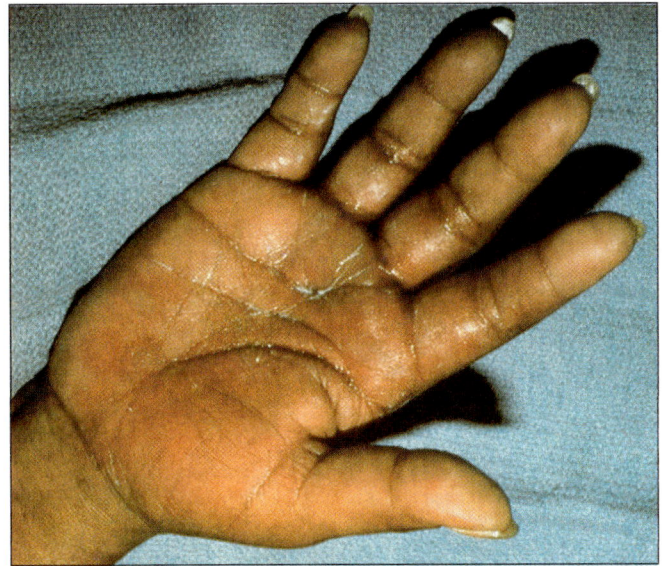

FIGURE 19-20 Chemotherapy-induced acral erythema lesions characterized by tender, red palms and fingers with superficial desquamation. (*From* Cohen [23]; with permission.)

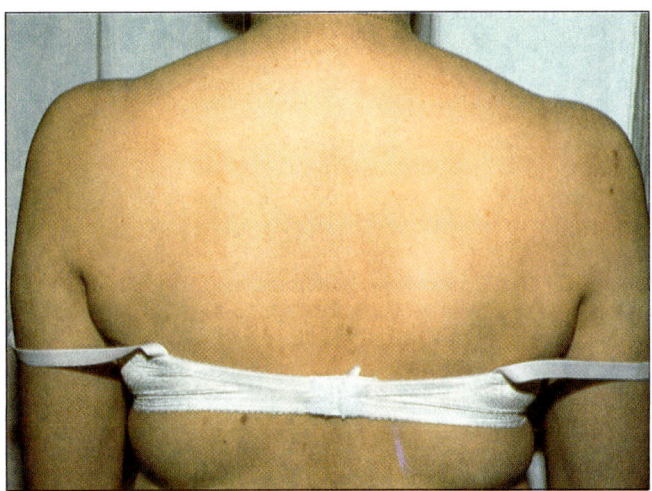

FIGURE 19-21 The "flagellate" (whip-like), linear, hyperpigmented streaks (which are most prominent in this patient over the scapulae and the posterior shoulders) that appeared after treatment with systemic bleomycin are a specific pattern of chemotherapy-induced hyperpigmentation. (*From* Cohen [21••]; with permission.)

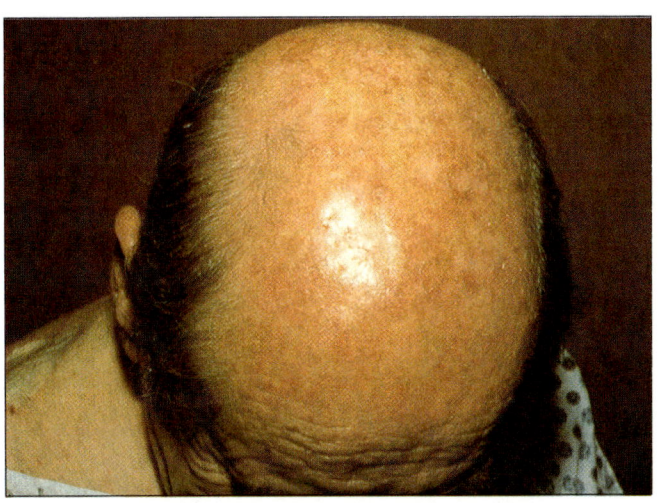

FIGURE 19-22 Multiple actinic keratoses on the scalp of a man with metastatic colon carcinoma that became inflamed 1 week after systemic chemotherapy with continuous-infusion fluorouracil and daily interferon alpha was started. (*From* Cohen [21••]; with permission.)

REFERENCES AND RECOMMENDED READING

Recently published papers of particular interest have been highlighted as:
• Of interest
•• Of outstanding interest

1.•• Cohen PR: Cutaneous metastases. *Am Fam Physician*, in press.

2.• Lookingbill DP, Spangler N, Sexton FM: Skin involvement as the presenting sign of internal carcinoma: a retrospective study of 7316 cancer patients. *J Am Acad Dermatol* 1990, 22:19–26.

3. Cohen PR, Buzdar AU: Metastatic breast carcinoma mimicking an acute paronychia of the great toe: case report and review of subungual metastases. *Am J Clin Oncol (CCT)* 1993, 16:86–91.

4. Manteaux A, Cohen PR, Rapini RP: Zosteriform and epidermotropic metastasis: report of two cases. *J Dermatol Surg Oncol* 1992, 18:97–100.

5. Cohen PR, Rapini RP, Beran M: Infiltrated blue-gray plaques in a patient with leukemia: Chloroma (granulocytic sarcoma) [off-center fold]. *Arch Dermatol* 1987, 123:251–254.

6.•• Cohen PR: Genodermatoses with malignant potential. *Am Fam Physician* 1992, 46:1479–1486.

7.• Cohen PR, Kohn SR, Kurzrock R: The association of sebaceous gland tumors and internal malignancy: the Muir-Torre syndrome. *Am J Med* 1991, 90:606–613.

8. Cohen PR: Sebaceous carcinoma of the ocular adnexa and the Muir-Torre syndrome [letter]. *J Am Acad Dermatol* 1992, 27:279–280.

9. Cohen PR: Neurofibromatosis type 1. *N Engl J Med* 1993, 329:1549.

10. Cohen PR: Muir-Torre syndrome in patients with hematologic malignancies. *Am J Hematol* 1992, 40:64–65.

11.•• Cohen PR: Cutaneous paraneoplastic syndromes. *Am Fam Physician* 1994, 50:1273–1282.

12. Kurzrock R, Cohen PR: Erythromelalgia: review of clinical characteristics and pathophysiology. *Am J Med* 1991, 91:416–422.

13.• Kurzrock R, Cohen PR: Paraneoplastic erythromelalgia. *Clin Dermatol* 1993, 11:73–82.

14. Cohen PR: Hypertrophic pulmonary osteoarthropathy and tripe palms in a man with squamous cell carcinoma of the larynx and lung: report of a case and review of cutaneous paraneoplastic syndromes associated with laryngeal and lung malignancies. *Am J Clin Oncol (CCT)* 1993, 16:268–276.

15. Cohen PR, Talpaz M, Kurzrock R: Malignancy-associated Sweet's syndrome: review of the world literature. *J Clin Oncol* 1988, 6:1887–1897.

16.• Cohen PR, Kurzrock R: Sweet's syndrome and cancer. *Clin Dermatol* 1993, 11:149–157.

17. Cohen PR, Kurzrock R: Malignancy-associated tripe palms. *J Am Acad Dermatol* 1992, 27:271–272.

18.• Cohen PR, Grossman ME, Silvers DN, Kurzrock R: Tripe palms and cancer. *Clin Dermatol* 1993, 11:165–173.

19.• Kurzrock R, Cohen PR: Vasculitis and cancer. *Clin Dermatol* 1993, 11:175–187.

20. Cohen PR, Grossman ME, Almeida L, Kurzrock R: Triple palms and malignancy. *J Clin Oncol* 1989, 7:669–678.

21.•• Cohen PR: Cancer chemotherapy-associated mucocutaneous reactions. In *Medical Oncology: A Comprehensive Board Review. University of Texas MD Anderson Cancer Center.* Edited by Pazdur R. Huntington, NY; PRR 1993; 491–500.

22. Kerker BJ, Hood AF: Chemotherapy-induced cutaneous reactions. *Semin Dermatol* 1989, 8:173–181.

23. Cohen PR: Acral erythema: a clinical review. *Cutis* 1993, 51:175–179.

SELECT BIBLIOGRAPHY

Callen JP: Skin signs of internal malignancy. *Australas J Dermatol* 1987, 28:106–114.

Cohen PR, Kurzrock R, eds: Cutaneous paraneoplastic syndromes. *Clin Dermatol*, 1993, 11:1 187.

Cohen PR, Kurzrock R: Genodermatoses with malignant potential. *Dermatol Clin* 1995, 13:1–230.

Hood AF: Cutaneous side effects of cancer chemotherapy. *Med Clin North Am* 1986, 70:187–209.

Poole S, Fenske NA: Cutaneous markers of internal malignancy: I. Malignant involvement of the skin and the genodermatoses. *J Am Acad Dermatol* 1993, 28:1–13.

Poole S, Fenske NA: Cutaneous markers of internal malignancy: II. paraneoplastic dermatoses and environmental carcinogens. *J Am Acad Dermatol* 1993, 28:147–164.

Worret W-IF: Skin signs and internal malignancies. *Int J Dermatol* 1993, 32:1–5.

Immunobullous Diseases 20

Grant J. Anhalt

Key Points

- Autoantibody-mediated skin diseases are infrequent but have significant morbidity and mortality.
- Diagnoses are established by histologic examination of lesions and immuno-fluorescent examination of perilesional skin and serum.
- The most common disease is bullous pemphigoid, manifest by pruritic skin blisters in the elderly.
- The most serious disorder is pemphigus vulgaris, manifest by painful erosions of the mouth and skin.
- Oral corticosteroids, immunosuppressive agents, and select other drugs are used to control these diseases.

Although immunobullous diseases are not common, they are the cause of significant morbidity and mortality, hence their importance in a specialty that predominantly deals with less serious disorders. Additionally, study of the autoantibodies that cause these diseases has provided critical reagents for identifying important cell adhesion molecules [1••]. This chapter concentrates on practical points for recognition and diagnoses of immunobullous disorders. Prompt identification is important because in these disorders early therapeutic intervention can greatly reduce morbidity. The disorders covered are presented in approximate order of their prevalence and not in terms of their traditional immunopathologic categories.

BULLOUS PEMPHIGOID

Clinical Presentation

By far the most common bullous disease and the one most likely to be seen in a general medical practice is bullous pemphigoid (BP) [2], although its precise incidence or prevalence is not known. BP is primarily a disease of the elderly, with the vast majority of patients over 60 years of age at the time of eruption. With the aging of the general population in this country, the incidence seems to be increasing. It occurs very rarely in children or young adults.

The cutaneous eruption can have a prolonged prodrome manifested by very pruritic urticarial patches and plaques, or the condition may erupt rather abruptly with pruritus and blisters (Figs. 20-1 through 20-3). The blistering eruption primarily affects the trunk and flexures of the extremities. Unlike other bullous diseases, the mucous membranes are not affected, which is an important clinical finding.

The prodromal phase of the disease deserves some discussion. Prolonged generalized pruritus is a common complaint in the elderly and is most often attributable to dry skin or xerosis, eczematous dermatitis, or unidentified causes. A few patients with BP will have prolonged periods of intractable pruritus, without the typical plaques and blisters of BP. Typical immunopathologic changes also appear on biopsy result (Fig. 20-4). These cases should be included in the differential diagnosis of pruritus in the elderly. Their response to specific therapy is usually gratifying.

Diagnostic Techniques

It is known that BP is an autoimmune disease, and detection of the characteristic autoantibodies is crucial to an accurate diagnosis. The basis of diagnostic procedures is founded on the following established immunopathologic features of the disease: 1) all cases (once sampling error is excluded) have IgG autoantibodies and complement bound in the skin both in and around lesions (perilesional); 2)

these autoantibodies are also present in the serum of approximately one half of cases and bind to an adhesion organelle on the basilar surface of the basal epidermal cell, the hemidesmosome; and 3) it is now proven that binding of autoantibodies to the hemidesmosome with subsequent complement activation and consequent inflammatory events causes detachment of the epidermis from the underlying basement membrane [3].

Once blistering is apparent, the diagnosis is confirmed by fulfilling the following three criteria: 1) histologic changes that include subepidermal blistering (detachment of the entire epithelium from the basement membrane) and an inflammatory infiltrate rich in eosinophils (Fig. 20-5); 2) direct immunofluorescence of perilesional skin that shows linear deposition of IgG and complement components

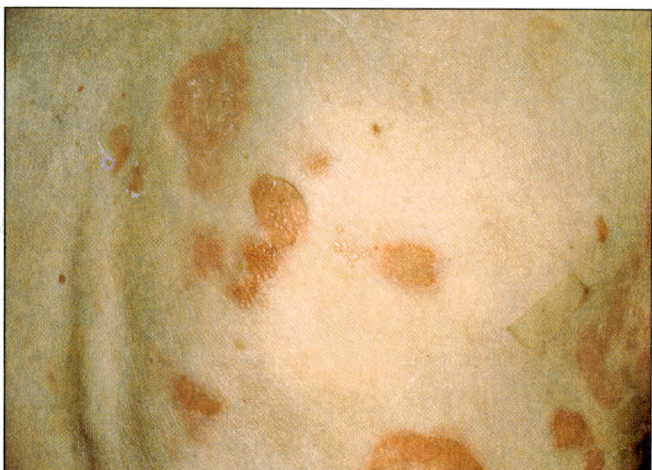

FIGURE 20-2 This lesion is representative of more chronic bullous pemphigoid, in which the blisters have ruptured leaving denuded areas and erosions.

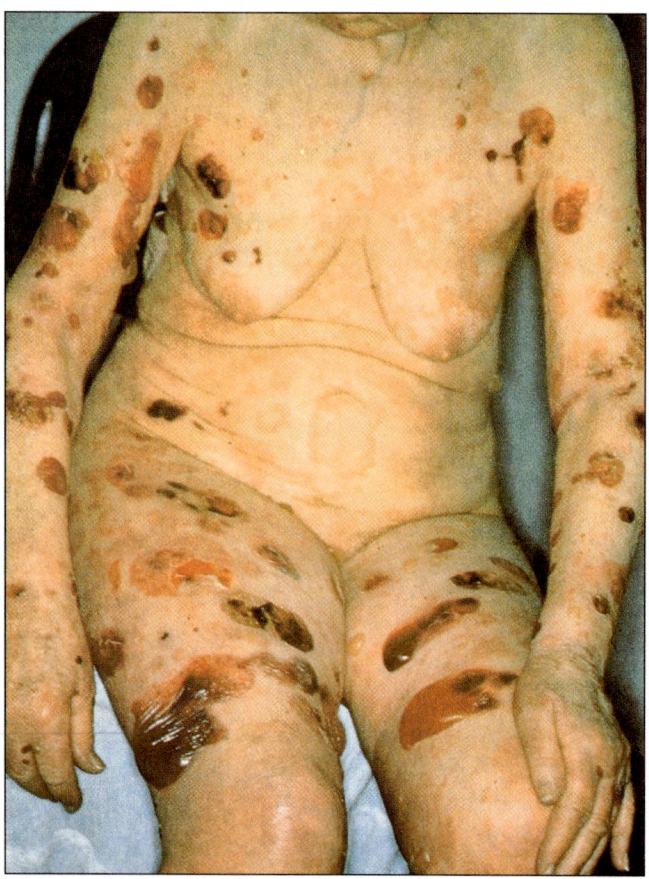

FIGURE 20-1 An elderly woman with explosive onset of bullous pemphigoid. There are numerous tense and hemorrhagic blisters that are distributed centrally on the trunk and on the flexures of the extremities. In the central trunk, there are also annular and urticarial lesions present. This is a very typical example of extensive bullous pemphigoid.

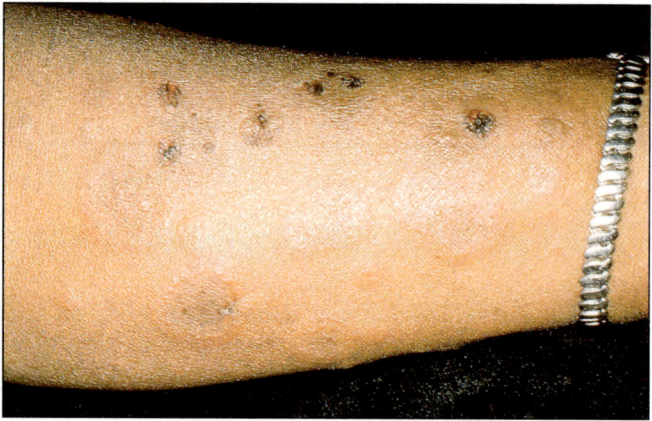

FIGURE 20-3 Acute onset of bullous pemphigoid may sometimes mimic other disorders. This elderly black man had an abrupt onset of pruritic annular lesions with central blistering. Clinically, these lesions closely resembled erythema multiforme, but were in fact evolving lesions of bullous pemphigoid.

along the basement membrane zone at the level that blistering is observed histologically (Fig. 20-6); and 3) indirect immunofluorescence of serum showing circulating autoantibodies that bind *in vitro* to the basement membrane zone of frozen sections of normal skin.

In practical terms, the patient's skin biopsy specimen should include the edge of a blister in formalin for histology and perilesional skin—an urticarial plaque or inflamed skin adjacent to the blister—in immunofluorescent transport media (Fig. 20-7) [4]. Biopsy results of the blister alone will frequently give false-negative immunofluorescence because the IgG and complement components are destroyed or obscured by the intense inflammatory reaction. A biopsy of skin too distant from a lesion may also cause a

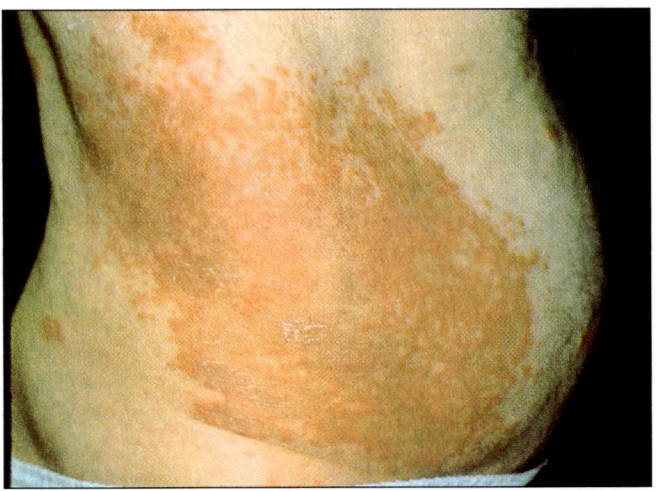

FIGURE 20-4 A typical presentation for the prodromal phase of bullous pemphigoid, in which urticarial patches and plaques predominate. This elderly man had large intensely pruritic erythematous plaques bilaterally on the flanks. Biopsy results showed these to be consistent with bullous pemphigoid. Persistent pruritic urticarial lesions in an elderly individual should alert one to the possibility of evolving bullous pemphigoid.

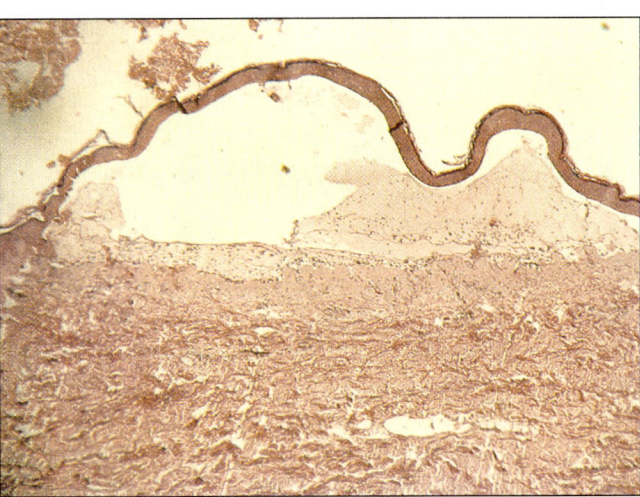

FIGURE 20-5 A low-power histologic picture of an intact blister of bullous pemphigoid. Bullous pemphigoid is a subepidermal blistering disorder, and the entire thickness of the epidermis forms the roof of the blister. The blister cavity is filled with a fibrin clot that is rich in eosinophils.

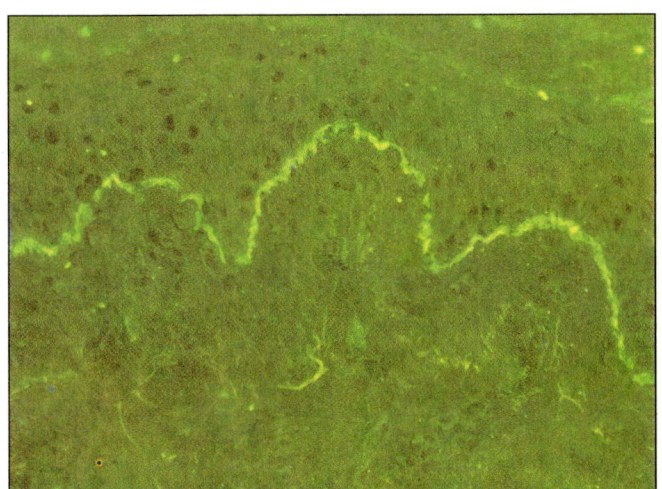

FIGURE 20-6 Direct immunofluorescence of perilesional inflamed skin in bullous pemphigoid reveals linear deposits of IgG and complement components along the basement-membrane zone at exactly the same level that histologic separation occurs. These findings confirm the diagnosis of bullous pemphigoid. Similar findings are seen in the variance of pemphigoid, herpes gestationis, and mucosal or cicatricial pemphigoid.

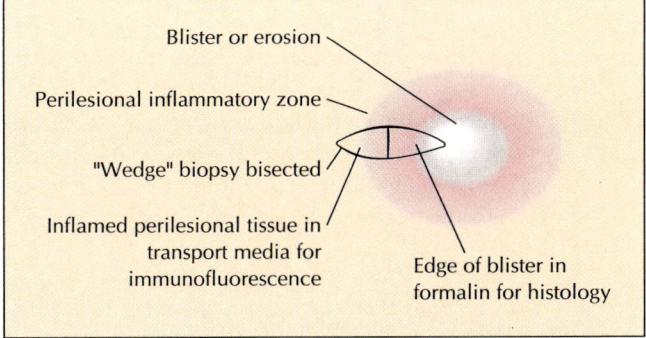

FIGURE 20-7 A biopsy technique that is appropriate for the vast majority of immunobullous disorders. The physician should identify a blister or erosion and perform a "wedge" biopsy, as indicated. The proximal half of the biopsied specimen that includes the edge of the blister or erosion should be submitted in formalin for histologic examination. The portion of the specimen that is distal to the lesion but still encompasses some clinically inflamed skin in the perilesional area should be placed in immunofluorescent transport media and can subsequently be tested by direct immunofluorescence. Alternatively, if the physician is uncomfortable performing a "wedge" biopsy, two individual 3-mm punch biopsies can be performed on the edge of the lesion and the perilesional skin. This technique gives an optimum chance for completing the diagnostic criteria in the majority of bullous diseases.

false-negative result, as the immunoreactants will only be weakly detected. Biopsy specimens immersed in formalin cannot be used for detection of immunoreactants. The immunofluorescent transport media is a stable solution of ammonium sulfate. Once the specimens are immersed in the transport media they are stable for weeks and can be mailed or transported to a laboratory without concern for stability. This transport media is inexpensive to prepare and should be available without cost from any laboratory that performs the test. Because the detection of autoantibodies in the serum can be negative in almost 50% of cases, this test is not critical for the diagnosis; demonstration of tissue-bound antibodies alone is often sufficient.

Therapy

Fortunately, BP is usually relatively easy to manage; anticipated morbidity is low, and mortality is rare. The disease is very responsive to oral corticosterioids (Table 20-1). The physician can anticipate that approximately one half of patients will experience a remission, and one half will require chronic therapy.

Despite this fact, a minority of patients with BP will have disease activity that will require prohibitively large doses of corticosteroids, and a second steroid-sparing agent is indicated [5]. The most effective drug in this scenario is azathioprine, 1 to 3 mg/kg/d. It has a high rate of success, does not produce significant neutropenia, and is generally well tolerated. Use of azathioprine carries with it a small increase in incidence of lymphoreticular malignancies, but in an elderly patient the risk for this event would often be expected to peak beyond the expected life span of the patient. Some patients are intolerant of azathioprine because of nausea or hepatotoxic reactions, and alternative drugs must be considered. These drugs include, in decreasing order of efficacy, cyclophosphamide, methotrexate, cyclosporine, dapsone, and gold therapy. Cyclophosphamide is effective, but the risk of neutropenia or hemorrhagic cystitis in the elderly is very high. Cyclosporine is extremely expensive and difficult to monitor in most cases. The response to methotrexate, dapsone, and gold therapy is unpredictable.

Rarer Variants of Pemphigoid

Herpes gestationis or gestational pemphigoid
Pruritic skin eruptions in the second or third trimester of pregnancy are relatively common, and most are caused by unknown factors (*eg*, pruritic urticarial papules and plaques of pregnancy). Rarely, a blistering eruption that is immunopathologically identical to BP can occur, and this eruption is called *herpes gestationis*. The disease resolves after delivery, often will flare with the return of menses or in the immediate postpartum period, and can be reproduced by challenge with oral estrogen. The incidence of disease is estimated at one in every 50,000 births, so a physician would not expect to see many cases.

Cicatricial Pemphigoid
Cicatricial pemphigoid is a serious disease of the elderly with peak incidence occurring in the sixth or seventh decade. Unlike BP, in which skin is involved and mucosal lesions are absent, cicatricial pemphigoid has scarring blisters that predominantly affect mucous membranes, and skin lesions are rare. Mucosal blisters and erosions are immunopathologically similar to BP [6•], but recurrent scarring may lead to profound morbidity or mortality. If lesions are found only on the gingiva or buccal mucosa, no serious morbidity will ensue. However, involvement of other structures can be disastrous. Specifically, if not aggressively treated, scarring of the conjunctiva leads to blindness, esophageal scarring leads to stenosis and asphyxiation from food, and laryngeal stenosis can also lead to asphyxiation. The physician must be alert to patients with chronic oral ulcerations or erosions or chronic conjunctival inflammation. Diagnosis is established by histologic and direct immunofluorescence (IF) examination of affected mucosa or conjunctiva. Lesions restricted to the oral cavity are treated with topical steroids, intralesional triamcinolone injections, or oral dapsone with variable response. If the eyes, esophagus, or larynx is involved, aggressive treatment with cyclophosphamide or prednisone for a period of 18 to 24 months will induce a remission in the majority of cases [7]. Early diagnosis is critical to a good prognosis.

PEMPHIGUS VULGARIS

Clinical Presentation

Pemphigus vulgaris (PV) is less common than BP but is a serious form of bullous disease. It is most common in middle-aged patients, but young adults and the elderly are also affected. The disease has a specific immunogenetic basis. The genes that encode this susceptibility appear to be overrepresented in the Jewish population, especially those of Eastern European origin. The incidence is highest in this population, although every race and ethnic group is affected

TABLE 20-1 DRUG REGIMEN FOR TREATMENT OF BULLOUS PEMPHIGOID
• Initial dosage of 0.5–0.75 mg/kg/d prednisone
• After a few weeks, slow taper of oral steroids, switch to alternate-day regimen
• Over 3–6 mo, dosage may be reduced by increments every 2–3 wk
• Drug may be discontinued after this time
• In case of recurrence Severe: low-dose prednisone, 5–10 mg every other day Mild: combination of potent topical steroid (fluocinonide 0.5% cream, three times daily) or intralesional injections with triamcinolone suspension (10 mg/cc) for limited areas

to some extent. PV usually presents with slowly progressive ulcerations of the oropharynx that often are misdiagnosed for weeks or months. Later, fragile cutaneous blisters and erosions occur on the head and neck, then spread acrally (Fig. 20-8). Without intervention, progressive skin loss and poor oral intake because of pain cause progressive debilitation, sepsis, and death. Prior to the introduction of oral corticosteroids, the mortality of this disease was 50% at 2 years and 100% at 5 years. The presence of persistent cutaneous and oral erosions should be a clinical red flag that prompts consideration of a serious immunobullous disease such as PV.

Diagnostic Techniques

The following is known about the pathophysiology of the disease, and this knowledge forms the basis for diagnostic maneuvers: 1) PV is an autoimmune disease caused by IgG autoantibodies against a cell-adhesion molecule of squamous epithelium (skin and mucosa); 2) binding of the antibody to the cell surface causes cell–cell detachment, resulting in an intraepidermal blister; and 3) there is a good correlation between levels of circulating autoantibodies and disease activity. Therefore, the diagnosis is established by fulfilling the following criteria: 1) clinically, there are erosions or blisters on both skin and mucous membranes; 2) histologically, there is an intraepidermal blister caused by epithelial

cells detaching from each other (Fig. 20-9); 3) direct IF shows IgG bound to the cell surface of affected oral epithelium or skin (Fig. 20-10); and 4) circulating antibodies that bind to the cell surface of squamous epithelium on frozen sections of skin or esophagus are detectable. Unlike BP, circulating antibodies are always

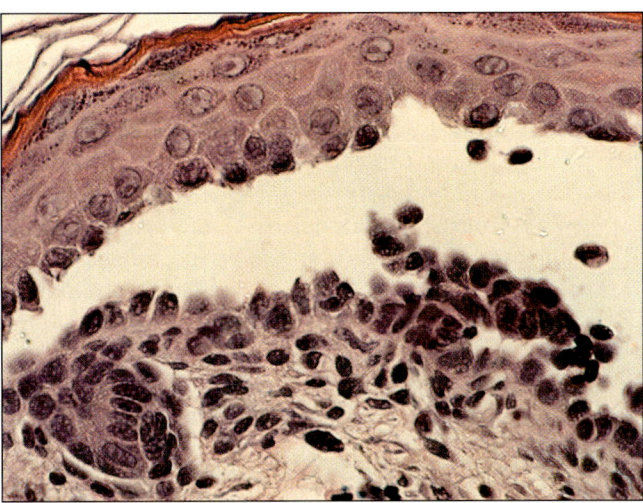

FIGURE 20-9 Histologic examination of the edge of a blister in pemphigus vulgaris shows a blister that forms just above the lower-most cells of the epidermis. Pemphigus, therefore, is a disorder in which the blister is intraepidermal. Note the epidermal cells have detached and rounded up and are floating free in the blister cavity. This loss of cell-cell detachment (acantholysis) is characteristic of all forms of pemphigus.

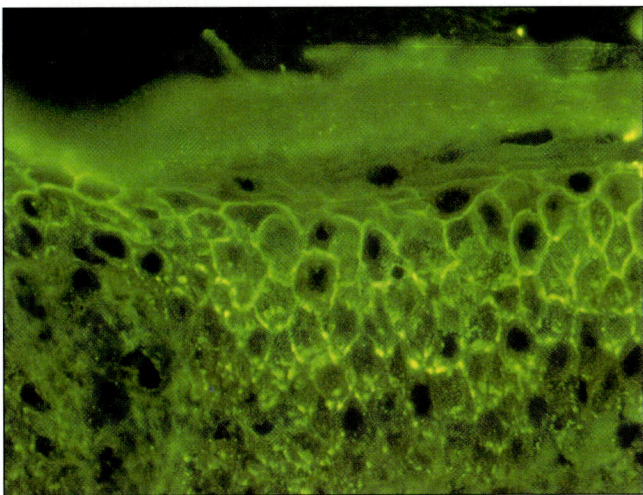

FIGURE 20-10 Direct immunofluorescence from perilesional skin in pemphigus vulgaris shows immunoglobulin G and complement components bound to the surface of the epithelial cells. Binding of the antibody to the cell surface adhesion molecules that are the target antigens in this disease cause the cell–cell detachment seen in the previous figure. It is easy to note the difference between the intraepidermal blistering disorders (pemphigus) and the subepidermal blistering disorders (pemphigoid) on the basis of these two criteria.

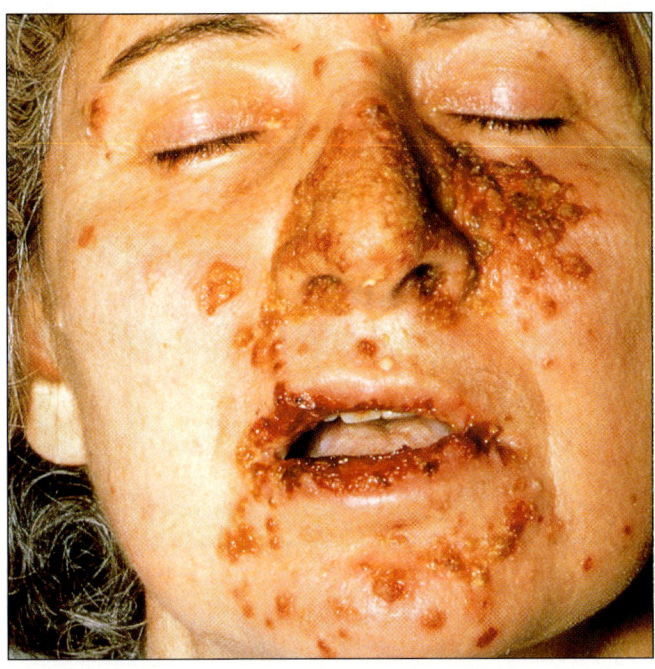

FIGURE 20-8 A typical presentation for pemphigus vulgaris. Note the mucosal lesions on the tongue and the lips. After these intraoral lesions have been present for a period of weeks or months, blisters and erosions start to appear on the central part of the face and then spread acrally. The combination of cutaneous and oral blistering must alert the clinician to the possibility of a serious immunobullous disease, such as pemphigus vulgaris.

detectable. Given the fact that the disease is potentially life-threatening, circulating autoantibodies must be demonstrated to fulfill the diagnostic criteria. Again, these criteria can be fulfilled by performing a biopsy on the edge of a blister for histology, and on adjacent perilesional skin for direct IF, and by obtaining a serum tube for indirect IF.

Therapy

Therapy must be directed at reducing autoantibody synthesis because as long as significant amounts of antiepithelial antibodies are present the disease will persist. Unlike BP, topical treatments are of secondary importance, and long-term improvement will only occur by treatment of the hematopoietic system. Again, unlike BP, remissions are very rare, and most individuals require therapy for life (Table 20-2). Approximately one half of patients will respond well to oral corticosteroids alone. Maintenance therapy with low-dose, alternate-day corticosteroids is required in all patients [8]. Patients that have resistant disease or are intolerant of corticosteroids should receive a second steroid-sparing agent. In decreasing order of efficacy these agents are cyclophosphamide [9•], azathioprine, chlorambucil, methotrexate, and gold. Management of difficult cases of PV is best handled by physicians with experience in its treatment.

Rarer Variants of Pemphigus
Pemphigus foliaceus and paraneoplastic pemphigus

Pemphigus foliaceus (PF) is a superficial form of pemphigus that is differentiated by two major criteria: 1) clinically, lesions are superficial and mucous membranes are never affected; and 2) histologically, cell-cell detachment occurs only in the most superficial layer of the epidermis. Otherwise, direct and indirect IF features of PV and PF are virtually identical.

In contrast to PV, PF has far less morbidity and only very rare mortality, so therapy is generally less problematic. It is important to note that certain drugs have been shown to induce PF and, less commonly, PV. Implicated drugs include D-penicillamine, gold sodium thiomalate, and angiotensin-converting enzyme inhibitors such as captopril and enalapril.

Paraneoplastic pemphigus

Paraneoplastic pemphigus is a recently described bullous disease associated with specific neoplasms [10]. These neoplasms include non-Hodgkin's lymphomas, chronic lymphocytic leukemia, thymomas, Castleman tumors, and Waldenström's macroglobulinemia. The presence of persistent mucosal erosions and a polymorphous skin eruption in patients with these neoplasms should prompt referral for evaluation of this syndrome. Treatment is difficult and when the syndrome is associated with malignant neoplasms, the mortality rate is approximately 90%.

DERMATITIS HERPETIFORMIS

Clinical Presentation, Diagnosis, and Therapy

Dermatitis herpetiformis is a rare IgA-mediated skin disease. It presents with intense pruritic papules and

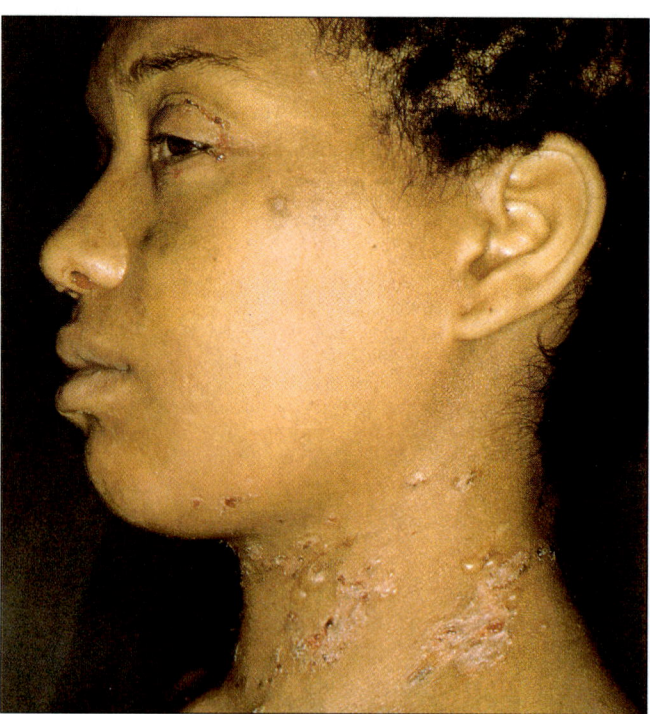

FIGURE 20-11 This young woman presented with a high fever, cerebritis, and blistering erosions of mucous membranes and flexural areas of the skin. She was subsequently found to have subepidermal blisters with dense IgG and complement components in the epidermis. This case was of epidermolysis bullosa acquisita that presented in a patient with bullous systemic lupus erythematosus. This presentation is typical for the inflammatory variety of epidermolysis bullosa acquisita seen in the context of acute lupus erythematosus. Once again, the combination of both mucosal and cutaneous blistering is a critical clinical feature of an evolving serious immunobullous disease.

TABLE 20-2 TREATMENT OF PEMPHIGUS VULGARIS IN VARYING CASES
50% Of patients diagnosed respond well to oral corticosteroids alone (prednisone, 1 mg/kg/d) tapered slowly over 6–9 mo
All patient responders require maintenance therapy with low-dose, alternate-day corticosteroids
Patients with resistant disease or intolerance to corticosteroids should receive a second steroid-sparing agent (ie, cyclophosphamide, azathioprine, chlorambucil, methotrexate, or gold)

vesicles distributed symmetrically over the shoulders, extensor elbows, and knees and on the scalp and sacrum. Peak incidence is in young adults; it is associated with a specific immunogenetic inheritance and asymptomatic gluten-sensitive enteropathy [11]. The disease affects white people and is extraordinarily rare in black people. The burning pruritus is typically disproportionate to the severity or extent of the skin lesions. Diagnosis is based on histologic evidence of coalescent subepidermal vesicles filled with neutrophils and granular IgA deposition in the upper dermis of perilesional skin. Circulating antibodies are not detectable. A dramatic elimination of pruritus within 24 to 48 hours of treatment with oral dapsone is an accepted clinical diagnostic sign. However, individuals who are glucose-6-phosphate-dehydrogenase-(G6PD)–sensitive cannot receive dapsone or massive hemolysis could ensue. Complete elimination of gluten from the diet for a period of months to years will reduce or eliminate maintenance requirements for dapsone, but complete avoidance of gluten is very difficult in North American diets.

VERY RARE BULLOUS DISEASES

Epidermolysis Bullosa Acquisita

This disease is an autoimmune disease that may mimic BP. Inflammatory blisters on mucous membranes and skin or trauma-induced blisters on the extremities are typical for this condition. IgG and complement components are present along the basement-membrane zone, but the target antigen is type VII collagen, and the subepidermal blister is actually located in the uppermost zone of the dermis [12]. Similar autoantibodies to type VII collagen and inflammatory blistering are seen in bullous systemic lupus erythematosus (Fig. 20-11).

Linear IgA Dermatitis

Linear IgA dermatitis, previously referred to as chronic *bullous disease of childhood*, presents as pruritic blisters on the trunk and extremities. It can occur in infants, young children, and adults. Subepidermal blisters are seen, and linear IgA is deposited along the basement membrane in contrast to the granular IgA deposition of dermatis herpetiformis.

REFERENCES AND RECOMMENDED READING

Recently published papers of particular interest have been highlighted as:

- Of interest
- •• Of outstanding interest

1.•• Stanley JR: Cell adhesion molecules as targets of autoantibodies in pemphigus and pemphigoid, bullous diseases due to defective epidermal cell adhesion. *Adv Immunol* 1993, 53:291–325.

2. Anhalt GJ, Morrison L: Pemphigoid: bullous, gestational and cicatricial. In *Bullous Diseases*. Edited by Provost TT, Weston WL. St. Louis: Mosby-Year Book; 1992:63–112.

3. Lui Z, Diaz DA, Troy JL, *et al.*: A passive transfer model of the organ-specific autoimmune disease, bullous pemphigoid, using antibodies generated against the hemidesmosomal antigen BP180. *J Clin Invest* 1993, 92:2480–2488.

4. Fine JD, Briggaman RA, Gammon WR: Laboratory approach to the evaluation of vesiculbullous disorders. In *Topics in Clinical Dermatology: Bullous Diseases*. Edited by Fine JD. New York: Igaku-Shoin; 1993:3–22.

5. McDonald CJ: Cytotoxic agents for use in dermatology. *J Am Acad Dermatol* 1985, 12:753–775.

6.• Chan LS, Yancey KB, Hammerberg C, *et al.*: Immune mediated subepidermal blistering diseases of mucous membranes. *Arch Dermatol* 1993, 129:448–455.

7. Jabs DA, Anhalt GJ: Cicatricial pemphigoid. In *Current Therapy in Dermatology*, edn 2. Edited by Farmer ER, Provost TT. Philadelphia: BC Decker; 1988:56–57.

8. Morrison L, Anhalt GJ: Pemphigus. In *Current Therapy in Allergy and Immunology*. Edited by Liechtenstein L, Fauci A. Philadelphia: BC Decker; 1988:186–189.

9.• Pandya AG, Sontheimer RD: Treatment of pemphigus vulgaris with pulse intravenous cyclophosphamide. *Arch Dermatol* 1992, 128:1626–1630.

10. Anhalt GJ, Kim SC, Stanley JR, *et al.*: Paraneoplastic pemphigus: an autoimmune mucocutaneous disease associated with neoplasia. *New Engl J Med* 1990, 323:1729–1735.

11. McCord M, Hall III RP: IgA mediated autoimmune blistering diseases. In *Topics in Clinical Dermatology: Bullous Diseases*. Edited by Fine JD. New York: Igaku-Shoin; 1993:97–120.

12. Gammon WR, Fine JD, Briggaman RA: Autoimmunity to type VII collagen: features and role in basement membrane injury. In *Topics in Clinical Dermatology: Bullous Diseases*. Edited by Fine JD. New York: Igaku-Shoin; 1993:75–98.

21 Cutaneous Manifestations of Endocrine and Metabolic Disorders

Victoria P. Werth
Lynn McKinley-Grant

Key Points

- There are many inflammatory and infectious skin dermatoses associated with diabetes mellitus. Prevention, evaluation, and treatment of infected leg and foot ulcers are particularly important concerns.
- The presence of xanthomas indicates the need for evaluation of serum cholesterol and triglyceride levels.
- Hyperandrogenemia, as manifest by hirsutism, acne, and androgenetic alopecia, can indicate either ovarian or adrenal pathology, and may warrant screening tests for elevated hormone levels.
- Porphyria cutanea tarda has recently been found to be associated with hepatitis C infection in some individuals, and can be aggravated by alcohol use and various medications.
- Other metabolic diseases affecting the skin include amyloidosis, hemochromatosis, cutis calcinosis, and acrodermatitis enteropathica.

ENDOCRINE DISORDERS

Diabetes Mellitus Disorders

Many inflammatory and infectious skin dermatoses are seen in patients with diabetes mellitus (Table 21-1). None are pathognomonic of diabetes, as is the case with granuloma annulare, but their occurrence should lead the clinician to consider whether diabetes is present (Fig. 21-1). In addition, the vascular changes seen in diabetics result in secondary cutaneous changes.

Inflammatory dermatoses

Necrobiosis lipoidica diabeticorum occurs in three in every 1000 diabetics, but only two thirds of those affected will eventually have diabetes. Clinically, erythematous to yellowish papules and plaques, atrophic in the center, occur most often on the legs (Fig. 21-2). About one third of these lesions ulcerate. Treatment includes topical and intralesional corticosteroid therapy, but care must be taken because the lesions are atrophic and tend to ulcerate.

Diabetic dermopathy is manifest by multiple, discrete, brown, slightly atrophic macules on the anterior lower legs. The origin of this condition is unknown, but it is seen in about 50% of patients with diabetes. No known therapy exists for this disorder. The bullous eruption of diabetes (bullous diabeticorum) is represented by the spontaneous formation of painless, tense blisters on the feet, lower legs, and occasionally, arms and hands, in patients with longstanding diabetes. The lesions heal in 2 to 5 weeks without scarring and can recur over a period of several years. The diagnosis can be made only after traumatic and chemical causes are excluded, cultures are sterile, and both uropor-

TABLE 21-1 SKIN CONDITIONS ASSOCIATED WITH DIABETES MELLITUS

Noninfectious, inflammatory	Infectious
Acanthosis nigricans	Bacteria
Diabetic dermopathy	Pyodermas (especially *Staphylococcus aureus*): folliculitis, impetigo, furuncles
Diabetic bullae	Malignant external otitis (*Pseudomonas aeruginosa*),
Granuloma annulare	Necrotizing fasciitis (gram-positive, gram-negative, anaerobic)
Lipodystrophy (from insulin or as part of syndrome)	Erythrasma
Necrobiosis lipoidica diabeticorum	Fungal
Perforating cutaneous disease of diabetes	Dermatophytosis
Pruritus	Candidiasis: balanitis, vaginitis, paronychia, intertrigo, finger webs
Scleredema	Mucormycosis
Stiff hand syndrome	**Vascular insufficiency**
Xanthomas	Ischemic ulcer
Vitiligo	Digital gangrene
	Erysipelas-like erythema

phyrin and direct immunofluorescence study results are negative [1].

Scleredema adultorum of Buschke is manifest by a diffuse erythema and induration of the skin over the posterior neck, the upper back, and occasionally, the face and trunk (Fig. 21-3). It occurs in patients with long-standing diabetes, but the cause of the increased dermal extracellular matrix is unknown. No effective therapy exists.

Pruritus may occur in diabetics, even without renal disease. Topical corticosteroids, antipruritic preparations containing phenol and menthol, and antihistamines may relieve the symptoms.

Infections

Many infections occur with an increased frequency in diabetics. Malignant external otitis results from *Pseudomonas aeruginosa* and includes severe ear pain, facial swelling, and a purulent, erythematous otitis. It occurs in elderly patients with diabetes. If untreated, it can progress rapidly to osteomyelitis and purulent meningitis. Multiple cranial nerve palsies are common. Prompt treatment with mezlocillin, ceftazidime, and tobramycin, as well as surgical débridement and drainage, is important [2].

Necrotizing fasciitis results from a mixed aerobic and anaerobic infection in the fascial plane, leading to a rapidly evolving, red, edematous induration of the skin. Crepitus can develop, along with blisters, purpura, and tissue necrosis, and the patient develops a high fever and prostration. Early diagnosis, possibly with a surgical biopsy, is important. Treatment includes surgical débridement of the involved fascia and intravenous antibiotics appropriate to destroy the causative organisms.

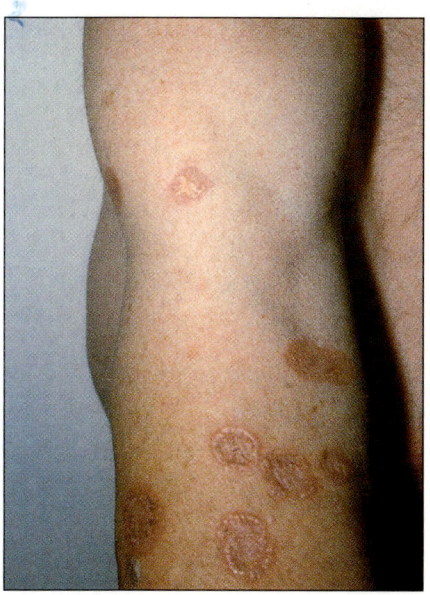

FIGURE 21-1
Granuloma annulare in a diabetic patient. Note multiple erythematous individual papules coalescing into annular and expanding lesions on the arm. (*Courtesy of* B. Witmer, Philadelphia, PA).

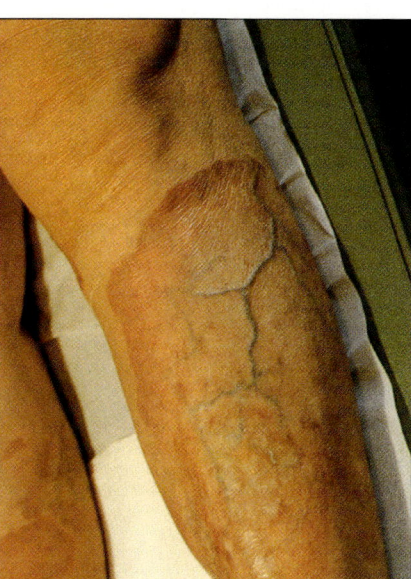

FIGURE 21-2
Necrobiosis lipoidica diabeticorum. Note atrophic yellow plaques on the anterior lower legs. (*Courtesy of* B. Witmer.)

Chapter 21: Cutaneous Manifestations of Endocrine and Metabolic Disorders

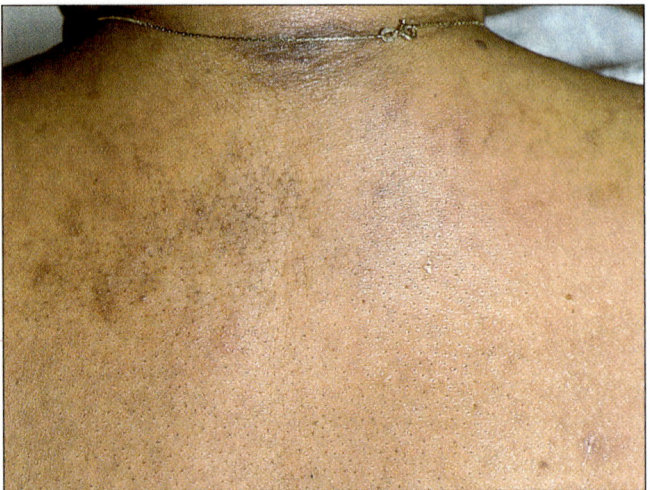

FIGURE 21-3 Scleredema. Note skin thickening and hyperpigmentation on the upper back of this diabetic patient. (*Courtesy of* B. Witmer.)

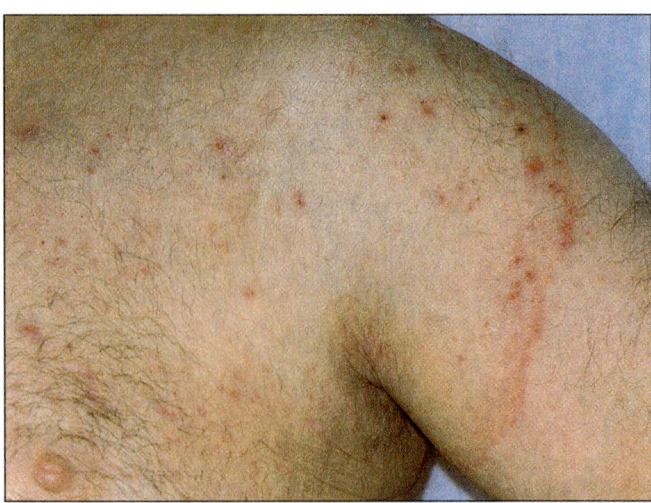

FIGURE 21-4 Tinea corporis. Note erythematous, scaly border on arm extending from large patch of tinea on trunk. (*Courtesy of* B. Witmer.)

Superficial *fungal infections* due to tinea or *Candida* are common (Figs. 21-4 and 21-5). These can be diagnosed with potassium hydroxide preparations or fungal cultures, and treated with topical antifungal creams (*see* Elewski, Common Fungal Infections of the Skin). Resistant infections may be treated with systemic therapy. Chronic daily treatment with antifungal creams may be necessary, particularly if onychomycosis is present, to prevent recurrences (Fig. 21-6). The abnormal skin barrier seen with fungal infections may allow for the entry of bacteria, which can then result in bacterial infections of the skin. It is thus important to examine the skin, especially the feet, of diabetics to prevent this

complication. Patients presenting with *Candida balanitis* should be screened for underlying diabetes.

Leg and foot ulcers

About 20% of hospitalized diabetics are admitted for foot problems. The causes of leg and foot ulcers in diabetics include neuropathy, ischemia, and infection. It is especially important for these patients not to smoke. Open wounds in these patients become colonized with bacteria, but uninfected ulcers do not require antibiotics (Fig. 21-7). Special orthotic shoe devices can prevent the neuropathic trauma that leads to ulcers. Ischemia needs to be evaluated with noninvasive vascular studies pertinent to the wound. If

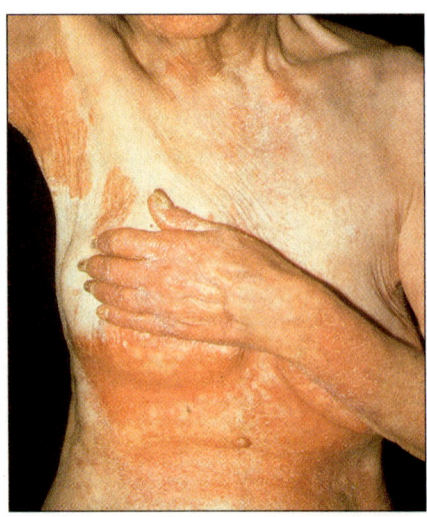

FIGURE 21-5 Candidal infection. Note inflammatory eruption with numerous satellite pustules occurring in multiple intertriginous areas. (*Courtesy of* B. Witmer.)

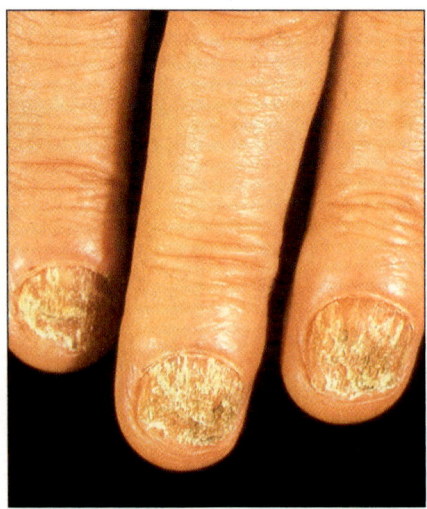

FIGURE 21-6 Onychomycosis due to tinea. Note yellow, dystrophic fingernails. (*Courtesy of* B. Witmer.)

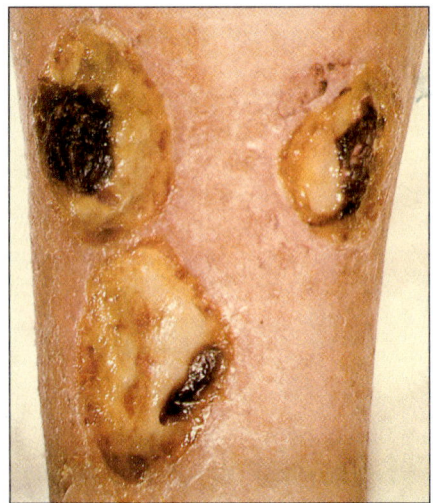

FIGURE 21-7 Multiple leg ulcers in a diabetic patient. Note multiple, somewhat crusted ulcers over the lower leg. (*Courtesy of* B. Witmer.)

severe atherosclerosis is present, revascularization may be necessary to heal an ulcer.

Evaluation of infected leg and foot ulcers

Purulent discharge or the presence of two or more of the signs and symptoms of inflammation (induration, redness, warmth, and tenderness) usually suggests infection. Cultures should be obtained from most soft tissue infections to select the appropriate specific antibiotic treatment. Swabs of purulent discharge are unreliable because anaerobes are inhibited by cotton swab and because the culture does not distinguish between pathogens and colonization [3]. Possible methods of specimen collection for quantitative assessment of bacteria in the wound include curettage specimen, biopsy, or needle aspiration. The curettage specimen is obtained after the surface of an open wound is cleaned with saline-soaked gauze, betadine, or alcohol. A sterile dermal curette or scalpel blade is used to scrape tissue from the base and edges of the ulcer [4••].

Organisms causing ulcers

Ulcers are commonly colonized by *Staphylococcus aureus*. Aerobic gram-negative bacilli are commonly isolated, including *Proteus*, *Escherichia coli*, *Klebsiella-Enterobacter* species, and *Pseudomonas*. Obligate anaerobes may also be important pathogens in these infections.

Treatment of infected leg and foot ulcers

Treatment of mild infections should include oral dicloxacillin, erythromycin, cephalexin, or clindamycin for 1 to 2 weeks. If gram-negative bacilli are involved, trimethoprim-sulfamethoxazole, amoxacillin-clavulanate, or ciprofloxacin should be administered. If the infection has a foul odor or the gram-stained smear shows several types of organisms, obligate anaerobes may be present. In these cases, clindamycin alone or metronidazole and an antistaphylococcal drug should be given [4••]. If the infection does not respond in 2 to 3 days, parenteral treatment should be given and the wound cultures used to determine therapy. Local care of ulcers should include elevation of the feet; local débridement of any eschar; soaks with saline; application of antimicrobial ointments, such as polysporin or bacitracin; and a nonadherent dressing. Once the infection is cleared, a whole range of new wound-care dressings is available to expedite healing. It is important to avoid desiccation of the wound, often caused by using wet-to-dry dressings.

Xanthomas and Dysproteinemias

Xanthomas can occur with or without elevated blood lipids. When a hyperlipidemia is present, the type of hyperlipidemia can be predicted from the type of xanthoma present (tuberous, tendon, eruptive, or planar; Table 21-2) [5]. Secondary causes of the hyperlipidemia must be sought. Xanthelasmas, and xanthomas associated with various

TABLE 21-2 CLINICAL DISORDERS IN WHICH XANTHOMAS OCCUR	
Xanthoma	**Clinical disorders**
Tuberous	Types II and III hyperlipoproteinemia
Tendon	Types IIa, IIb, and III hyperlipoproteinemia
	Obstructive liver disease
	Hypothyroidism
	Diabetes mellitus
	Cerebrotendinous xanthomatosis
Eruptive	Types I, IV, and V hyperlipoproteinemia
	Diabetes mellitus
	Pancreatitis
	Hypothyroidism
	Nephrotic syndrome
	Medications: isotretinoin, estrogen, glucocorticoids
Xanthoma striatum palmare	Type III, IV hyperlipoproteinemia
	Biliary cirrhosis
	Diabetes mellitus

dysproteinemias, inflammatory skin disorders, and lipid storage disease can occur in the setting of normal blood lipid levels [6].

Tuberous xanthomas appear as yellow-to-red grouped papules and nodules, often located on elbows, extensor forearms, knuckles, palms, knees, heels, and buttocks. This condition is particularly associated with increased serum cholesterol levels but can be seen with increased very-low-density lipoprotein (triglyceride-rich) and intermediate-density lipoprotein levels.

Tendinous xanthomas are deep, firm, variably sized nodules with normal overlying skin that are present in tendons, ligaments, and fascia. They occur in the Achilles tendons and extensor tendons of the knees, elbows, and dorsa of the hands, and can be painful. The differential diagnosis includes rheumatoid nodules and gouty tophi. These xanthomas are seen with hypercholesterolemia.

Eruptive xanthomas are 1- to 4-mm erythematous papules usually found on the buttocks and extensor thighs, knees, and arms (Fig. 21-8). They may be pruritic and often occur in response to trauma. This form of xanthoma occurs with hypertriglyceridemia.

Planar xanthomas include several discrete entities. Xanthelasmas are yellow infiltrative macules and papules found on the eyelids. These are associated with increased serum cholesterol in 50% of people, and those under 40 to 50 years of age are particularly at risk. Xanthoma striatum palmare occurs as yellow, soft, often linear patches in the creases of the palms and fingers. This condition is associ-

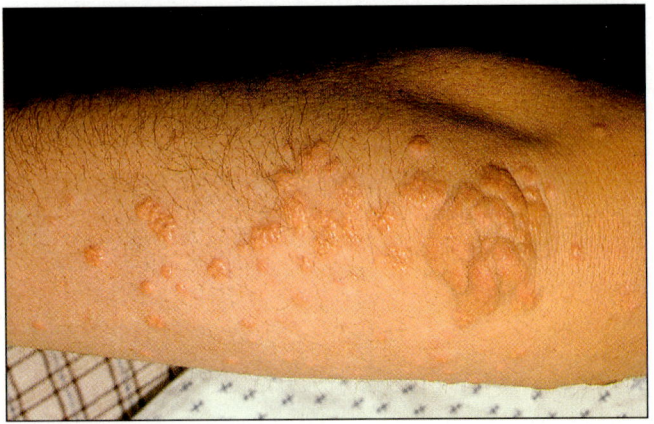

FIGURE 21-8 Eruptive xanthomas in a diabetic patient whose blood glucose level is poorly controlled. Note yellow papules and plaques on the extensor surface of the elbow and arm. (*Courtesy of* B. Witmer.)

TABLE 21-4 DERMATOLOGIC DISEASES ASSOCIATED WITH THYROID DISEASE

Dermatitis herpetiformis
Alopecia areata
Pemphigus foliaceus and vulgaris
Bullous pemphigoid
Herpes gestationis
Dermatomyositis
Lupus erythematosus, chronic cutaneous and systemic
Scleroderma
Vitiligo
Pustulosis palmoplantaris
Sweet's syndrome
Urticaria
Cowden's disease

ated with increased triglyceride or intermediate-density lipoprotein levels. Extensive, yellow-orange infiltrative plaques on the face, neck, upper trunk, and arms are seen in association with several dysproteinemias, including myeloma, lymphomas, chronic leukemias, cryoglobulinemias, Waldenström's macroglobulinemia, and benign monoclonal gammopathy.

Evaluation and treatment of xanthomas

A skin biopsy helps confirm the diagnosis of xanthoma if the diagnosis is uncertain. The clinical appearance of xanthelasma is usually distinctive enough to render a biopsy unnecessary. Any patient with xanthomas deserves serum cholesterol and serum fasting triglyceride level testing to screen for hyperlipidemia. Any abnormalities need further evaluation as to the type of hyperlipidemia, any possible secondary causes, and then treatment of the secondary cause or the primary disorder.

Control of the hyperlipidemia leads to rapid resolution of eruptive xanthomas and slower regression of tuberous xanthomas. Tendinous xanthomas and xanthelasmas seldom resolve with treatment.

Thyroid Disorders

Many nonspecific findings occur in the skin, hair, and nails in hyperthyroidism and hypothyroidism (Table 21-3) [7]. Other findings are more specific, as discussed later. In addition, many dermatologic diseases, such as vitiligo, are associated with thyroid disease (Table 21-4, Fig. 21-9).

Pretibial myxedema is seen in 0.5% to 4% of patients with Graves' disease, and rarely, in patients with Hashimoto's thyroiditis. Bilateral, asymmetric, pink to purple-brown firm plaques and nodules occur most frequently on the lower legs (Fig. 21-10*A*). The lesions may exhibit hypertrichosis or become verrucous (Fig. 21-10*B*). Pretibial myxedema is often associated with exophthalmos

TABLE 21-3 NONSPECIFIC GENERAL DERMATOLOGIC FINDINGS IN HYPERTHYROIDISM AND HYPOTHYROIDISM

	Manifestations	
Affected area	**Hyperthyroidism**	**Hypothyroidism**
Skin	Warm, moist, smooth	Cold, pale, decreased sweating
Hair	Facial, palmar erythema	Xerosis, ichthyosis, keratoderma
Nail	Generalized hyperhidrosis	Carotenemia (yellow palms, soles, nasolabial folds)
	Increased pigmentation (palms, soles, oral mucosa)	Poor wound healing
	Pruritus	Dry, course, brittle
	Fine, soft	Diffuse thinning
	Diffuse, nonscarring alopecia	Loss of lateral third of eyebrows
	Plummer's nails (concave contour with distal onycholysis)	Thick, brittle
		Longitudinal striations
		Slow growth

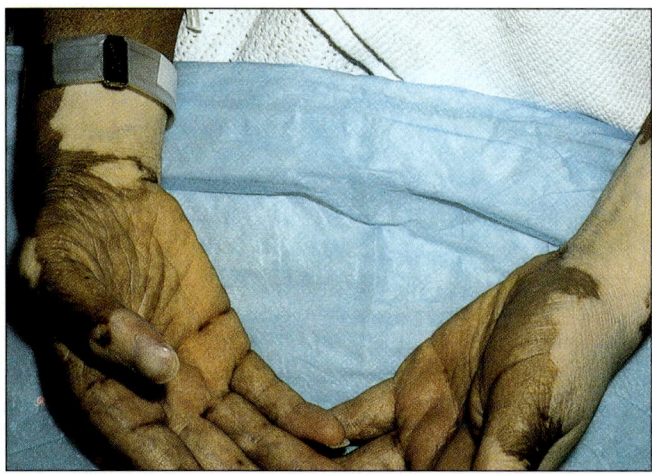

FIGURE 21-9 Vitiligo in a patient with hypothyroidism. Note hypopigmented patches on the wrists and hands.

(Fig. 21-11), and results from the accumulation of hyaluronic acid in the dermis and sometimes the subcutaneous tissue. The diagnosis is confirmed with a skin biopsy. If the patient is not known to have thyroid disease, thyroid function tests should be obtained. This process is most often found in euthyroid patients whose hyperthyroidism has been treated with surgery or radioactive iodine. Treatment with topical or intralesional corticosteroids is sometimes effective.

Thyroid acropachy is seen in 0.1% to 1% of patients with Graves' disease and rarely in those with Hashimoto's thyroiditis. It consists of digital clubbing, soft-tissue swelling of the hands and feet, and periosteal proliferation of the shafts of the fingers, toes, and other distal long bones (Fig. 21-12). It is often associated with exophthalmos or pretibial myxedema and most often occurs after treatment

of the thyroid disease. No treatment is necessary, and the findings may slowly resolve.

Generalized myxedema occurs in patients with hypothyroidism and is manifest as diffusely edematous, waxy, and firm skin. Patients often have a puffy appearance, with thickening of the lips, a broad nose, and macroglossia. These changes result from dermal deposition of acid mucopolysaccharides in the skin. Thyroid hormone replacement generally leads to resolution of the cutaneous changes.

Adrenal Cortex Disorders

Skin disorders are associated with several hypersecretion syndromes of the adrenal, including those in which increased cortisol (Cushing's syndrome), androgens (virilization), and estrogens (feminization) occur. In addition, adrenocortical failure results in skin changes.

Cushing's syndrome results from an increase in endogenous cortisol production from an adrenal tumor or from exogenous glucocorticoids. The associated cutaneous findings include increased fat deposition in the supraclavicular fossae, upper back, and abdomen. The face is round and puffy, and the skin is thinned, leading to easy bruising and delayed wound healing (Fig. 21-13). Other changes include acne, facial erythema, lanugo hair, and hair loss [8].

Hyperandrogenemia can lead to hirsutism, acne, and androgenetic alopecia (Figs. 21-14 and 21-15). Other cutaneous signs include loss of breast tissue and clitoral enlargement. The sources of elevated androgens include the adrenal and ovary glands [9]. Ovarian causes of increased androgens include polycystic ovarian syndrome, insulin resistance, and ovarian tumors. Adrenal causes include Cushing's disease, androgen-producing tumors, and congenital adrenal hyperplasia. Some drugs can cause hirsutism by a mechanism unrelated to androgens. These

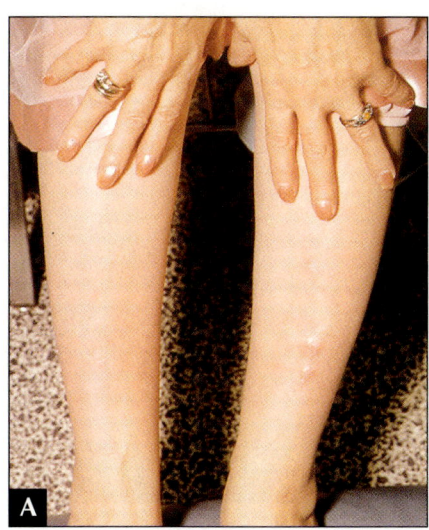
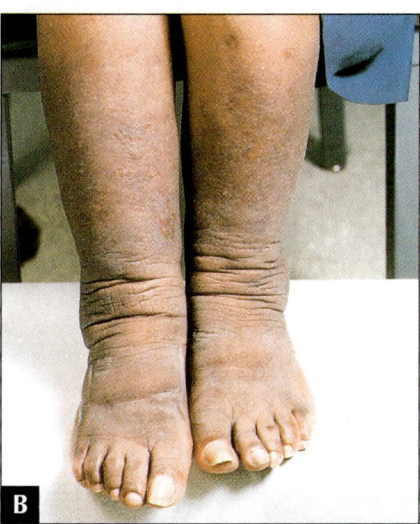

FIGURE 21-10 **A**, Pretibial myxedema. Note pink nodules on legs with diffuse, nonpitting edema. **B**, Nonpitting edema with prominent hair follicles and "cobblestone" pattern to lesions on legs. (*Courtesy of* F. Sterling; Philadelphia, PA.)

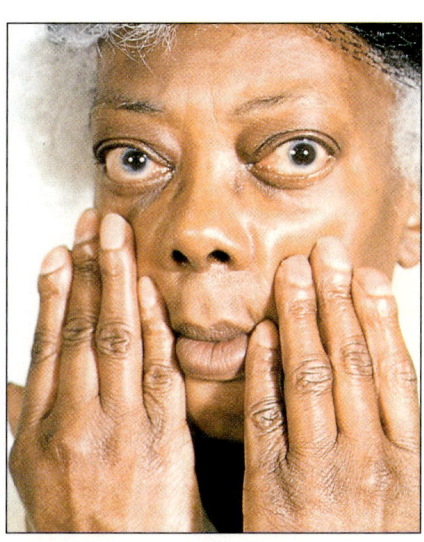

FIGURE 21-11 Graves' ophthalmopathy. Prominent proptosis of the eyes is seen. (*Courtesy of* F. Sterling.)

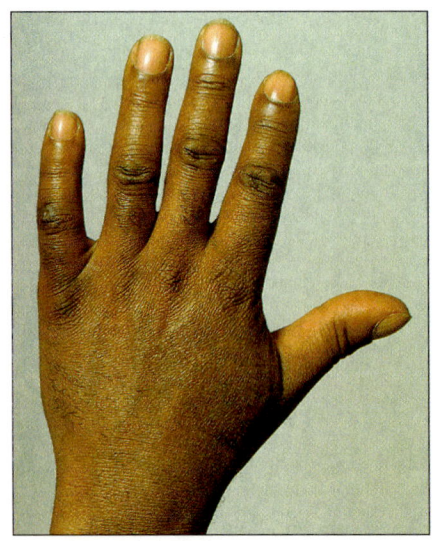

FIGURE 21-12 Thyroid acropachy with clubbing of the digits. (*Courtesy of* F. Sterling.)

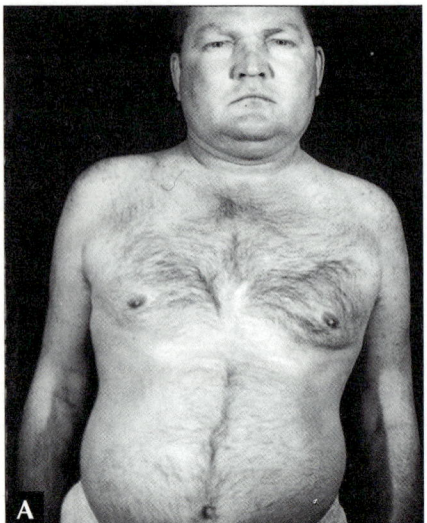

FIGURE 21-13 Cushing's disease, before (*panel A*) and after (*panel B*) bilateral adrenalectomy. There is truncal obesity and cushingoid facies before surgery. (*Courtesy of* F. Sterling.)

drugs include minoxidil, diazoxide, phenytoin, glucocorticoids, and cyclosporine.

In evaluating patients for hyperandrogenemia, it is important to obtain a history, including the age and rapidity of onset, other symptoms of virilism, other symptoms of Cushing's disease, drug history, and menstrual history. The physical examination should evaluate the amount and distribution of hair, clitoral enlargement, presence of acne refractory to treatment, pelvic and abdominal exam, skin qualities, and muscle strength. Screening tests should include a total and free serum testosterone and dehydroepiandrosterone sulfate (DHEAS) level. If the total testosterone level is

greater than 200 ng/dL or the DHEAS level is over 700 μg/dL, then evaluation should include pelvic ultrasound, and computed tomography or magnetic resonance imaging of the adrenals, in search of tumors. Free testosterone level is a more sensitive indicator of hyperandrogenism than total testosterone level. Intermediate elevations of DHEAS level suggest an adrenal etiology of hyperandrogenemia and can be evaluated with an corticotropin stimulation test to detect mild, late-onset congenital adrenal hyperplasia [10••]. Intermediate elevations of testosterone can be seen with hyperandrogenemia of adrenal or ovarian cause. If menstrual dysfunction exists with other signs of hyperandrogenism,

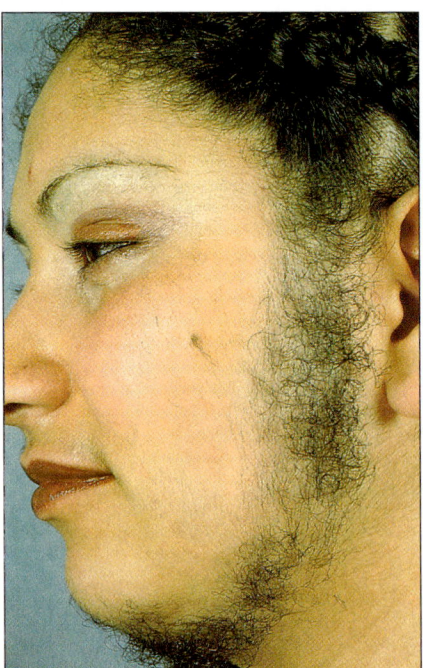

FIGURE 21-14 Hirsutism in a patient with ovarian thecoma. There is prominent facial hair, especially in the beard and mustache areas.

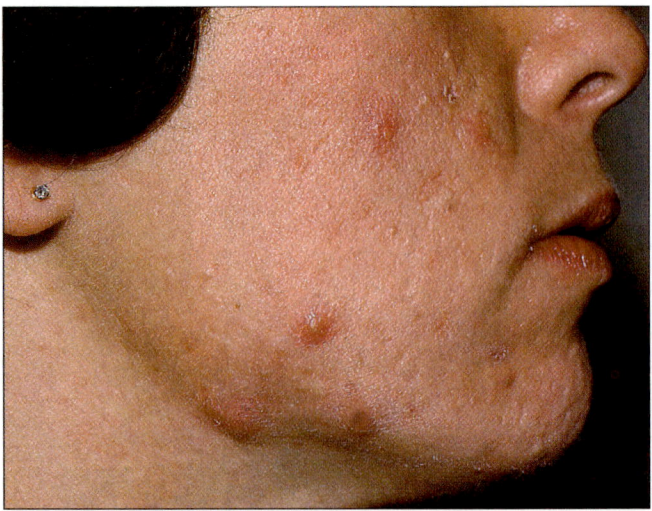

FIGURE 21-15 Acne in a patient with hyperandrogenemia. There are active erythematous cysts, as well as many areas with pitted scarring owing to previous acne lesions. (*Courtesy of* B. Witmer.)

then a serum prolactin level and luteinizing hormone–follicle-stimulating hormone ratio should be checked. If the serum prolactin level is greater than 20 ng/dL, then a prolactinoma should be excluded with magnetic resonance imaging or computed tomography. Mild prolactin elevations have been reported in up to 30% of women with polycystic ovary disease. If the luteinizing hormone–follicle-stimulating hormone ratio is greater than three, polycystic disease should be suspected, and a gynecologic consult and ultrasound of the ovaries should be obtained. If symptoms of Cushing's syndrome exist, a dexamethasone suppression test should be performed: 1 mg of dexamethasone given at midnight and the morning serum cortisol level measured. If the cortisol level is greater than 0.5 μg/dL, then Cushing's syndrome must be ruled out.

Treatment of hyperandrogenemia

First, any medications that may be contributing to the condition must be stopped. Polycystic ovary disease can be treated with low-dose oral contraceptives. Insulin resistance has been treated with oral contraceptives or a long-acting luteinizing hormone-releasing hormone analogue. Ovarian tumors are treated with surgery, and Cushing's disease is treated with pituitary surgery. Androgen-producing tumors are treated with surgery. Congenital adrenal hyperplasia is treated with small evening doses of prednisone (2.5 to 5.0 mg) for 1 year. During treatment, the serum testosterone or DHEAS level should be obtained every 3 months to assess the effectiveness of therapy. After treatment ends, glucocorticoids should be restarted after serum androgen levels increase or if the patient becomes symptomatic. Idiopathic hirsutism is usually ovarian in etiology and can be treated with oral contraceptives. Other therapy includes antiandrogens that work mainly at the end-organ tissue level, and these can be used alone or with other therapies. These agents include spironolactone, 50 to 200 mg/d, and flutamide, neither of which is approved for use in hyperandrogenemia. Mild symptoms of hyperandrogenemia can be treated directly with such treatments as bleaching, depilation, epilation, and electrolysis to treat increased facial hair.

Adrenocortical failure

Adrenocortical failure can result from autoimmunity, chronic infections, bilateral tumors, or vasculitis. Secondary failure can result from hypopituitarism. The findings include hyperpigmentation of the skin, especially involving the oral mucosa and palmer creases (Fig. 21-16). Nevi darken and flat pigmented macules called lentigos can develop. Body hair can decrease. Fifteen percent of patients, usually those with autoimmune disease, develop vitiligo.

Multiple endocrine neoplasia

The multiple endocrine neoplasia type 3 syndrome includes mucosal neuromas, bumpy lips, pheochromocytoma, and medullary thyroid carcinoma. The mucosal neuromas involve the tongue, lips, buccal mucosa, and other sites. The

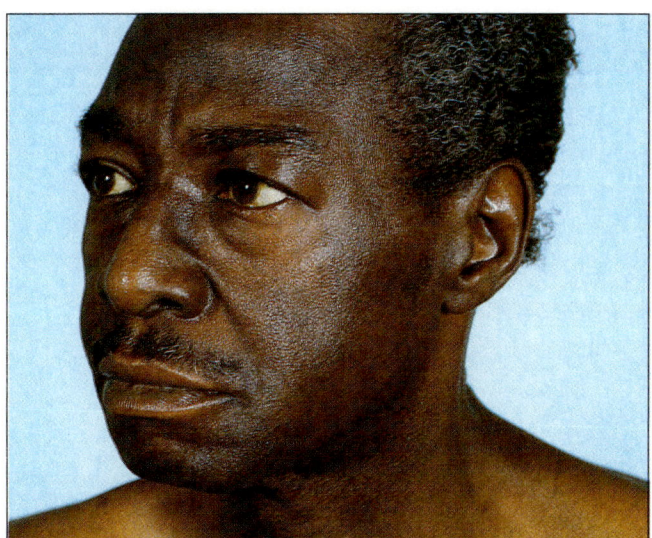

FIGURE 21-16 Addison's disease. There is marked hyperpigmentation of the face. (*Courtesy of* B. Witmer.)

neuromas begin in the first decade of life, and the syndrome is inherited in an autosomal dominant fashion [11]. Pituitary gland disorders, such as acromegaly, Cushing's disease, and panhypopituitarism each have associated skin findings (Table 21-5).

METABOLIC DISORDERS

Porphyrias

The porphyrias are a group of defects in heme synthesis that affect the skin, the nervous system, and the gastrointestinal system. Only two porphyrias do not have photodermatoses: acute intermittent porphyria and aminolevulinic acid dehydrase deficiency. The diagnostic test for porphyria depends on the type of porphyria present.

Porphyria cutanea tarda, the most common porphyria, involves decreased production of the enzyme uroporphyrinogen decarboxylase. Variegate porphyria, which results from a defect in protoporphyrin oxydase, presents with the same skin lesions as porphyria cutanea tarda but also causes gastrointestinal and neurological symptoms. Clinically, these patients present with bullae, erosions, scarring, hyperpigmentation and hypopigmentation, and sclerodermoid changes of sun-exposed areas of the hands, face, and legs (Fig. 21-17). Hypertrichosis of the face is common (Fig. 21-18). Porphyria cutanea tarda is associated most frequently with excessive alcohol intake. In addition, several drugs may exacerbate the disease (*eg*, estrogens). Hemochromatosis, carcinomas, lymphomas, and chronic renal failure may also be associated with porphyria cutanea tarda [12]. Recently, multiple reports of porphyria cutanea tarda, HIV infection [13•] and hepatitis C antibodies [14] have been published. HIV, hepatitis antigen and anti-hepatitis C virus should be checked as part of a routine evaluation.

TABLE 21-5 PITUITARY GLAND DISORDERS

Affected area	Manifestations
Acromegaly	
Skin	Enlarged hands, feet
	Thickened eyelids
	Cutis verticis gyrata
	Hypertrichosis
	Hyperhidrosis
	Skin tags
	Acanthosis nigricans
	Abscesses: axillae, buttocks
	Hyperpigmentation
Mouth	Macroglossia
Nail	Thick, hard
Hair	Loss of body hair
	Scalp hair fine, silky
Cushing's disease	
Skin	Hyperpigmentation
	Changes of hypercorticism (Cushing's syndrome)
Panhypopituitarism	
Skin	Dry, smooth, soft, pale
	Fine wrinkles
Hair	Hair loss: axillae, pubic, beard
	Scalp hair: fine, dry, thin

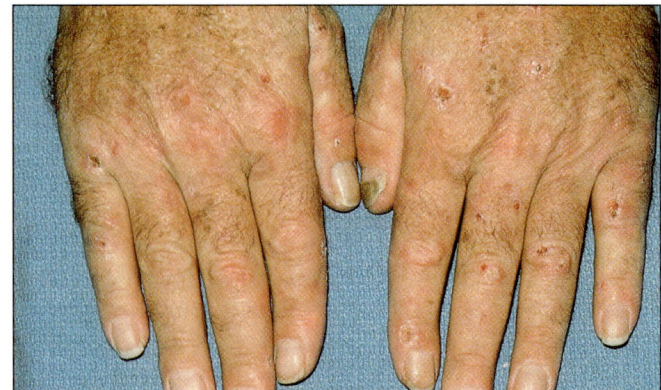

FIGURE 21-17 Bullae and erosion on the dorsal surface of the hands resulting from porphyria cutanea tarda.

The diagnosis of porphyria cutanea tarda can be suggested by demonstration of pink coral fluorescence of the urine with a Wood's lamp; however, a 24-hour urine specimen is required to measure uroporphyrins and coproporphyrins. The treatment is to remove any drugs, which exacerbate the disease. Iron stores are removed by repeated phlebotomy [15].

Erythropoietic porphyria is a rare porphyrin disorder that presents in childhood with severe photosensitivity, even through window-glass, resulting initially in erythematous urticarial plaques. Chronic erythropoietic porphyria leads to scarring, very thick skin over the finger joints, severe photodamage, and atrophy of the rim of the ears. Patients can also develop liver involvement, and rarely even fatal cirrhosis. The diagnosis is made through measurement of erythrocyte protoporphyrin and fecal protoporphyrin levels. The urine does not fluoresce. Treatment includes administration of oral β-carotene, antimalarials, antihistamines, and cholestyramine. To prevent photosensitivity in all porphyrias, physical sunscreens, protective clothing, and sun avoidance are advised [16].

Amyloidosis

Amyloidosis is a group of disorders in which amyloid is deposited in tissue. The classification of amyloidosis is as follows: primary localized cutaneous amyloidosis (which includes papular or lichen amyloidosis, macular amyloidosis, and nodular amyloidosis), secondary localized cutaneous amyloidosis, systemic immunoglobulin-related amyloidosis, and familial amyloidosis [12]. All types of amyloid have the same biochemical configuration and appear as an amorphous eosinophilic material on routine pathologic staining. When tissue is stained with Congo red, a green birefringent appears under a polarizing microscope.

Primary systemic amyloidosis can present with skin findings early in the disease. Spontaneous purpuric lesions develop in areas of trauma, body folds, eyelids, sides of the nose, neck, axilla, umbilicus, and the anogenital region. The hemorrhage results from amyloid infiltration in blood vessel walls. Macroglossia, mucosal lesions, waxy translucent papules, sclerodermoid plaques, alopecia, and bullous lesions may occur [17]. Patients with these findings should have serum and urine immunoelectrophoresis, and an evaluation for end-organ involvement.

The cutaneous types of amyloidosis do not need a systemic evaluation. Lichen or papular amyloid consists of

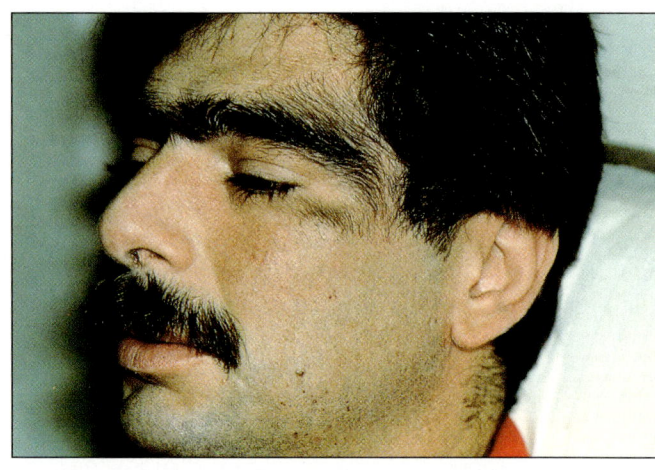

FIGURE 21-18 Hypertrichosis of the lateral forehead resulting from porphyria cutanea tarda.

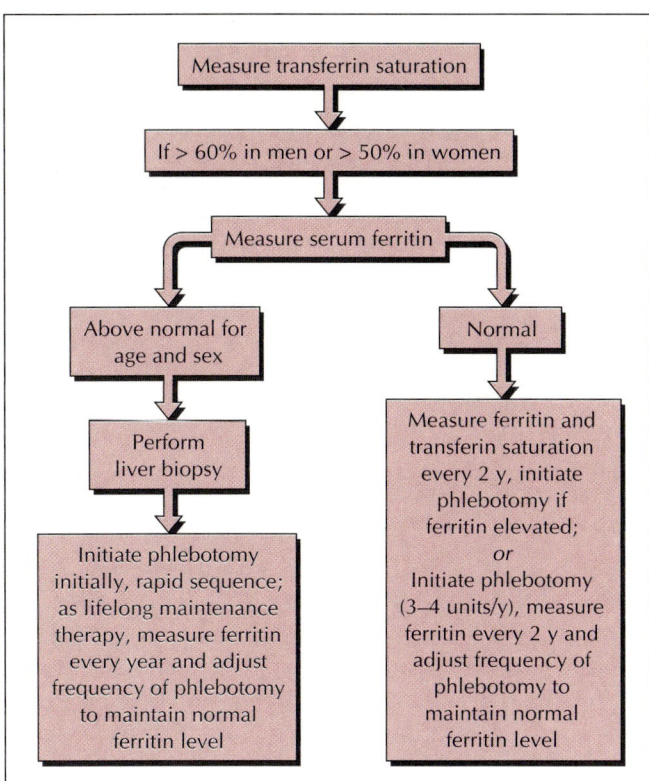

FIGURE 21-19 Protocol for hemochromatosis screening and treatment. (*From* Edwards and Kushner [19]; with permission.)

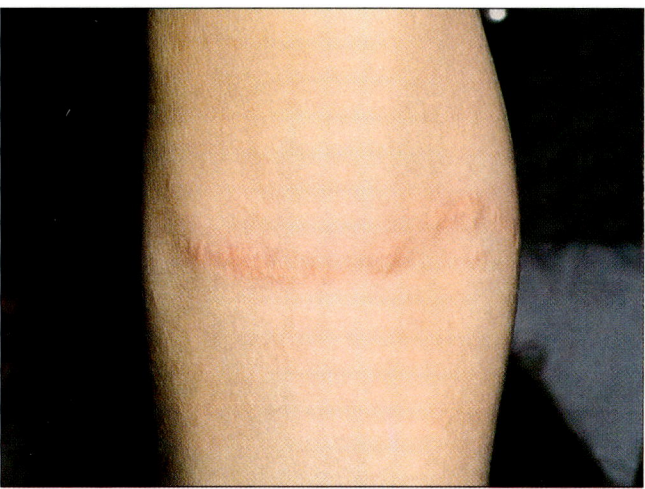

FIGURE 21-20 Cutis calcinosis due to renal failure and secondary hyperparathyroidism. Note yellow-white, firm papules in a linear distribution on the arm.

very pruritic papules and plaques on the shins of adults and can be treated with topical steroids. Macular amyloid presents with reticulated hyperpigmentation on the trunk and extremities [18]. Nodular amyloid is rare, with waxy brown yellow nodules occurring anywhere. Secondary localized cutaneous amyloidosis can occur in previous areas of inflammation, such as near basal cell carcinomas.

Hemochromatosis

Hemochromatosis is an inborn error of intestinal iron absorption. The dermatologic manifestations are a distinct gray-to-brown coloration of the face, extensor surfaces of the forearms, dorsum of the hand, and genital areas. Mucosal hyperpigmentation is also seen. It occurs mostly in men and is rarely seen in homozygous persons under the age of 20 years. Xerosis, diabetes, endocrine failure, heart failure, and arthropathy are also seen. Recently, a screening test that detects hemochromatosis before symptoms appear was described (Fig. 21-19) [19]. This test would measure transferrin saturation and serum ferritin levels. Therapy with phlebotomy can remove iron and lead to an improvement in liver function.

Cutis Calcinosis

There are three main types of calcium deposits in the skin: metastatic calcinosis (hypercalcemia or hyperphosphatasemia), dystrophic cutis calcinosis (no metabolic disorder), and idiopathic calcinosis (no metabolic disorder) [20]. There are two causes of metastatic calcinosis: hypercalcemia or hyperphosphatasemia, or deficient end-organ response to parathyroid hormone. Clinically, these conditions occur in normal skin as subcutaneous nodules or plaques around the joints. Linear cutaneous nodules and plaques can also be present. The differential diagnosis for metastatic calcinosis includes secondary hyperparathyroidism, uremia, vitamin D toxicity, milk alkali syndrome, and sarcoidosis (Fig. 21-20). Dystrophic cutis calcinosis occurs in areas of previous trauma or inflammation. This condition occurs in two types: localized and generalized. The localized type occurs in areas of trauma and old inflammation, such as acne cysts and calcium infusion [21]. A generalized type of dystrophic calcinosis is found in hereditary disorders, such as pseudoxanthoma elasticum, Ehlers-Danlos syndrome, or Werner's syndrome. Calcinosis is also seen in dermatomyositis and

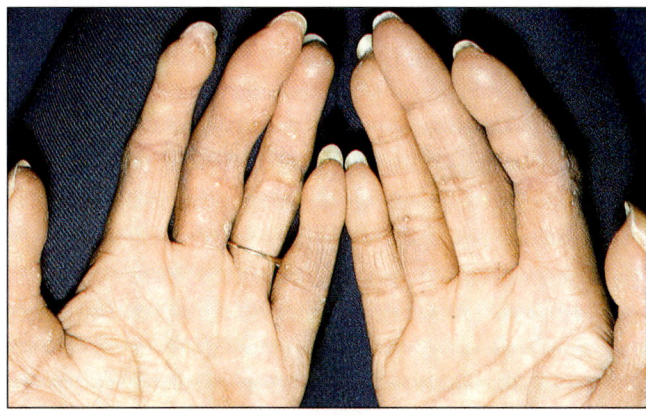

FIGURE 21-21 Cutis calcinosis in a patient with scleroderma. Note firm, whitish papules on the fingers.

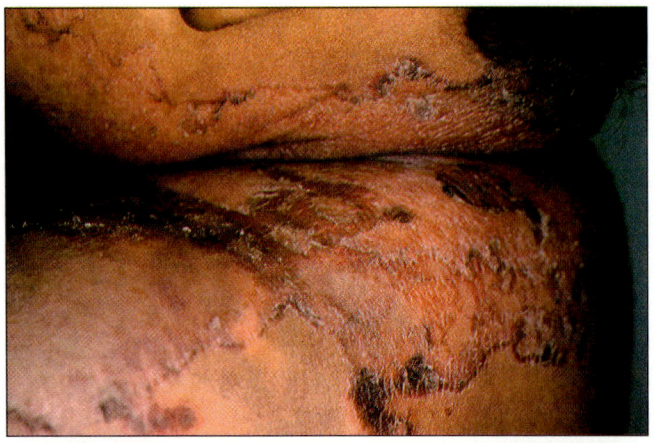

FIGURE 21-22 Acrodermatitis enteropathica in a child. Note desquamating, eczematous eruption on the neck and upper back.

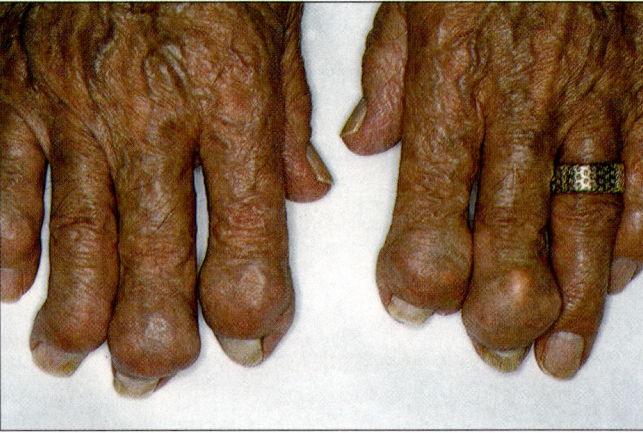

FIGURE 21-23 Gouty tophi of hands. Note white to skin-colored firm papules on distal interphalangeal joints of hands.

scleroderma, but only rarely in lupus erythematosus (Fig. 21-21). Idiopathic cutis calcinosis occurs most commonly in the scrotum and is asymptomatic. Treatment of calcinosis cutis is generally directed toward the underlying metabolic disorder, or the lesion is excised.

Acrodermatitis Enteropathica

Two types of acrodermatitis enteropathica exist: an autosomal recessive disorder and an acquired zinc deficiency. The clinical findings are similar in adults and children, and present with early acral and periorificial erythema and scale with serpiginous borders, alopecia, gastrointestinal symptoms, anorexia, immune dysfunction, growth retardation, and central nervous system symptoms (Fig. 21-22).

Borderline zinc deficiency can occur in patients with any malabsorption disorder, liver disease, chronic alcohol abuse, those on total parenteral nutrition, and those with other nutritional deficiencies. Recently, cases of acrodermatitis enteropathica have been described in anorexia nervosa [22•] and immunodeficiency syndrome [23•]. Response to treatment is very rapid, with lesions clearing in approximately 10 days with oral zinc sulfate, 250 mg, administered once or twice a day. The diagnosis of zinc deficiency is most accurately made by obtaining a serum concentration of zinc. Before the level is drawn, consultation should be made with the laboratory that will interpret the results. Urine and hair concentrations of zinc are not reliable methods of measuring zinc levels.

Gout

Gout is a disorder of uric acid, where there is either a defect in absorption and production, or a defect in excretion of the acid. It results in a group of diseases that are caused by the deposit of monosodium urate monohydrate crystals in the tissues around the joints of the extremities, the ears, and the kidney.

A positive family history is present in some patients with gout. Gout is commoner in men and in patients taking thiazide diuretics. Acute gouty arthritis commonly involves the first metatarsal of the foot. Patients can develop tophaceous gout, in which deposits in the subcutaneous tissues of the skin, gouty nephropathy, and urolithiasis occur (Figs. 21-23 and 21-24). Therapy for acute gouty arthritis is discussed in the rheumatology section, but nonsteroidal anti-inflammatory agents and antiurate agents are used as preventive therapy. Allopurinol is probably the best inhibitor of the enzyme xanthine oxidase, and thus inhibits uric acid production and prevents tophaceous gout. Many patients develop an allergy to allopurinol. Patients with maculopapular eruptions and not life-threatening dermatoses can be desensitized to allopurinol by use of an oral desensitization method, but this method should be used with extreme caution [24•].

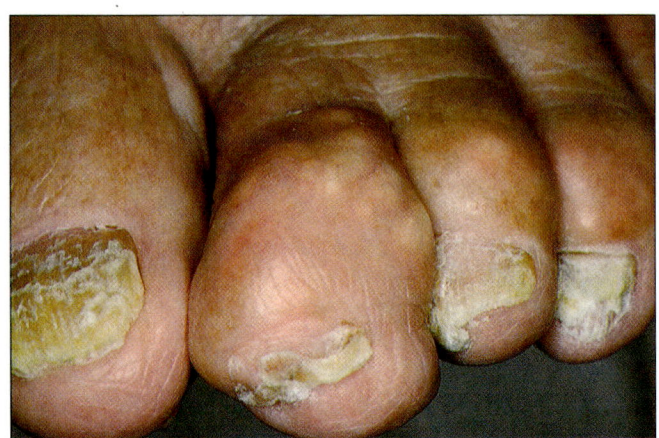

FIGURE 21-24 Gouty tophi of feet. Note yellow- to skin-colored firm papules on distal joints of feet. Nail changes are typical of onychomycosis.

REFERENCES AND RECOMMENDED READING

Recently published papers of particular interest have been highlighted as:
* Of interest
** Of outstanding interest

1. Oursler JR, Goldblum OR: Blistering eruption in a diabetic. *Arch Dermatol* 1991, 127:247–252.

2. Johnson MP, Ramphal R: Malignant external otitis. *Rev Infect Dis* 1990, 12:173–180.

3. Wheat LJ, Allen SD, Henry M, *et al.*: Diabetic foot infections. Bacteriologic analysis. *Arch Intern Med* 1986, 146:1935–1940.

4.•• Lipsky BA, Pecoraro RE, Wheat LJ: The diabetic foot: soft tissue and bone infection. *Infect Dis Clin North Am* 1990, 4:409–432.

5. Parker F: Xanthomas and hyperlipidemias. *J Am Acad Dermatol* 1985, 13:1–30.

6. Feingold KR, Castro GR, Ishikawa V, *et al.*: Cutaneous xanthoma in association with paraproteinemia in the absence of hyperlipidemia. *J Clin Invest* 1989, 83:796–802.

7. Heymann WR: Cutaneous manifestations of thyroid disease. *J Am Acad Dermatol* 1992, 26:885–902.

8. Werth VP: Management and treatment with systemic glucocorticoids. *Adv Dermatol* 1993, 8:81–103.

9. Sperling SC, Heimer WL: Androgen biology as a basis for the diagnosis and treatment of androgenic disorders in women. *J Am Acad Dermatol* 1993, 26:669–683.

10.•• Sperling SC, Heimer WL: Androgen biology as a basis for the diagnosis and treatment of androgenic disorders in women: II. *J Am Acad Dermatol* 1993, 26:901–916.

11. Khairi MRA, Dexter RN, Burzynski NJ, Johnston CC: Mucosal neuroma, pheochromocytoma and medullary thyroid carcinoma: multiple endocrine neoplasia, type 3. *Medicine* 1965, 54:89–112.

12. Finkel LJ: Cutaneous mucinoses and amyloidosis. In *J Dermatology*, edn 3. Edited by Moschella S, Hurley HJ. Philadelphia: WB Saunders; 1992:1597–1604.

13.• Blauvelt A, Harris H, Hogan D, *et al.*: Porphyria cutanea tarda and human immunodeficiency virus. *Int J Dermatol* 1992, 31:474–479.

14. LaCour J, Bodokh I, Castanet J, *et al.*: Porphyria cutanea tarda and antibodies to hepatitis C virus. *Br J Dermatol* 1993, 128:121–123.

15. Paslin D: The porphyrias. *Int J Dermatol* 1992, 31:517–539.

16. Parker F: Disorders of metabolism. In *Dermatology*, edn 3. Edited by Moschella S, Hurley HJ. Philadelphia: WB Saunders; 1992:1667–1678.

17. Robert C, Aractin G, Prost S, Verola C: Bullous amyloidosis: report of three cases and review of the literature. *Medicine* 1993, 72:38–44.

18. Bourke JF, Berth-Jones J, Burns DA: Diffuse primary cutaneous amyloidosis. *Br J Dermatol* 127:641–644.

19. Edwards C, Kushner J: Screening for hemochromatosis. *N Engl J Med* 1993, 328:1616–1620.

20. Orlow S, Watsky K, Bolognia J: Skin and bones II. *J Am Acad Dermatol* 1991, 25:447–462.

21. Werth S, Latour D, Wilson D: Yellow plaques and ulcerations in a cardiac transplant patient. *Arch Dermatol* 1992, 128:547–552.

22.• Voorhees A, Riba M: Acquired zinc deficiency in association with anorexia nervosa. *Pediatr Dermatol* 1992, 9:268–271.

23.• Reichel M, Mauro T, Ziboh V, *et al.*: Acrodermatitis enteropathica in a patient with the acquired immunodeficiency syndrome. *Arch Dermatol* 1992, 128:415–416.

24.• Fam AG, Lewtaf J, Stein J, Patton TW: Desensitization allopurinol in patients with gout and cutaneous reactions. *Am J Med* 1992, 93:299–302.

SELECT BIBLIOGRAPHY

Decastro M, Sanchez J, Herrera JF, *et al.*: Hepatitis C virus antibodies and liver disease in patients with porphyria cutanea tarda. *Hepatology* 1993, 17:551–557.

Fatourechi V, Pajouhi M, Fransway AF: Dermopathy of Graves' disease (pretibial myxedema)—review of 150 cases. *Medicine* 1994, 73:1–7.

Meola T, Lim HW: The porphyrias. *Dermatol Clin* 1993, 11:583–596.

Reiber GE, Pecoraro RE, Koepsell TD: Risk factors for amputation in patients with diabetes mellitus: a case control study. *Ann Intern Med* 1992, 117:97–105.

Rosenfield RL, Lucky AW. Acne, hirsutism, and alopecia in adolescent girls. Clinical expressions of androgen excess. *Endocrinol Metab Clin North Am* 1993, 22:507–532.

Stevens B, Fleischer A, Piering F, Crosby D: Porphyria cutanea tarda in the setting of renal failure. *Arch Dermatol* 1993, 129:337–339.

Index

Page numbers followed by "f" indicate figures; those followed by "t" indicate tables

Growths, *continued*
    algorithms for, 2f
Guttate psoriasis, 60, 60f

*H*and(s)
    gouty tophi of, 176, 176f
Hand, foot, and mouth disease, 27
Hand dermatitis, 72–73, 72f, 72t
Hartnup disease, 102, 102t
Hemangioma
    versus melanoma, 47t
Hematoma
    subungual
        versus melanoma, 47t
Hemochromatosis
    cutaneous manifestations of, 175, 175f
Hemodialysis
    chronic
        pruritus in, 84, 85f
Herpes gladatorum, 23
Herpes simplex virus (HSV) infections, 8f, 22–25
    complications of, 24, 24f
    described, 22–23, 23f
    diagnosis of, 23–24
    erythema multiforme due to, 119, 119f, 119t
    genital, 23, 23f
        treatment of, 24t
    orolabial
        treatment of, 24t
    treatment of, 24–25, 24t
Herpesvirus type 6, 26
Herpetic proctitis, 23
Herpetic whitlow, 23, 23f
Hirsutism
    ovarian thecoma and, 172f
History
    in skin disorders, 1, 3
Hodgkin's disease
    cutaneous involvement of, 148
Hot tub folliculitis, 16
Howel-Evans syndrome, 149
HSV infections. *see* Herpes simplex virus (HSV) infections
Human papillomavirus infections, 20–22
    common warts, 20–21, 21f, 21t
    flat warts, 21–22, 21f
    plantar warts, 21, 21f, 21t
Human parvovirus, 26–27, 27f
Hyperandrogenemia, 171–173, 172f
    treatment of, 173
Hyperpigmentation
    appearance of, 3t
    mucocutaneous
        chemotherapy-induced patterns of, 156t
Hyperplasia
    sebaceous, 52, 52f
Hypertrichosis lanuginosa acquisita
    malignancy-associated
        site and clinical characteristics of, 152t
Hypertrophic pulmonary osteoarthropathy
    malignancy-associated
        site and clinical characteristics of, 152t
Hypertrophic scars, 52–53, 53f, 53t
Hypopigmentation
    appearance of, 3t

*I*chthyosis
    acquired
        malignancy-associated
            site and clinical characteristics of, 152t
Imidazoles
    for dermatophytoses, 33t
Immunobullous diseases, 159–165
    key points, 159
Impetigo, 8f, 12–15
    Bockhart's, 15–16, 15t
    bullous, 13, 13f, 13t
    diagnosis of, 12–13, 13f
    nonbullous, 12–13, 13f, 13t
    prevention of, 15
    treatment of, 14–15, 14t
    types of, 13t
Infection(s)
    bacterial, 12–19. *see also* Bacterial infections
    in diabetes mellitus, 167–168, 168f
    fungal, 29–36. *see also* Fungal infections
    viral, 20–28. *see also* Viral infections
Inflammatory acne, 78–80, 79t
Insect bites, 83f
Intertrigo, 75, 76t
Isotretinoin
    for acne, 79–80
Itching, 82–86. *see also* Pruritus
    defined, 82
    in skin disorders, 1

*K*aposi's sarcoma, 6f
Kaposi's varicelliform eruption, 24f
Kawasaki syndrome, 143, 143t
Keloids, 52–53, 53f, 53t
Keratoacanthoma, 39
Keratolytic acid paintings
    for warts, 21t
Keratoses
    actinic, 4f
        described, 37–38, 38f
    seborrheic, 5f, 47f, 50–51, 51f
        described, 50
    solar
        described, 37–38, 38f
Ketoconazole
    for dermatophytoses, 33t

*L*aboratory tests
    in skin disorders, 9–10
Laser vaporization
    CO$_2$
        for warts, 21t
            genital, 22t
Leg
    ecthyma on, 15f
    superficial folliculitis on, 16f
    ulcers of. *see* Leg ulcers
Leg ulcers, 87–95
    arterial, 88t, 89–90, 89f, 90f
        treatment of, 94
    causes of, 88–93, 94t
    classification of, 87t